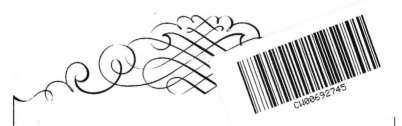
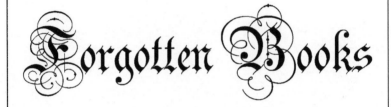

ISBN 978-1-331-25054-8
PIBN 10164370

English
Français
Deutsche
Italiano
Español
Português

www.forgottenbooks.com

Mythology Photography **Fiction**
Fishing Christianity **Art** Cooking
Essays Buddhism Freemasonry
Medicine **Biology** Music **Ancient
Egypt** Evolution Carpentry Physics
Dance Geology **Mathematics** Fitness
Shakespeare **Folklore** Yoga Marketing
Confidence Immortality Biographies
Poetry **Psychology** Witchcraft
Electronics Chemistry History **Law**
Accounting **Philosophy** Anthropology
Alchemy Drama Quantum Mechanics
Atheism Sexual Health **Ancient History**
Entrepreneurship Languages Sport
Paleontology Needlework Islam
Metaphysics Investment Archaeology
Parenting Statistics Criminology
Motivational

LECTURES AND ESSAYS

ON

FEVERS AND DIPHTHERIA

LECTURES AND ESSAYS

ON

FEVERS

AND

DIPHTHERIA

1849 TO 1879

BY

SIR WILLIAM JENNER, BART., G.C.B. 1815-18

M.D. LOND. AND F.R.C.P., D.C.L. OXON., LL.D. CANTAB. AND EDIN.,
F.R.S., PRESIDENT OF THE ROYAL COLLEGE OF PHYSICIANS FROM 1881 TO 1888
PHYSICIAN IN ORDINARY TO H.M. THE QUEEN AND TO H.R.H. THE PRINCE OF WALES
CONSULTING PHYSICIAN TO UNIVERSITY COLLEGE HOSPITAL

London

RIVINGTON, PERCIVAL & CO

1893

DEDICATED

TO THE MEMORY OF

WILLIAM SHARPEY, M.D.
PROFESSOR OF PHYSIOLOGY IN UNIVERSITY COLLEGE, LONDON

OF

EDMUND ALEXANDER PARKES, M.D.
PROFESSOR OF CLINICAL MEDICINE AT UNIVERSITY COLLEGE, LONDON,
AND SUBSEQUENTLY PROFESSOR OF MILITARY HYGIENE IN VICTORIA HOSPITAL, NETLEY

AND OF

SIR JAMES CLARK, BART.
PHYSICIAN IN ORDINARY TO H.M. THE QUEEN

THREE OF THE MOST ABLE, HONOURABLE AND

KIND-HEARTED MEN

THE AUTHOR HAS EVER KNOWN IN

THE MEDICAL PROFESSION

PREFACE

SEVERAL years since I collected from the Journals to which I had originally sent them my papers on Fever. I now publish together all the papers I have written on Fever, because many of my medical friends have from time to time urged me to do it, and also because all the facts detailed and analysed were observed and recorded at the bedside and in the dead-house by *myself*. While collecting some of these facts in 1847 I caught typhus fever, and three or four years later typhoid fever. I mention this because it was said at the time, 'Before typhus and typhoid fevers can be said to be absolutely different diseases some one must be found who has suffered from both,' and I was the first, so far as I know, who at that time could be proved to have suffered from both. Dr. E. A. Parkes attended me in both illnesses, and had no doubt about the diagnosis in each case.[1]

When I had written the paper which subsequently appeared in the *Edinburgh Monthly Journal*,

[1] The late Dr. A. Tweedie most carefully attended me, with Dr. E. A. Parkes, for my attack of Typhus fever, and in acknowledgment of their great kindness I dedicated my first published pages to them.

before sending it for publication I asked Dr. Parkes to read it; having done so, he advised me to place the conclusions to which I had come at the beginning in place of at the end of the paper. 'If you place the conclusions first, whoever is interested in the subject will read them carefully, and then will read what follows to see how you prove the points which interest him.'

Dr. Sharpey, after the papers had appeared and were attracting some attention, advised me never to reply to criticism, 'unless a critic should affirm that you had said something which you have never said. Others will answer mere criticism.'

That advice of Dr. Parkes and that of Dr. Sharpey have influenced me throughout my life in writing and in lecturing.

The papers I am now publishing are identical with those I originally published in various Journals and in the Transactions of Societies. The only alterations or additions I have now made are contained in a brief note or two appended to some of the pages.

I cannot conclude without heartily thanking Dr. Sidney Coupland and Dr. T. Barlow for the care and attention with which they have superintended the arrangements of the publication of these papers.

W. J.

Greenwood, Bishops Waltham.
September 1893.

CONTENTS

b

Typhoid Fever.

Relapsing Fever.

Febricula.

ON DIPHTHERIA
1861.

1875.

ON THE IDENTITY OR NON-IDENTITY
OF TYPHOID AND TYPHUS FEVERS

1849-50

NOTE.

This essay was republished in book form in 1850, with the addition of a preface, which is here reproduced, as it indicates the prevalent views on the subject at that time :—' A few words only are needed as preface to the following pages. The reader must not suppose that the importance of the labours of others on the subject there considered is underrated, because no special references have been made to them. I am deeply sensible of the value of the writings of Gerhard, Shattuck, Valleix, Louis, Stewart, Bartlett, etc. ; but, notwithstanding their researches, the question of the specific difference of Typhoid and Typhus Fevers was considered by some of those who had most closely criticised the papers referred to as settled, or likely ultimately to be settled, in the negative. "We venture," said the reviewer of Dr. Bartlett's book, in the *British and Foreign Medical Quarterly* of April 1844, " to prognosticate that the ultimate issue of the investigation will show the truth of a remark of Dr. Southwood Smith that ' there is but one kind of idiopathic fever' : " and again, "We remain, then, of the same opinion, that the continued fever of England and France are the same species of disease." I considered, therefore, that it was necessary to begin *de novo*, and consult only the voice of nature, —convinced that, although the most intellectual might fail at first to comprehend her often ambiguous language, yet that her most humble votaries might, by patience and daily watching, by keeping honest record of every sound she uttered—by joining letter to letter, adding word to word, and line to line—at last spell out her meaning, and so reach that rank which the great master of induction tells us man may legitimately hope to attain, namely, that of her interpreter. The consciousness of his ability to gain this title ought to stimulate man to exertion—the certainty that he is able to reach no higher cannot fail to annihilate his pride.'

ON TYPHOID AND TYPHUS FEVERS[1]

INTRODUCTION.

IT is beyond dispute that there are large groups of diseases arranged under the same heads in systematic works on medicine, of which the only bonds of union are, that their nature is unknown, and that they present in common certain pretty constant and striking symptoms.

Of these ill-defined anomalous groups, continued fever is one of the most remarkable and important. To trace the relations, and to detect the differences of the incongruous mass of diseases united together under this name, only the most careful analysis of daily recorded clinical observations can suffice.

The memory is too treacherous to be depended on in the science of medicine, in which the effects of primary are complicated by the effects of secondary lesions, and in which observation has to be corrected by observation.

For the elucidation of its obscurer points, no loose or general statements are of use—the most rigid induction can alone avail.

It would be a great point gained towards the right understanding of the true value of the differences observed in cases known as continued fever, if the question raised by Louis could be positively answered—no matter whether in the affirmative or negative—as to the identity of typhus and typhoid fevers; that is to say, have or have not British physicians confounded under the term continued fever, two

1 Published in the Edinburgh Monthly Journal of the Medical Sciences, 1849-50.

essentially distinct diseases ?—the one characterised by an anatomical lesion peculiar to it, and distinguishing it from all other acute diseases, the other exhibiting no certain anatomical character, and each presenting symptoms by which it can with more or less facility be distinguished from the other.

It will be necessary, before proceeding further, briefly to explain what is meant by the terms identity and non-identity, as applied to cases of typhus and typhoid fevers.

A given case of any disease always differs more or less from all other cases of the same disease, and therefore it may be said that no two are identical ; but it is not with this kind of identity that we have here to do. It is not regarding differences in degree, but in kind, that question is here made.

Whether the primary affection is identical in typhus and typhoid fevers is the problem to be solved. Are the differeuces allowed to exist between them due simply to individual peculiarities, atmospheric differences, epidemic constitutions or hygienic conditions, giving rise to local complications in the one which are absent in the other, and to variations in the symptoms as a consequence of these local complications ? Or are they distinct diseases, as are scarlet fever and small-pox ?—distinct as to their primary or exciting cause, their essential symptoms, and anatomical lesions. It may be as well, before proceeding further, to anticipate a little, and to state that the conclusion necessarily drawn from the analysis about to be submitted to the reader of sixty-six fatal cases of fever, is in opposition to the opinion of the principal writers on the subject of continued fever in this country. With few exceptions, British physicians have laboured to prove that typhoid and typhus fevers are identical. The results obtained by this analysis justify the assertion, that they are essentially distinct diseases. This difference from the opinion of others, I should be slow to express if I was not supported by a larger body of facts than, so far as I am aware, has ever been offered in evidence to prove the identity of the two fevers. To those who delight to dwell on the imperfections common to all analysis of cases, who smile at any attempt to improve medicine by rigid induction, the value of the figures presented for their consideration may be increased by the following general assertion, that for two years, in distinguishing the two diseases by the eruption alone, not a single error has been made, so far as could be proved by examination after death of the fatal cases, or by the progress of the non-fatal cases after their diagnosis was recorded.

Two cases cannot seem to differ more, to a superficial observer, than a slight sore throat, the result of exposure to the poison of scarlet fever, and a case of scarlatina anginosa, or than a mild case of scarlatina simplex and one of scarlatina maligna; yet no one now doubts the identity of the two, *i.e.* as we here use the word, or that however much they may differ, it is in degree and not in kind, for we find every variation in the severity of the throat affection, and in the intensity of the rash uniting the two extremes; the latter may be present or absent, but if present is similar in character, though more vivid in the one case than in the other. The former is trifling or absent in the one, fearfully severe in the other; and it may be remarked that these two symptoms of the disease bear no necessary relation in severity the one to the other. In like manner, how different is a mild case of modified smallpox from one of variola maligna; yet that they are varieties of the same disease is undoubted. No one, however, questions the non-identity of scarlet fever and small-pox, although there are some symptoms common to the two diseases, and others which, more frequently in the one, are occasionally present in the other—*e.g.* rigor, chilliness, followed by heat of skin, headache, delirium, somnolence or coma, hoarseness, sore throat, dysphagia—one or all of which symptoms may be present in either disease. In both there is an eruption of the skin, and though the usual period of its appearance differs, that of scarlet fever may not make its appearance till the third day, and the first symptoms of smallpox may have been so mild, that the patient will assert that he has been ill only two days when the skin affection appears.[1] The duration of the two generally differs; but the

[1] So like too is the rash, which often precedes by a day the eruption of the pustules in smallpox, to the rash of scarlet fever, that those conversant with the two diseases may be led to form an erroneous diagnosis. Cases are constantly sent in to the London Fever Hospital, with certificates stating they are suffering from scarlet fever, the true nature of the case not appearing till the day after their admission.

illness of the person attacked by either may be prolonged by local complications to an indefinite period, and so the duration of the disease, which is the shorter, may in some cases appear to be the longer.

On what grounds, then, do we assert that they are two diseases ?

1st, In the vast majority of cases the general symptoms differ.

2nd, The eruptions, the diagnostic characters if present, are never identical.

3rd, The anatomical character of smallpox (in this particnlar case also the eruption) is never seen in scarlet fever.

4th, Both being contagious diseases, the one, by no combination of individual peculiarities, atmospheric variations, epidemic constitution, or hygienic conditions, can give rise to the other.

5th, The epidemic constitution favourable to the origin, spread, or peculiarity in form or severity of either, has no influence over the other, excepting that which it exercises over disease in general.

By the anatomical character of a disease I intend to signify that lesion, or those lesions of structure which are the invariable concomitants of a disease if it has continued for a given time, which time must be determined by a separate series of observations for every distinct affection. The anatomical character is not, be it remarked,—and this is of immense importance,—necessarily the cause of the disease, for it may be merely a symptom ; but then, if the disease be not cut short by death, it is an invariable symptom. Thus the anatomical character of smallpox is the distinctive pustule ; but the patient may die before that lesion of structure has been developed, and yet die of smallpox—the condition of the blood or nervous system, induced by the absorption of poison, having been incompatible with a duration of life sufficiently long for the change of structure to take place. But the anatomical character may be the cause of death, and that before the primary disease has run its full course ; or it, or its effects, may remain after the original disease has disappeared, and retard recovery, or even finally prove fatal to the patient. Again, the anatomical character being merely the invariable concomitant of a disease, and not necessarily its cause, it is evident that the extent of the lesion of structure constituting that character, need bear no relation to the violence of the essential symptoms of the disease. It must not be supposed that the question of the identity or non-identity of typhus and typhoid fevers is merely one of words —that its solution has no practical bearing—that it is a matter of indifference whether the latter be regarded as typhus with abdominal complication, or as a distinct disease. If continued fever be one disease, the *essential* treatment must be the same in every case, modified only by the presence of local complications; if two diseases,[1] then the essential treatment *may be* totally different for the one from that required by the other, and this without regard to local complications. The very groundwork of the treatment, so to speak, may for the one be diametrically opposed to that necessary for the other.

To illustrate the extreme practical importance of the point, we need only remember that, until a comparatively late date, scarlet fever and measles were viewed as the same disease. Of what value would any dissertation on the general treatment of the two have been, so long as they were thus confounded, even though the local complication of scarlet fever— i.e. the throat affection—had been taken into consideration ? The cold sponging or douche, so beneficial in scarlet fever, might be death to a patient suffering from measles.

London alone, of all the cities of Europe, from the fact of fever with and without intestinal disease being almost constantly present within its bounds, afforded a field for observation capable of setting the vexed question at rest.

In Edinburgh, writes Dr. Christison, the intestinal lesion is seen often enough only to prevent physicians being ignorant of its characters. In Dublin it appears to be equally infrequent. While on the Continent fever without lesion of the agminated glands is so rare, that many eminent practitioners have doubted the existence of such an affection.

---

[1] From observations made on from 1000 to 2000 cases of continued fever, admitted into the London Fever Hospital, I think it probable that there are in this country at least four distinct continued fevers.

The London Fever Hospital, by collecting within its walls cases of continued fever from all parts of the great metropolis, offered peculiar facilities for its study; and I am indebted to the medical officers of that institution for permission to avail myself of the advantages it presented. To Dr. Tweedie, the senior physician to the hospital, so long known and so highly appreciated by the profession for his researches on fever, I beg especially to acknowledge my obligations. To my talented friend, Mr. Sankey, M.B., I am also greatly obliged for his readiness to assist me on all occasions, and for many valuable suggestions and observations.

In examining the subject of this paper—one beset with extreme difficulties, not so much from its own intricacy as from the mode in which fever has been treated of by the hosts who have chronicled its symptoms and its phases—I have endeavoured to bear the following rules constantly in mind:—

That the facts known with absolute certainty were to be kept distinct from those only approximatively ascertained.

That the question at issue—*i.e.* of the identity or non-identity of typhus and typhoid fevers—involving not only a consideration of symptoms but also of internal lesions, it was absolutely necessary that the latter should be demonstrated, and the former recorded, in every case that was to be admitted as evidence in determining the judgment.

I have during the last two years made notes of nearly one thousand cases of acute disease, chiefly of patients under the care of Dr. Tweedie, at the London Fever Hospital—of these, sixty-six were cases of continued fever, which proved fatal, and were examined by me after death.

For the reasons before stated—*i.e.* the absolute necessity of the condition of the intestinal mucous membrane being demonstrated, and not surmised, with however great an amount of probability that might be—I have excluded from my present calculations all those cases which did not prove fatal; all those cases which, although they died, were not examined after death; and all those which I examined after death, but whose symptoms I had not noted during life.

These sixty-six fatal cases I have divided into two groups, placing in the one the cases in which disease of Peyer's patches existed; in the other, those in which, so far as the unassisted eye could determine, the agminated glands were in a healthy condition. Of these sixty-six cases, forty-three belonged to the latter group, or were cases of typhus fever; the remaining twenty-three being cases of typhoid fever.

I propose, in the first place, to take certain general conditions and the symptoms presented by either disease, and compare them with those which existed in the other; and then, in like manner, to collate the appearances found after death.

YEARS AND MONTHS IN WHICH THE SIXTY-SIX CASES HERE ANALYSED WERE ADMITTED.

Typhoid Fever.		Typhus Fever.	
1847.		**1847.**	
Months.	Cases.	Months.	Cases.
January	1	April	1
February	1	May	4
August	4	June	1
November	1	July	5
		September	3
		October	3
		November	1
1848.		**1848.**	
June	3	May	5
July	2	July	3
August	2	August	1
September	3	September	3
October	2	October	2
November	1	November	5
December	2		
1849.		**1849.**	
January	1	January	5
		February	1

PREVIOUS HEALTH, GENERAL BODILY CONDITION, AND SIZE.

Typhoid and Typhus Fevers.—The patients, as a general rule, had enjoyed uninterrupted health before the attack from which they died, and were, in the large majority of cases, of robust bodily conformation, and, if admitted soon after the commencement of either disease, moderately stout.

The size of patients suffering from the two was nearly equal; thus, in *typhoid fever*—

Of the Males,	Of the Females,
The mean height was 5 f. 5¼ in.	The mean height was 5 f. 1½ in.
The tallest ,, ,, 5 f. 10½ in.	The tallest ,, ,, 5 f. 5 in.
The shortest,, ,, 5 f. 2 in.	The shortest,, ,, 5 f.

In *typhus fever*—

Of the Males,	Of the Females,
The mean height was 5 f. 4¼ in.	The mean height was 4 f. 7¼ in.
The tallest ,, ,, 5 f. 10½ in.	The tallest ,, ,, 5 f. 6 in.
The shortest,, ,, 4 f. 10 in.	The shortest,, ,, 4 f. 6 in.

COMPLEXION.

Typhoid Fever.—Twelve out of fifteen of the patients, or 80 per cent., were noted as of fair complexion.

Typhus Fever.—Eight only out of twenty-six of the patients, or 30·7 per cent., of whom notes on the point were made, were fair; but here a fallacy exists, as will be shown when speaking of the aspect of the patients while suffering from this disease. Many whose complexions were extremely dark when admitted with typhus fever, became comparatively fair as the disease disappeared. Of course, this could only be observed in patients who recovered.

SEX.

Of the patients labouring under *typhoid fever* whose cases are here considered, thirteen were males; ten females.

Of forty-three cases of *typhus fever*, twenty were males twenty-three females.

AGE.

Typhoid Fever.—The average of the ages of the twenty-three patients affected with this disease was 22·08 years. The youngest was ten years old; the eldest thirty-six.

There were—

Between the ages of 10 and 19, both years inclusive, 8 patients.
,, ,, 20 and 29, ,, ,, 12 ,,
,, ,, 30 and 36, ,, ,, 3 ,,

Typhus Fever.—The mean age of the forty-three patients suffering from this affection was 41·8 years. The youngest was eight years old, the eldest seventy.

There were—

Between the ages of 8 and 19, both years inclusive, 5 patients.
,, ,, 20 and 29, ,, ,, 4 ,,
,, 30 and 39, ,, ,, 9 ,,
,, 40 and 49, ,, ,, 12 ,,
,, ,, 50 and 59, ,, ,, 6 ,,
,, ,, 60 and 69, ,, ,, 6 ,,
Of the age of 70, 1

MODE OF ATTACK, AND THE DATE OF THE DISEASE ON WHICH THE PATIENTS WERE FIRST CONFINED TO BED.

Typhoid Fever.—No data to determine the mode of attack could be obtained in six of the twenty-three cases. The disease, in seven only of the remaining seventeen cases, began so suddenly that the exact day of its commencement could be ascertained; six out of the seven took to their beds respectively on the 1st, 1st, 2nd, 3rd, 10th, and 16th days;[1] the last two patients, however, were obliged to lie down for part of the day from an early period in the disease. No note was taken of the time when the seventh first kept his bed.

In the remaining ten of the seventeen cases, the disease began gradually. Of these, four were ailing for a few days, and then became suddenly worse; three of the four took to their beds respectively on about the 7th, 8th, and 11th days of the disease. The other six of the ten in whom the disease began insidiously, could fix on no particular day as that on which their illness began, but only stated that they became gradually ill from about a given day; of these, four took to bed severally on about the 3rd, 7th, 12th, and 17th days of the disease; when the others first kept their bed was uncertain. So that only 28·5 per cent. took to bed before the 7th day.

Typhus Fever.—Of sixteen of the forty-three cases, no

[1] In reckoning the day of the disease, both the day on which it commenced and the day on which the event referred to happened, whatever that may be, have constantly been included in the calculations. Thus, a patient who entered the hospital on the 9th of a month, and whose illness began on the 4th, would be stated to have been admitted on the 6th day of the disease.

particulars as to whether the disease began suddenly or
insidiously could be obtained.

Of the remaining twenty-seven cases, twenty-three were
taken ill suddenly; nineteen of these twenty-three cases first
kept their beds as follows:—

4 On the 1st day of the disease.		' 3 On the 4th day of the disease.	
6 ,, 2nd day ,, ,,		1 ,, 6th day ,, ,,	
5 ,, 3rd day ,, ,,			

Thus all these patients were confined to their beds before
the 7th day. Of these twenty-three cases, when four took
to their bed was not learned. In four of the twenty-seven
cases of which a correct history was obtained from the
patients or their friends, the disease began insidiously, so that
the day of its commencement could not be exactly ascertained, but they took to their beds on about the 2nd, 3rd,
4th, and 6th days; so that, if this group be added to the first,
every patient may be said to have been confined to bed by
the 6th day; while, as we have seen, 28·5 per cent. only of
the patients affected with typhoid fever took to bed before
the 7th day.

DURATION.

Typhoid Fever.—Seven cases were received into the
hospital respectively on the 4th, 5th, 6th, 8th, 10th, 12th,
and 16th days of the disease, the average day of admission
being the 8·7th.

Of thirteen patients, the exact duration of whose illness
before they entered the hospital could not be ascertained—

1 was admitted about the 7th day of the disease.				2 were admitted on about the 15th day of the disease.					
1	,,	,,	,,	9th ,,	1	,,	,,	,,	19th ,,
1	.,	,,	,,	12th ,,	2	,,	,,	,,	21st .,
1	.,	,,	,,	13th ,.	1	,,	,,	,,	27th ,,
3	,	,,	,,	14th ,,					

These thirteen cases were thus admitted on about the
14·5th day of the disease; one as early as about the 7th day,
and one as late as about the 27th day.

The disease began gradually in these thirteen cases, so
that the date of its commencement could not be accurately

fixed; but four out of the thirteen cases became suddenly much worse after from three to eleven days' indisposition; and it is singular that, if the disease be reckoned to have commenced from the time of the sudden increase in the severity of the symptoms, and to which moment the patients themselves usually referred the beginning of their illness, the average day of the disease on which these four cases entered the hospital will exactly agree with the average day of the disease on which the patients were admitted, the precise commencement of whose illness was clearly ascertained—*i.e.* both sets will have been admitted on the 8·7th day.

If the dates of the disease on the admission of the latter group of cases (being considered as nearly correct) are added to those of the first group of cases, it will be found that 23·5 per cent. only were admitted before the 9th day of the disease.

I omit one patient who had been ill, probably more than three weeks when admitted, and lived till after the 21st day from her entrance; and two cases in which the duration of the disease, prior to the day they first came under observation, was unknown. These patients remained in the hospital three and eight days before the fatal termination.

Of the seven cases, the exact date of whose illness on admission was known, three survived till after the fever had run its course. The other four died respectively on the 12th, 17th, 20th, and 27th days of the disease—the average day of death of these four cases being the 19th. This is probably below what a larger number of cases would give, because one case proved fatal on the 12th day from severe pneumonia.

Of the thirteen cases in which the duration of the disease before the patients were received into the hospital was only more or less nearly ascertained, six lived some time after the termination of the typhoid fever, and the remaining seven died severally on about the 16th, 17th, 23rd, 25th, 27th, 28th, and 30th day of the disease. The average day of death, dating from the commencement of illness, being for these seven cases 23·7, this average probably, for the reason above stated, is nearer the truth than that obtained from the first group of cases, or those in which the exact date of the illness was ascertained.

This close relation between the average day on which the disease proved fatal in the two groups—*i.e.* the group in which the exact date of the disease on admission was accurately fixed, and that in which it was only approximately ascertained—renders it probable that, in spite of the late date of the disease at which the second group entered the hospital, the mildness of their first symptoms, and then their sudden increase in severity, I have done right in dating the commencement of the illness from the moment when the patients first felt themselves ailing, and not from the time when they became suddenly worse.

If the two groups be added together, it will be seen that ten out of the eleven cases—*i.e.* 90·9 per cent.—survived till after the 15th day, the only exception being the patient who died of pneumonia on the 12th day of the fever.

Twelve[1] of the twenty-three cases here analysed proved fatal during the progress of the fever. The average day of residence in the hospital on which these patients died was the 10·5th. One case proved fatal on the 3rd day; and one lived till the 20th day after admission.

Ten survived the fever; but the duration of the disease in one of these cases was too uncertain for it to be taken into calculation.

Dating from the commencement of illness, the remaining nine cases proved fatal, on an average, about the 47th day—one of the patients dying on the 32nd, and one as late as the 86th day; or, counting from their entrance into the hospital, one lived till the 20th day, and one till the 79th day—or they died, on an average, on the 32nd day of their residence in the hospital.

Typhus Fever.—The exact day of the disease on which the patients were admitted into the hospital (omitting one case, that of a nurse who resided in the institution), was ascertained in twenty-two cases to be as follows:—

1 was admitted on the 5th day of the disease.				5 were admitted on the 9th day of the disease.				
2	,,	,,	6th ,,	2	,,	,,	12th ,,
4	,,	,,	7th ,,	1	,,	,,	14th ,,
7	,,	,,	8th ,,				

[1] One case is here omitted, because I have not the data to determine whether it proved fatal before or after the fever had run its course.

The day of the disease on which nine of the forty-three patients were admitted, was only approximately learned. Of these—

1 was admitted on about the 4th day of the disease.	1 was admitted on about the 9th day of the disease.
1 ,, ,, 5th ,,	1 ,, ,, 10th ,,
2 ,, ,, 7th ,,	2 ,, ,, 14th ,,
1 ,, ,, 8th ,,	

So that the twenty-two patients, the commencement of whose illness was clearly made out, were, on an average, admitted into the hospital on the 8th day of the disease—one entering as early as the 5th, and one as late as the 14th day: and the nine patients, the exact date of whose illness was not quite accurately ascertained, were, on an average, admitted on about the 8·6th day of the disease—one entering as soon as about the 4th day, and two as late in the disease as about the 14th day. Or, if the two groups be added together, it will be seen that as many as 61·29 per cent. were admitted before the 9th day of the disease, whereas only 23·5 per cent. of the cases of typhoid fever were admitted before the 9th day.

The duration of the disease, prior to the patient's entrance into the hospital, was entirely unknown in eleven cases. Of these, four survived after the fever terminated. Out of the twenty-three cases in which the exact day of the commencement of the disease was accurately fixed, five recovered so far as the fever was concerned. Of the remaining eighteen patients—

1 died on the 10th day of the disease.	1 died on the 15th day of the disease.
2 ,, 11th ,, ,,	2 ,, 16th ,, ,,
2 ,, 12th ,, ,,	2 ,. 17th ,, ,,
3 ,, 13th ,, ,,	1 ,, 19th ,, ,,
3 ,, 14th ,, ,,	1 ,, 20th ,, ,,

The average day of the disease on which death in these eighteen cases occurred was the 14·27th; one dying on the 10th day, and one not till the 20th day.

Of the nine cases in which the day that the disease began was only approximately ascertained, two died after the fever had run its course. Of the seven cases which proved fatal during the progress of the fever—

1 died on about the 9th day.	1 died on about the 15th day.
1 ,, ,, 11th ,,	1 ,, ,, 16th ,,
1 ,, ,, 13th ,,	2 ,, ,, 17th ,,

The average day of the disease on which these seven cases died, being about the 14·4th day—one terminating fatally on about the 9th day, and one as late as about the 17th day. Or, if the two groups of cases be taken together, it will be seen that 36 per cent. only proved fatal after the 15th day of the disease, and not one after the 20th day; presenting in this particular a striking contrast to the cases of typhoid fever, of which, as we have seen, 90·9 per cent. proved fatal after the 15th day, and nearly one-half after the 20th day.

Thirty-two cases proved fatal during the progress of the fever. The average day of residence in the hospital on which these patients died was the 7th—two dying on the 3rd day after their admission, and one surviving till the 16th day.

The six patients (omitting one who died of smallpox) that recovered from the attack of typhus, and the date of the commencement of whose illness was ascertained, or nearly so, died respectively on the 22nd, 23rd, 24th, 29th, 44th, and 148th days, reckoning from the outset of the disease; the day of death of these patients being respectively the 19th, 18th, 17th, 17th, 31st, and 141st of their residence in the hospital.

The four patients, the duration of whose illness before admission was unknown, and who died of disease that supervened during the progress of the typhus, and continued after that had run its course, or that began after its termination, died severally on the 11th, 12th, 16th, and 30th days after they were admitted into the wards.

ERUPTION.

Description of the Rose Spots peculiar to Typhoid Fever.— The eruption in the cases of typhoid fever here analysed was papular. The papulæ, called by Louis *taches roses lenticulaires*, possessed the following characters :—

They were slightly elevated. To detect the elevation the finger had to be passed very delicately over the surface, as they had none of the hardness of the papulæ of lichen, or of the first day's eruption of smallpox. Their apices were never acuminated, never flat, but invariably rounded—their bases gradually passed into the level of the surrounding cuticle. No trace of a vesicle or white spot of any kind was ever detected on them. They were circular and of a bright rose colour, the latter fading insensibly into the natural hue of the skin around. They never possessed a well-defined margin.

They disappeared completely on pressure, resuming their characteristic appearances as soon as the pressure was removed, and this was true from first to last, from their first eruption to their last trace. They left no stain of the cuticle behind; they never passed into anything resembling petechiæ —the characters they presented on their first appearance continned till they vanished. Their ordinary size was about a line in diameter, but occasionally they were not more than half a line, and sometimes a line and a half in diameter.

The duration of each papula was three or four days; fresh papulæ made their appearance every day or two. Sometimes only one or two were present at first, ran the course above described, and then one or more fresh ones made their appearance, vanished in three or four days, and were followed by others to last as long.

The number of papulæ seen at one time on the surface was ordinarily from six to twenty—though occasionally there was only one, and sometimes more than one hundred.

They usually occupied the abdomen, thorax, and back, but were occasionally present on the extremities. One was frequently noticed on the thorax over the cellular interval, at the upper border of the pectoralis major on either side.

A *very pale and delicate* scarlet tint of the skin sometimes preceded the eruption of the papulæ, but never lasted more than a day or two—the skin resembling in tint that of a person shortly after leaving a hot bath.

Rose spots were present in nineteen of the twenty-three fatal cases here analysed.

There was no eruption detected in four cases.

The date of the first appearance of the papulæ was ascertained in three cases, which commenced suddenly, and was the 8th, 12th, and 20th days; the patients being admitted respectively on the 4th, 5th, and 10th days of the disease.

In a fourth case, in which the papulæ first appeared on the 19th day, the patient, a strong-made butcher's man, left his work only eight days before the eruption appeared, but had been ailing for ten days before he left his work.

The papulæ were present in thirteen cases when the patients first came under observation—three of these cases being seen for the first time on the 9th, 13th, and 18th. day of the disease ; five on about the 8th, 10th, 12th, 16th and 22nd day ; and two on about the 15th, and two on the 28th day. In one case no clew to the duration of the disease before the patient's admission could be obtained. In two cases the date of the first appearance of the spots was not noted.

Of the four cases in which no spots were detected, three had been ill before they entered the hospital more than fourteen days, and one probably more than three weeks.

The longest time any given papula remained visible was six days, the shortest time one day. The average duration of each spot, calculated from repeated observations on nine of the cases here analysed, each observation including several spots, was 3·14 days.

In three cases which proved fatal on the 32nd, 34th, and 86th days, fresh spots made their appearance as late as the 29th, 21st, and 24th [1] days. The first of these cases proved fatal from peritonitis, the other two died of erysipelas.

In the seven cases which proved fatal on about the 23rd, 25th, 28th, 30th, 44th, 46th, and 71st days, fresh spots were observed to appear, respectively, as late as about the 19th, 15th, 24th, 24th, 23d, 24th, and 30th days of the disease. Of these patients, the first three, or those who expired as nearly as could be ascertained before the 30th day, died chiefly from the abdominal lesion.

The last four died respectively of pneumonia, sloughing, erysipelas, and pleuro-pneumonia and sloughing.

No second crop of papulæ was observed in seven cases, the patients dying on the 2nd, 3rd, 3rd, 5th, 6th, 7th, and 15th days, after they came under observation.

In the two cases in which the date of the first appearance of the spots was not noted, the presence or absence of more than one crop of papulæ was not recorded.

To sum up—

1. Rose spots were detected during the progress of all the cases admitted before the 14th day of the disease.

---

[1] This patient had a relapse after convalescence was partially established, and then spots reappeared and continued as late as the forty-ninth day.

2. The spots usually appeared between the 7th and 14th days after the first symptoms of the disease showed themselves.[1]

3. The ordinary duration of each spot was three days.

4. Fresh spots generally appear every day or two after their first eruption, till from the 21st to the 30th day.

5. One case relapsed, and in that fresh papulæ appeared every day or two till the 24th day, then no more were seen till the 37th day, after which fresh spots were again noted daily till the 49th day, reckoning from the first outset of the disease.

6. The fever terminated by the 30th day, as proved by no fresh spots appearing after that day, unless in the case of a relapse, and by the presence of local complications sufficient to account for death in all cases that proved fatal after that date.

Description of the Mulberry Rash[2] peculiar to Typhus.—In the case of typhus fever, the eruption was never papular. Its characters varied with its duration. On the first appearance of the rush, it consisted of very slightly elevated spots of a dusky pink colour. Each spot was flattened on the surface, irregular in outline, had no well-defined margin, but faded insensibly into the hue of the surrounding skin, disappeared completely on pressure, and varied in size from a point to three or four lines in diameter. The largest spots appeared to be formed by the coalescence of two or more smaller ones, and the shape of the former accordingly was more irregular than that of the latter.[3]

[1] I would here remind the reader, that as these particulars are deduced from a limited number of fatal cases, the exact days of the first and last appearance of the eruption seem to be a little more irregular than they really are. It is well known that fatal cases of smallpox and scarlet fever are not the best fitted for exhibiting the regular course of the eruption in the two diseases.

[2] I have ventured to use a new term for designating the rash peculiar to typhus, because I consider it unadvisable to retain any of the names now in use, limited as each of those names is to a peculiar modification of the one rash here described. In consequence of the eruptions in scarlet and typhoid fevers having received names from their colour, and the rash of typhus fever often resembling the hue of the stain of the mulberry, I have been led to adopt the above term.

[3] In some cases it was doubtful if the spots on their *first* appearance had not the characters here assigned to them as their second stage.

Second Stage.—In one, two, or three days, these spots underwent a marked change; they were no longer elevated above the surrounding cuticle, their hue was darker and more dingy than on their first appearance, their margins rather more, but still imperfectly defined, and now they only faded on pressure.[1]   In this stage they were usually darker, less affected by pressure, and their margins more defined on the posterior than on the anterior surface of the body.   In some cases the spots after this grew paler, passed into faintly marked reddish-brown stains, and then disappeared.

Third Stage.—In others a third stage was reached, the centres of the spots became dark purple, and remained un-altered by pressure, although their circumferences still faded; or the entire spots, the circumferences as well as the centres, changed into true petechiæ, *i.e.* spots presenting the following characters—a dusky crimson or purple colour, quite unaffected by pressure, a well-defined margin, and total want of elevation above the level of the cuticle.   This alteration was most fre-quently observed to take place on the back, at the bend of the elbow, and in the groin.   At the bend of the elbow they were generally oval, their long axis lying in the direction of the long axis of the arm.

In a large majority of the cases the spots were very numer-ous, close together, sometimes almost covering the skin.   In a few instances, however, they were comparatively few in number, very pale, and situated at some distance from each other.[2]

The usual situation of the spots was the trunk and extremities, but occasionally they were limited to the trunk, and now and then were observed on the face.

---

[1] By the term 'faded on pressure,' I intend to signify, that however firmly the finger was pressed on the spots, they could not be entirely obliterated, but some trace of the spots or stain of the cuticle remained.

[2] In these cases, on the first day of their appearance they occasionally bore so close a resemblance to the rose spots, that although they were never alto-gether identical with the best-marked specimens of the latter, yet the most tutored eye might be in some doubt as to which order they belonged; and when the general symptoms were at the same time equivocal, the diagnosis was impossible till a day or two had elapsed, when some or all of the spots passed into their second stage; whereas, if they had been the spots peculiar to the typhoid fever, they would have retained the characters they presented on the first day, till they disappeared altogether on the third or fourth day after their eruption.

Their number reached its maximum on the first, second, or third day, no fresh spots appearing after the latter date, and each spot remained visible from its first eruption till the whole rash vanished.

When very numerous, the whole of the spots seen together on the surface had not an equal depth of colour, many were much paler than the others, and had a dull appearance as if seen through the cuticle. In my notes I have been in the habit of distinguishing these collectively as the 'subcuticular rash.' *It often, by its abundance, gave a mottled aspect to the skin, on which ground the darker spots were seated.*

Variations in the absolute or relative amount of the sub-cuticular rash, and of the spots, as well as in the depth of their respective colours, cause much difference in the general appearance of the rash. Sometimes it resembles measles so closely as to be distinguished from it with difficulty ; at others, it presents that appearance which has been called the spotted rash ; and again, it is sometimes so pale, that unless carefully looked for it might be passed over altogether. When the spots on the back were of a much deeper hue than those on the anterior surface of the trunk, the skin covering the posterior surface was generally considerably congested. Slight pressure of the finger left a white mark, which slowly returned to its previous dusky red colour.

The eruption (mulberry rash) characteristic of typhus fever, was observed in all of the forty-three cases of that disease here analysed.

The rash appeared in two cases after the patient's admission into the hospital ; the date of its first eruption in these two cases was the seventh and ninth days. In the remaining forty-one cases, the rash was developed before the patients came under observation.

Of these forty-one cases—

1 was first seen on the 6th day of disease.				1 was first seen on about the 5th day of disease.		
2	were	,,	7th ,,	2	,, ,,	8th ,,
5	,,	,,	8th ,,	2	,, ,,	9th ,,
5	,,	,,	9th ,,	1	,,	10th ,,
5	,,	,,	10th ,,	2	,,	15th ,,
1	,,	,,	12th ,,			
1	,,	,,	13th ,,			
	,,	,,	15th ,,			

And in twelve cases it was uncertain how long the disease had existed prior to the presence of the rash being noted.

In eleven of the forty-three cases, the eruption disappeared before death, a mere trace of the spots only existing in four cases on the 14th day, in two on the 20th, and in one there was no trace of the spots on the 24th day, no note of their condition having been taken for some days preceding; these seven patients were first seen on the 7th, 8th, 9th, 9th, 9th, 10th, and 15th days of the disease, the eruption being present on all at these times.

The four patients from whom the rash disappeared on the 14th day died on the 23rd, 24th, 32nd, and 148th days, after the first symptoms of fever showed themselves. Of these the first died of asthenic laryngitis; the second of phlebitis, which began after the patient had left his bed and was considered convalescent; the third of smallpox, caught during convalescence; and the fourth of erysipelas, sloughing of the back, and pneumonia. The diseases that caused death in the first and last supervened during the progress of the fever, and continued after that had run its course.

Of the three patients from whom the rash disappeared on the 20th, and before the 24th days of the disease, the two former died on the 22nd and 29th days of circumscribed gangrene of the lung, and of sloughing abscess and pleuro-pneumonia; and the third on the 44th day, of gangrenous abscess of the lung. These fatal complications also arose during the course of the primary disease, and caused the patients' death some time after the specific fever had termiuated. It was uncertain how long the disease had existed prior to the admission of the remaining four patients (i.e. of the eleven from whom the eruption disappeared before death), but a mere trace only of the spots was to be seen on the 8th, 9th, 9th, and 13th days of their residence in the hospital, the patients dying on the 11th, 12th, 30th, and 16th days respectively, of pus in the joints, cerebral congestion, pleuro-pneumonia, and erysipelas; all commencing before the fever had finished its course, and continuing and proving fatal to the patient after its termination.

In one case, some difficulty was experienced in determining the nature of the spots, i.e. whether they were true

typhus spots; they were in fact so imperfectly marked, that
the diagnosis between typhus and typhoid fever could not
in this case have been positively formed from the eruption
alone.

In the remaining thirty-one cases, the rash was distinctly
visible till death. In four of these cases, it became somewhat
paler the last two or three days of life; in four others, no
note of its condition was made for a day or two before the
fatal termination—these eight patients survived beyond the
14th day of the disease; in twenty-three of these thirty-one
cases, the rash continued to grow darker, and to be less
affected by pressure, till death.

Of the thirty-one cases in which the mulberry rash was
distinctly visible till death—

1 died on the 10th day of the disease.	1 died on about the 9th day of disease.
2 „ 11th „ „	1 „ 11th „ „
2 „ 12th „	1 „ 13th „ „
3 „ 13th „	1 „ 15th „ „
3 „ 14th „	1 „ 16th „ „
1 „ 15th „	2 „ 17th „ „
2 „ 16th „	
2 „ 17th „	
1 „ 19th „	
1 „ 20th „ „	

The date of the disease on admission in six cases was entirely
unknown; two of the six died on the third day of their
residence in the hospital, the other four respectively on the
4th, 6th, 7th, and 8th days. To sum up—

1. The mulberry rash was present in all the cases.

2. The rash usually appeared from the 5th to the 8th
day of the disease.[1]

3. Fresh spots never appeared after the 2nd or 3rd days
of the eruption.

4. The duration of each spot was from its first appearance
till the death or recovery of the patient from the attack of
typhus.

5. The rash disappeared between the 14th and 21st days
of the disease; when death ensued after the latter date, it
was the result of local disease, which either complicated
the progress of the fever, and continued after that had run

[1] See note [2], p. 19.

its course, or sprang up anew, connected or not with the enfeebled state of constitution, the consequence of the fever.

6. In no case was there any return of the eruption, and therefore *no true relapse.*

MILIARY VESICLES—HYGROMETRIC AND THERMOMETRIC CONDITIONS OF THE SKIN.

Typhoid Fever.—Miliary vesicles were noted to be present during life in three of the twenty-three cases here analysed. In one they appeared on the 84th day of the disease,[1] and continued till the death of the patient on the 27th day ; in one of the three there were none present on the 9th day, but a great number were observed on the 11th, and continued till the 14th or 15th, the patient dying on the 25th day; in the third case there was an abundant crop on the 26th day. In all the three cases they were preceded and accompanied by a warm skin and profuse sweating.

In four of the remaining twenty cases, miliary vesicles were detected after death ; two of the four sweated profusely just before death ; the condition of the skin in the other two at that time was not recorded. Therefore, seven of the twenty-three had miliary vesicles—*i.e.* in the proportion of 30·4 per cent., or nearly one-third.

The skin during the first week of the disease was hot and dry in two cases, warm and perspiring in one case. None of these cases were seen before the 4th day of the disease.

During the second week it was hot and dry in one case: hot and sweating in three ; cool or cold in one.

During the third week it was hot and dry in three cases ; hot and sweating in one ; warm and dry in two ; cool and dry in five cases.

During the fourth week it was hot and dry in three cases ; hot and sweating in one; warm and dry in two : and warm and sweating in one case.

[1] From the calculation made when treating of the duration of the two diseases, it appeared probable that I had ascertained very nearly the date of the disease on which those said to have been admitted on about a given day of the disease were received into the hospital. I shall, therefore, henceforth, make no distinction between the two groups, but speak of all as admitted or seen on a given day of the disease.

The variations in the temperature of the skin in the same patient were considerable; and in several instances where the typhoid fever was prolonged, these changes were observed to have no relation to the duration of the disease. Thus the skin hot on the 8th day was in one case warm on the 9th, hot on the 10th, warm on the 11th, 12th, and 14th, and again hot the six or seven succeeding days. And the same want of relation existed between the sweats and the duration of the disease. Thus in the case last referred to the patient perspired during the 10th, 12th, 13th, and 14th nights—the skin having been dry during the days; on the 17th day the skin was moist; while on the 15th, 16th, 18th, and 22d, there were no sweats either at night or during the day.

Typhus Fever.—Miliary vesicles were observed during life in two of the forty-three cases. In one the hygrometric condition of the skin was not noted at the time of their appearance—viz., the 12th day of the disease; they had disappeared before the patient was seen on the 16th day—the skin having been cool and dry the preceding day. This patient survived till the 148th day from the commencement of illness. In the other case the skin, hot and dry on the 11th day, was sweating profusely on the 12th and 13th—on neither of which days were any miliary vesicles present; but on the 14th day there were a few in the groin and under the clavicles. This patient died on the 15th day of the disease.

There were no miliary vesicles in eleven cases. The skin in three of the eleven perspired profusely; in one it was cool, in five warm and dry; and in two it was hot and dry.

No note of the presence or absence of miliary vesicles was made during life in the remaining thirty cases; but in three of the thirty some were discovered after death. The hygrometric state of the skin, which existed for some time before the fatal termination, was not recorded in these three cases.

During the first week of the disease the skin was hot and dry in two cases, and warm and dry in four—none of them being seen before the 5th day.

During the second week it was hot in seven cases, two of which sweated profusely, one on the 15th, and the other on the 13th and 14th days; it was warm and dry in fourteen cases, two of which sweated profusely on respectively the 9th and 10th day; it was cool in twelve cases, two of which perspired freely on the 15th day of the disease.

The profuse perspirations in the above six cases preceded the fatal termination one or two days, and continued till death.

During the third week of the disease the skin was warm and dry in one case, which survived till the 148th day of illness, and cool in three cases. After the temperature began to fall, it was exceedingly rare for it to rise again, unless the illness was prolonged by local disease beyond the termination of the typhus fever.

It is remarkable that of the five patients who sweated profusely, and on whom, nevertheless, no miliary vesicles were detected, four were more than forty years old, their mean age being fifty-five years; while the five patients on whose skin miliary vesicles were detected, either during life or after death, were all under forty, their mean age being thirty-one years.

Seventeen of the forty-three patients who laboured under typhus fever, and whose cases we are examining, were under forty years of age; five of the seventeen—*i.e.* in the proportion of 29·4 per cent.—had, as I have stated, miliary vesicles of their surface, either detected during life or discovered after death.

Twenty-six of the forty-three patients labouring under typhus fever were forty years of age and upwards; but on not one of these was a vesicle detected.

EXPRESSION—MANNER—HUE OF FACE, ETC.

Typhoid Fever.—The expression in two cases was nearly natural throughout the whole course of the disease.

In the majority of the cases here examined it was oppressed, heavy, and somewhat anxious; the expression of heaviness and prostration was, however, far less marked than in the cases of typhus fever; and in two patients, while delirious, the expression was highly vivacious.

The natural hue of the face—*i.e.* of the skin of the whole face—was unchanged, excepting in three cases, in which it had a very slightly marked dusky appearance.

There was no flush in three, and no note made of its presence in eight cases.

In twelve of the twenty-three cases the face was flushed; in eleven of the twelve the flush was pink, and limited to one or both cheeks; it varied in intensity, disappeared, and returned occasionally in the same day.

This limitation of the flush to the cheeks was not peculiar to any one period of the disease ; it was well marked in one case, when admitted on the 8th day of the disease, and continued so till the 23rd day, the patient dying on the 25th. In another, admitted on the 5th day, there was a circumscribed flush on the cheeks on the 7th day, which continued with little change till the 15th day, the patient dying on the 17th day.

This flush when conjoined, as it sometimes was, with extreme emaciation, sunken eyes, large pupils, quick breathing, sharp and somewhat anxious manner, forcibly recalled to the mind cases, not of typhus fever, but of phthisis.

Typhus Fever.—In none of the forty-three cases was the expression natural throughout the disease.

In a large majority of the cases both the expression and the manner of the patient were so peculiar, that from them alone the diagnosis might have been formed. They were dull, heavy, oppressed, confused, like those of a drunken man just disturbed from sleep. The mind was rarely intelligent enough after the commencement of the second week to be disturbed as to the final issue ; and, as the disease in itself is free from serious organic lesion, all automatic as well as mental expression of anxiety was absent.

The hue of the face, after about the 6th day, was, like the expression and manner, peculiar—it was thick and *muddy-looking*; the change from this condition to the clearness of health was most remarkable—it was well seen in the patient who recovered from the attack of fever and died of small-pox, before referred to.

This muddy hue had no relation to the flush of the face, for it was often present when the face was pale ; moreover, though only noted in the face, it affected more or less the whole skin.

The face was flushed in eighteen cases, and in every case the flush covered the whole face, though in some it might have been somewhat more intense on the cheek than elsewhere.

The colour of the face when flushed was dusky red, and never pink, as the cheeks were in the cases of typhoid fever.

In some cases the face was recorded to be pale throughout the disease. Its condition in the other cases was not noted.

HEADACHE.

Typhoid Fever.—In two cases, the histories of which were complete, and the duration of the disease lengthened, there was no headache.

In twelve cases, headache was one of the earliest symptoms; in five of these it disappeared respectively on about the 6th, 13th, 13th, 17th, and 17th day of the disease; in six, before they came under observation, severally on the 15th, 16th, 18th, 21st, 21st, and 28th day. In one case there was a little headache on the 14th day; but, from the subsequent mental confusion of the patient, it was uncertain when it ceased.

Of the previous histories of nine cases, with respect to the point we are investigating, no particulars could be obtained; but in three there was no headache on the 15th, 21st, and 21st day; in one there was only trifling headache on the 15th day; the state of mind in the remaining five was such when they entered the hospital, that I could not ascertain if headache existed at that time.

Thus headache was in a large majority of cases one of the earliest symptoms of these cases of typhoid fever; and in the majority of them it disappeared spontaneously at the latter end of the second, or during the third week of the disease.

The pain was generally seated in the forehead, and never in the occiput. It varied much in degree, some patients complaining of it severely, others scarcely noticing it. It had no definite character—*i.e.* the patients could rarely give it any name, as darting, bursting, etc.

Typhus Fever.—In two cases there was no headache.

In nineteen cases it was one of the earliest symptoms, and, in the majority, commenced the first or second day of the disease; in four of the nineteen it disappeared respectively on the 8th, 9th, 11th, and 12th day; in seven there was no headache present when the cases were severally taken on the 8th, 9th, 9th, 10th, 10th, 13th, and 14th day; in three others it was still very severe respectively on the 6th, 7th, and 9th day; in the remaining five of the nineteen there was so much mental confusion or actual delirium present when the patients came under observation, that no dependence could be placed on their answers to questions regarding their sensations; the fact of the existence of headache at an early period of the disease was in these cases obtained from the friends of the patients. In three cases, the histories of which were doubtful, the headache was trifling when they were first seen severally on the 8th, 8th, and 9th day; it had disappeared in all the three on the 10th day.

Of five patients in whom the duration of the disease before their admission into the hospital was unknown, and the histories of whose cases were uncertain, four had some headache when first seen; the fifth was at that time free from pain in the head.

No dependence could be placed on the replies of fourteen of the forty-three patients to questions regarding their sensations, in consequence of their mental confusion; but none of the fourteen while in the hospital complained of headache.

So that headache was one of the earliest symptoms in a large majority of the cases, and it usually disappeared spontaneously by the 10th day of the disease, and in every case before the termination of the second week.

The seat of the pain was generally the forehead, very rarely the vertex or temples, and in no case the occiput. It varied much in severity, was often extremely intense, but was sometimes so trifling, that unless inquiries had been made of the patients, they would not have mentioned it.

It was usually an undefinable pain, not to be characterised by such terms as stabbing, throbbing, etc.

DELIRIUM.

Typhoid Fever.—There was no delirium in three cases, but in one of the three there was considerable mental confusion.

Delirium was present in twenty cases; in ten of the twenty it began severally on the 3rd, 6th, 6th, 10th, 14th, 15th, 23rd, 26th, 28th, and 29th day; seven were delirious when first seen between the 13th and 21st days inclusive: in the remaining three of the twenty cases it was uncertain at what date of the disease the delirium set in.

The delirium continued till death in nine cases; in eight of these the fatal termination occurred on the 12th, 17th, 17th, 21st, 25th, 27th, 30th, and 30th day of the disease; in one of the nine the duration of the disease at the time of the patient's death was unknown.

In one case, which proved fatal on the 23rd day, there was no delirium after the 21st day, from which time till her death the patient lay in a state of profound stupor.

The delirium usually first showed itself at night, the patients sleeping during part of the day. It varied much in amount, sometimes being so violent that the patients left their beds, and even ran screaming through the wards; at others showing itself by slight delusions only discovered to exist by accident, or again by almost constant chattering.

Ten of eighteen patients—i.e. more than one-half, or in the proportion of 55·5 per cent. of those who were delirious after they entered the hospital, and of whom notes on the point were made—left their beds to wander about the ward.

Typhus Fever.—The mind of one patient of the forty-three, whose cases I am here examining, was perfect throughout the disease. This was a very mild case in every particular; the patient died of phlebitis after he had once left his bed. In another case there was only slight mental confusion; this patient also survived the fever. Although there was no actual delirium in thirteen other cases, yet there was in them such extreme mental confusion that the patients could give no account of their past state, 'felt bothered,' had no idea how long they had been in the hospital, nor in some cases where they were.

Delirium began in ten cases respectively on the 5th, 8th, 10th, 10th, 11th, 11th, 11th, 12th, and 13th day. It was present when five cases first came under observation, severally on the 6th, 8th, 9th, 9th, and 14th day.

In every instance in which the delirium commenced after

the patients entered the hospital, excepting one, it was preceded by a varying amount of mental confusion.

It was uncertain how long nine patients had been ill, who were delirious when I first saw them. Four patients were admitted into the wards in a state of complete stupor. The delirium continued till the death of the patients in thirteen cases, nine of which proved fatal severally on the 9th, 11th, 11th, 14th, 16th, 17th, 17th, 19th, and 20th day. The remainder of the forty-three patients either sank into a state of absolute coma, or survived the termination of the fever.

The character of the delirium was usually far less active than that of the delirium of typhoid fever, the patients displayed less vivacity, and fewer of them, seven only of the twenty-four, i.e. at the rate of 29·2 per cent. of those who were delirious after they were admitted into the hospital, attempted to leave their beds to roam in the wards.

SOMNOLENCE—COMA VIGIL.

Typhoid Fever.—There was no somnolence in twelve cases; one of these proved fatal after the patient had been ill an uncertain time; eleven on the 12th, 17th, 17th, 21st, 25th, 25th, 27th, 30th, 32nd, 46th, and 86th day after the illness commenced. These eleven cases were seen for the first time respectively on the 5th, 6th, 15th, 14th, 7th, 11th, 20th, 28th, 18th, 16th, and 9th day.

Somnolence was observed in eleven cases; of three of these I have no notes to show when it ceased, but it was profound when one was admitted on the 6th day; in four cases which proved fatal after the termination of the fever, somnolence began on the 15th, 22nd, 25th, and 26th day, and ceased on the 19th, 28th, 31st, and 27th day, the patients dying respectively on the 44th, 71st, 34th, and 46th day; in three cases somnolence commenced on the 14th, 23rd, and 27th day, and continued till the death of the patients severally on the 23rd, 28th, and 30th day; one patient was somnolent when the case was taken on the 15th day; continued so till the 23rd, and died on the 33rd of pleuro-pneumonia.

The intensity of the somnolence varied from mere

drowsiness to profound stupor. I have not included among
the cases affected with somnolence, those of the patients who
slept during a portion of the day, but who had been awake a
great part of the night. *Coma Vigil*, as described under the
head of typhus, was not present in a single case.

Typhus Fever.—There was no somnolence in sixteen
cases; six of these survived the fever. The duration of the
disease prior to the admission of four of the sixteen cases
could not be ascertained. The remaining twelve were admitted into the hospital, one on the 6th, four on the 7th,
four on the 8th, one on the 9th, one on the 12th, and one on
the 14th day of the disease, and (those that lived after the
termination of the fever being omitted) died, one each on
the 10th, 11th, 12th, and 14th days, and three on the 16th
day.

Somnolence occurred in twenty-seven cases; in eleven of
them on the 7th, 10th, 9th, 11th, 11th, 11th, 12th, 12th, 12th,
13th, and 13th day; in seven before the 10th, 10th, 13th,
14th, 14th, 14th, and 15th day.

It continued in twenty cases till death, which in eleven of
the twenty happened during the latter part of the second
week, *i.e.* from the 9th to the 14th day inclusive; in four
during the third week, *i.e.* between the 15th and 20th day;
in five of the twenty cases the duration of the disease was
unknown. In three cases the somnolence terminated in
coma vigil.

Coma Vigil.—By this term I intend to express that peculiar condition in which the patient lies with his eyes open,
evidently awake, but indifferent or insensible to all going on
around him, and not what some writers on fever have meant
by the expression, viz., that state in which a patient lies
asleep for hours, and yet declares on awakening that he has
never closed his eyes.

Nine patients, or more than one-fifth of the forty-three
patients, experienced coma vigil (as I have above defined the
expression) from one to four days immediately preceding
their death. These nine cases terminated fatally on from the
10th to the 19th day, and in two cases at an uncertain period
of the disease.

RELATION BETWEEN HEADACHE, DELIRIUM, SOMNOLENCE, AND COMA VIGIL.

Typhoid Fever.—The two patients who from the outset of the disease were free from headache, had violent and long-continued delirium, but were up to the time of their death exempt from somnolence.

In two cases only was there any headache after delirium commenced.

One patient, who died after the termination of the fever, was violently delirious on his admission on the 15th day of the disease, and profoundly comatose on the 16th; another, delirious and sleeping less than natural on his admission on the 15th day, continued in the same state till the 26th day, when he became very drowsy and remained so for twenty-four hours; after recovering from this slight somnolence he slept tolerably well till his death, on the forty-sixth day from the commencement of his illness.

The delirium continued after the somnolence began in all the cases, and did not disappear till the death of the patient, unless the somnolence passed into coma.

In one case the delirium was considerable and long-continued, the somnolence trifling.

There was headache in one case, in the course of which there was neither somnolence nor delirium.

Typhus Fever.—Of the two patients whose histories rendered it probable that they had no headache, even from the outset of the disease, and certainly they could have had but little, one suffered from violent delirium, and the other from somnolence terminating in coma vigil.

The headache disappeared before the delirium began in every case in which the latter commenced after the patient's entrance into the hospital.

Of ten cases accurate information was obtained respecting the date of the commencement of somnolence and delirium; in nine of the ten the delirium preceded the somnolence, in one only did the somnolence precede the delirium.

Delirium was unaccompanied by somnolence in five cases, but two of these had coma vigil. Somnolence without actual

c

delirium occurred in six cases ; coma vigil without delirium in three; somnolence and delirium conjoined in nineteen cases.

Delirium preceded coma vigil in five cases, the delirium in one being accompanied by somnolence; this peculiar condition was preceded by somnolence without delirium in one case, mental confusion not amounting to actual delirium preceded it in two cases, and it was present when one case entered the hospital.

SPASMODIC MOVEMENTS.

Typhoid Fever.—Spasmodic twitchings of the muscles of the face or arms occurred in six of twenty-one cases ; picking of the bed-clothes in two. In no case were there general convulsions.

Typhus Fever.—Involuntary twitchings of the muscles of the face, arms, or hands, were observed in twelve cases. In two of these the spasmodic action of the inferior recti muscles of the eyes, and of the levatores palpebrarum gave to the countenance a most remarkable aspect ; the spasmodic movements were in both cases excited at any moment by suddenly raising either arm—the patients at the time appearing totally insensible to all going on around.

Two patients suffered from general convulsions ; in both cases they were repeated twice, at intervals of one and three days.

RETENTION OF URINE, AND INVOLUNTARY DISCHARGE OF URINE AND STOOLS.

Typhoid Fever.—The urine was retained in one case only, and the catheter had to be introduced for its removal on the 23rd day of the disease.

The urine was passed involuntarily in ten cases ; for the first time on from the 9th to the 27th day of the disease. Thus about one-half of the cases experienced involuntary discharge or retention of urine. Ten patients passed stools into the bed ; this symptom was noted to be present for the first time on from the 13th to the 35th day of the disease. With one exception the urine was passed involuntarily into the bed at the same time as the stools.

Typhus Fever.—The urine was retained, and required the use of the catheter for its removal in eleven of the forty-three cases. The retention first occurred between the 10th and 21st days inclusive, and with two exceptions between the 10th and 16th days inclusive. It was passed involuntarily in twelve cases—this first took place on from the 8th to the 20th day; in two cases the retention of urine was preceded for a day by its involuntary discharge. Either retention or involuntary discharge of urine was a symptom in twenty-one or in nearly one-half of the patients; and as no notes on the point were taken in seven cases in which the prostration was extreme, it is probable that considerably more than one-half were thus affected.

The stools were passed involuntarily in seventeen cases; the day of the disease on which this symptom first occurred was from the 8th to the 21st; it was in every case accompanied by an involuntary discharge of urine.

LOSS OF MUSCULAR POWER AFTER THE PATIENT'S
ADMISSION INTO THE HOSPITAL.

Typhoid Fever.—Two patients were able to leave their beds unassisted and with facility throughout the whole course of the disease. One of these patients died on the 25th day of the disease, and the other five weeks after her admission.

Two were able to leave their beds with tolerable facility up to the 15th and 24th day of the disease respectively, but the former on the 16th and the latter on the 26th day, were unable, without assistance, to reach the close stool placed immediately adjoining the bed.

Five patients could, though with great difficulty, get out of bed unassisted, from the 13th to the 30th days, while ten were quite unable to do so from the 5th to the 26th days; there was extreme prostration in eight cases from the 14th to the 30th days.

Of four patients my notes were incomplete.

Two others were admitted in a state of extreme prostration after the disease had lasted an uncertain period.

Typhus Fever.—One patient only could leave his bed with

tolerable facility through the whole course of the disease; this was a very mild case in every respect, and the patient died of phlebitis some time after convalescence from the fever; two with difficulty from their admission on the 8th and 7th day of the disease, till the death of one on the 14th, and the recovery of the other, who eventually died of small-pox.

Twelve patients were unable to leave their beds unassisted from the 6th to the 14th day.

In thirty-four cases the prostration was extreme; in a large majority of these cases the prostration became extreme between the 9th and the 12th days. In one case the patient, though able to get out of bed unassisted, with difficulty, on the 5th day of the disease, was quite unable to leave her bed unassisted on the 6th, and on the 9th day was in a state of extreme prostration. In one case only the prostration was not extreme till as late as the 17th day of the disease.

Nine cases were at the time of their admission into the hospital in a state of extreme prostration; the duration of the disease, prior to the time they came under observation, being unknown.

SYMPTOMS FURNISHED BY THE ORGANS OF THE SENSES.

Typhoid Fever.—*Epistaxis* occurred in one-third of the cases, or in five out of fifteen, the particulars of which were obtained from the commencement of the disease; in neither of them was it excessive, and in one case only a few drops of blood were lost. The hemorrhage took place in these five cases respectively on the 4th, 8th, 11th, 12th, and 12th day; it was repeated in the last on the 14th day.

In six cases it was not known whether epistaxis had taken place prior to the patients' admission into the hospital, which in four of the six was on the 6th, 13th, 14th, and 21st day, and in two at an undetermined period of the disease.

Hearing.—Almost a fourth, or six of the twenty-three patients had deafness more or less complete after they entered the hospital; and three tinnitus aurium; one of these three subsequently became deaf. The difficulty in hearing made its appearance on from the 12th to the 25th days.

Eyes.—The conjunctivæ were injected in three cases, and in one of the three continued so from the time the patient was first seen, *i.e.* the 13th day of the disease, till the fatal termination on the 23rd day; the other two came under observation between the 21st and 27th days. In one case they were injected when the patient was first seen on the 9th day of the disease, but on the 11th day they were pale. In ten other cases the conjunctivæ were noted to be pale, the patients being under observation repeatedly at different periods of the disease; one of these ten cases was seen as early as the 5th, and one as late as the 30th day.

In two cases only were the pupils of the eyes noted to be smaller than natural, while in seven cases they were decidedly dilated; the pupils of the eyes in two patients, first observed on the 5th and 14th days of the disease, were in each, at those dates noted to be normal in size, but on the 8th and 22nd day respectively, they were larger than natural.

The exact day of the disease on which they were first observed to be greatly dilated, varied in six cases, respecting which notes on the point were taken, from the 8th to the 22nd day; a seventh case came under observation after the fever had continued an uncertain time.

Typhus Fever.—Epistaxis.—There was not a single instance of bleeding from the nose in twenty-three cases, the particulars of which, before they entered the hospital, were obtained; nor did one of the forty-three patients, whose cases we are examining, suffer from epistaxis after their admission into the hospital.

Hearing.—Nine, or rather more than a fifth of the forty-three patients labouring under typhus, had more or less complete deafness as a consequence of the fever, and one tinnitus aurium.

The difficulty of hearing was first observed from the 10th to the 13th day of the disease.

Eyes.—The conjunctivæ were more or less intensely injected in twenty-five cases; and in all of those in which the opportunity occurred of observing the date of the first appearance of this increased vascularity, it began during the second week. In one case only, seen during the first week, were they injected at that time; in eleven of the twenty-five cases in which the conjunctivæ were more vascular than natural, the pupils were contracted.

THE TONGUE.

Typhoid Fever.—Notes respecting the physical condition of the tongue were made in twenty of the twenty-three cases here considered.

In six it was moist during the whole time the patients were under observation, or respectively from the 10th, 11th, 12th, 15th, 18th, and 20th day, till their death; four of them dying between the 15th and 30th days, and two some time after the latter date. In four of these six cases it was clean or slightly furred, neither of the four dying before the 24th day of the disease; in the fifth it was brown and furred, and in the sixth yellow and furred.

In another case, first seen on the 20th day, and which proved fatal on the 27th day, the tongue, with the exception of the 25th day, when it was dry in the centre, was moist throughout the disease.

So that the tongue may be said to have been moist during the whole course of the disease in a third of the cases in which its condition in that respect was noted.

In twelve cases the tongue was entirely or partially dry and brown at some period of the disease; in two, however, the hue never exceeded in depth a pale yellow brown; in six it could never be said to be dark brown; while in two it was almost black; one of the two, however, was at the time suffering from extensive gangrene of one lower extremity.

In about one-third of the cases, *i.e.* seven of the twenty, it was more or less red; in one-fourth glazed entirely or partially; and in one-fifth of the twenty it was deeply fissured at some period of the disease.

In one case only was the patient unable to protrude the tongue when directed to do so.

There was no regularity in the order of the succession of these various conditions of the organ; thus, in one case seen on the 8th day, it was at that time covered with a thick layer of brown mucus, and rather moist; on the 9th and 10th days it was partially covered with yellowish brown flakes and fissured; on the 11th day moist, and covered with a thick white fur; on the 12th and 14th days it resumed the appearance it presented on the 9th and 11th days; on the 15th day it was again moist and white; on the 16th it presented a dry centre; on the 17th, 18th, and 19th days, it was pale brown over its whole surface, and fissured in the centre, while on the 22nd day its centre only was pale brown, its edges being white, on which day the last note of the tongue was made; the patient died on the 25th day of the disease.

Typhus Fever.—The varying physical conditions of the tongue were recorded in forty-one of the forty-three cases here analysed.

In one only was it moist during the whole time it was under observation; the patient, a female child, aged ten years, was first seen on the 15th day of the disease, the tongue being then moist and white; from the 18th to the 21st day it was moist and partially brown; the child eventually died from gangrenous tubercular abscess of the lung.

It was moist in ten cases when first seen on from the 8th to the 11th day, but grew darker as the disease advanced.

The tongue in thirty cases was dry when first under observation; the day of the disease on which twenty of the thirty were seen varied from the 6th to the 18th day; of the other ten, no history to determine the date of the disease could be obtained.

It was moist and slightly furred in a patient seen on the 9th day, dry and slightly furred in the same patient on the 10th, 11th, and 12th days; this was a very mild case, in which the fatal termination was caused by phlebitis.

In thirty-cases the tongue was completely dry and dark-brown at some period of the disease.

The patients, in whom it was dry and brown when they were first seen, and the date of whose disease on their admission was exactly or approximately ascertained, came under observation from the 6th to the 13th day.

It was moist and loaded in three patients on their admission the 8th, 8th, and 9th day of the disease, and became dry and brown in these three cases, respectively on the 10th, 10th, and 12th day.

In four only of the forty-one cases, or about one-tenth,

was the tongue fissured, and in five only, or about one-eighth, was there any redness of the organ. One-fifth of the patients were unable to protrude the tongue at some period of the disease.

ABDOMINAL PAIN, TENDERNESS AND PHYSICAL SIGNS.

Typhoid Fever.—Of eleven patients, respecting whose condition previous to their admission into the hospital pretty accurate histories with reference to the point were obtained, five, or nearly one-half, suffered pain in the abdomen, as one of the earliest symptoms of the outset of the disease.

Six of twenty-one patients, of whom notes on the point were made, suffered from pain in the abdomen after their admission into the hospital; these patients were received into the wards between the 8th and 16th day of the disease: in one case only was any pain complained of in the 4th week.

No tenderness existed in five cases while they were under observation, respectively from the 5th, 15th, 19th, and 21st day, till the 12th, 27th, 28th, and in two cases until after the 30th day.

Tenderness of the abdomen was present in three-fourths, or in fifteen of twenty cases, respecting which notes on the point we are considering were made.

In one of the fifteen, however, it did not arise till peritonitis, the consequence of perforation, had taken place.

The tenderness was sometimes limited to the right iliac fossa, and, though frequently extreme, was occasionally trifling.

Gurgling, generally situated in the right iliac fossa, was present in five cases, or nearly a fourth; the bowels being relaxed in every one of the five cases.

The abdomen was full in three cases, resonant in five, full and resonant in ten cases. In one instance only did it preserve its normal form, and afford a natural percussion note. The size of the abdomen was often extreme, but whether much or little distended, its shape was invariably the same, and somewhat peculiar; its convexity was from side to side, and not from above downward; the patient was never 'pot-bellied,' but tub-shaped. The cause probably was, that the flatus chiefly occupied the colon — ascending, descending, and transverse.

Typhus Fever.—One only out of twenty cases, of which histories on the point were obtained, had suffered pain in the abdomen among the first symptoms of the disease; this was a female, aged fifty-six, in whom the catamenia had for some time appeared at irregular intervals; she fainted suddenly nine days before her entrance into the hospital, and on recovery experienced severe headache and pain in the abdomen; on the following day the catamenia flowed freely, and all pain in the abdomen vanished.

Another admitted on the 8th day of the disease, had experienced griping pains in the abdomen from the 5th to the 7th day; there was no return of the pain in either case after admission.

Two patients, after they were received into the hospital, suffered from slight pain in the abdomen, respectively on the 8th and 9th day of the disease.

There was trifling tenderness of the abdomen in five of twenty-six cases seen during the second week of the disease; in two others there was tenderness at an uncertain period of the disease.

Of nine patients under observation, during the third week of the disease, and of whom notes were made with reference to the subject, one only experienced any tenderness of the abdomen.

Tenderness of the abdomen was then present at some period of the disease in nine cases, but in eight of them it was trivial and transient; in the ninth it was more decided, commenced gradually on the 12th day, and continued till the fatal termination on the 20th day; it was limited almost entirely to the hypogastric region. The subject of this anomaly suffered from retention of urine, and after death there was found minute capillary injection of the mucous membrane of the bladder, more marked on its anterior than on its posterior surface.

Gurgling was detected in one case only, and in that there existed at the time considerable diarrhœa.

The abdomen in twelve of forty-one cases, of which notes

on the point were made, was full and resonant; in three only of these twelve cases was it unnaturally distended, and in none of the three was it noted to possess the peculiar shape of the typhoid abdomen.

In twenty-two cases there was neither fulness, resonance, tenderness, nor gurgling; in these twenty-two cases the abdomen presented all the physical signs of health, and in two of them it was noted to be somewhat concave.

DISCHARGES FROM THE BOWELS.

Typhoid Fever.—Particulars were obtained from the patients or their friends, regarding the condition of the bowels before admission into the hospital, in sixteen of the twenty-three cases.

In two of the sixteen the bowels were confined, the patients being admitted respectively on the 9th and 15th day of the disease; in four, confined till after a dose of aperient medicine, from the moment of the action of which diarrhœa set in (these four were admitted into the hospital respectively on the 8th, 8th, 12th, and 29th day); in two cases which came under observation on the 4th and 13th day, the bowels were stated to have been regular up to those dates, one stool only having been passed daily.

The bowels were much relaxed before the admission of the remaining eight cases, in the majority from the outset of the disease, and in all before the administration of aperients.

The condition of the bowels was recorded frequently after the admission into the hospital in twenty-one of the twenty-three cases.

Of these twenty-one, two only needed aperients, one a single dose of castor oil, the second repeated doses of that and other aperients, while one case in the first week of the disease, three in the second, two in the third, and six during the fourth week, required the repeated exhibition of opiates to restrain diarrhœa. Of two patients seen during the first week of the disease, one passed from two to six watery stools daily, the other from three to four.

In the second week the number of stools passed each day varied from one to four. Of seven patients under observation during this time, five passed as many as three stools each, and one four stools in twenty-four hours. Of fourteen patients of whom notes were taken during the third week of the disease, nine passed three stools each, and two as many as four and six in one day, while in the fourth week fourteen out of fifteen patients passed three stools each on one day, and ten of fifteen from four to six stools. From the above calculations I have excluded the two cases which required an aperient after they came under observation. One of these, a male aged twenty-eight, entered the hospital on the 10th day of the disease. His bowels had been confined from the first, and for the twenty-four hours succeeding his admission he passed no stool; half an ounce of castor oil was given; on the following day he had three stools, on the 13th day two, on the 16th day he passed no stool, and from that time the bowels continued regular till the 25th day of the disease, when the patient died of profuse hemorrhage from the bowels. The other case was that of a female who entered the hospital on about the 15th day of the disease, but who had been under my observation for some days preceding her admission. From the first her bowels had been confined. On the 16th day she passed one stool, on the following day none, she then had half an ounce of castor oil, which acted three times; from this time till the 25th day, she scarcely had a stool without the aid of aperients. On the 28th she seemed nearly well, her bowels were quite regular, and she left her bed. On the 36th day she was suddenly seized with severe pain in the abdomen, took an aperient on the 37th day, and on the 38th passed four dark solid lumpy stools, on the 40th four equally solid stools; from this time she had one or more scanty solid stools till her death on the 46th day, from extensive ulceration and perforation of the agminated glands at the lower part of the ileum.

The consistence of the stools was watery in twelve cases at some period of the disease, and soft, pultaceous, or almost fluid in four others.

In eight cases only were stools of natural consistence passed after the patients came under observation, and in five of these the stools were watery during some period of the disease. Their colour varied from pale brown to almost black; when watery they were usually pale yellowish brown, with a sediment composed of small solid yellowish particles.

Seven out of twenty-one patients, particulars respecting whose stools were recorded, passed blood from the bowels. In one, discharges of blood took place on the 6th and 7th day of the disease. On the 10th the stools were healthy in appearance, and well formed, and although they afterwards became watery, there was no return of the hemorrhage. One man passed a small quantity of blood on the 8th, 9th, and 10th days of the disease, and again from the 28th to the 32nd —*i.e.* the day of death—the stools between the two attacks of hemorrhage being watery, but free from blood. In one case blood was mixed or passed with every stool from the 14th to the 21st day, the patient dying on the 25th day.

In four cases hemorrhage from the bowels occurred during the last day or two of life, the patients dying respectively on the 17th, 23rd, 25th, and 28th day of the disease.

The blood lost varied in quantity from an ounce or two to two or three pints; in hue from black to bright red; and in consistence from a reddish watery fluid to the consistence of treacle, and even solid clots.

Typhus Fever.—The bowels were stated to have been more or less confined from the commencement of the disease till the admission of the patients, in ten out of nineteen cases, the histories of which were obtained with as much accuracy as possible; in six of these nineteen cases they were regular from the first; five of the nineteen had taken one or more powerful doses of aperients, without producing any diarrhœa; three only of the nineteen had diarrhœa before their entrance into the hospital, and in two of the three it supervened after the use of aperient medicine; these nineteen cases were admitted between the 5th and the 12th days of the disease. Notes were taken of the condition of the bowels in the whole of the forty-three cases after the patient's admission into the hospital. Twenty-two needed, while under observation, the use of from one to four doses of aperient medicine, while in one case only was an opiate required for the purpose of checking diarrhœa.

In two of the four patients seen during the first week of the disease, the bowels were confined till an aperient was administered; and in neither of the other two did the number of stools passed in any one day exceed two.

Of ten patients seen during the second week who took no aperient, four only passed more than two stools on any one day; but one of these two had severe diarrhœa, passing from four to six watery stools daily.

Of nine patients under treatment during the third week, four required the use of aperient medicine, and in one only was there any diarrhœa.

Two of eleven patients admitted after the disease had lasted an uncertain time, required the use of aperients, and in one case only of the eleven was diarrhœa present; but in this case it was very severe, from two to six stools being evacuated daily for nearly a fortnight.

The consistence of the stools was noted in seventeen cases: in two only were they watery, in eight they were pultaceous, in seven solid. No note was made of their consistence in twenty-six cases; but in fourteen of these twenty-six aperients were required: so that in these the stools were at least as solid as natural, or scanty in quantity.

Hæmorrhage from the bowels did not occur in a single case.

APPETITE AND THIRST.

Typhoid and Typhus Fevers.—Loss of appetite was one of the earliest symptoms in both diseases, and continued till their termination. There was more or less thirst in every case of the two affections, but my notes do not enable me to state the relative quantities of fluids drunk by the two groups of patient, though the point is one of interest, with reference especially to the large quantity of urine passed in many cases of typhoid fever, compared with the amount of the same excretion in typhoid fever, even though deduction be made for the loss of fluid by purging in the latter.

THE PULSE.

Typhoid Fever.—The frequency of the pulse varied very greatly in different cases during the same period of the disease. During the first week it ranged from 110 to 132;

during the second from 80 to 128; during the third from 60 to 160; and during the fourth from 96 to a rate too rapid to count.

The pulse-frequency varied much from day to day in the same patient. To show these variations, I have arranged in the following table the number of its beats per minute on particular days in four cases;[1] these variations in its frequency were, so far as could be ascertained, independent of increase or diminution in the severity of local complications :—

Day of Disease.	Beats of Pulse.	Day of Disease.	Beats of Pulse.	Day of Disease.	Beats of Pulse.	Day of Disease.	Beats of Pulse.
13th	120	18th	76	5th	132	16th	108
14th	100	19th	96	7th	110	17th	108
15th	120	20th	78	8th	120	18th	96
16th	100	23d	96	9th	102	21st	96
18th	110	26th	108	10th	120	23d	100
20th	96	27th	96			25th	100
22d	120	28th	108			28th	90

In a man who came under observation on the 15th day of the disease, and whose pulse was at that time 120, by the 20th day it had fallen to 96, and by the 21st day to 60; it then gradually rose again till it reached 120 by the 30th day; the fall in the pulse was in this case accompanied by profound coma, which disappeared as the pulse rose again.

The pulse in one case, which was first seen on the 11th day, and proved fatal on the 25th from hemorrhage from the bowels, gradually rose from 80 to 96, and never exceeded the latter number in the frequency of its beats. The skin in this case was cool, and the mind unaffected, throughout the disease.

The pulse of one patient admitted delirious, on the 5th day, and who continued so till his death on the 17th day, varied from 102 to a rate too rapid to count.

In another case—that of a female, who on the day of her admission (the 12th day of the disease) was violently

[1] For the particulars of these, as well as other cases of the disease, I may refer to the series of papers originally published in the *Medical Times* (1849-51), and reprinted in the present volume.

delirious, and the following day deeply somnolent—the pulse, while she was delirious, was 120; the first day of somnolence, 120; the second, 144, gradually rose to 160, and was too rapid to count on the day of her death, although the somnolence still continued profound, and was uninterrupted by delirium.

The pulse was never hard or bounding : it was occasionally full and soft, but usually small and weak.

It was irregular in two of twenty-one cases. In one of the two, which proved fatal on the 12th day of the disease, the pulse was on the 5th day very weak but regular; on the 9th and 10th days it was 130, very weak and irregular in frequency and force; on the 11th day it was too rapid to count. After death, in addition to the intestinal ulceration common to all these cases, there was found a form of grey hepatisation of the lung. The substance of the right ventricle of the heart was flabby—of the left, firm and healthy.

In another case the pulse on the 16th day of the disease was 130, small, weak, and rather irregular; on the 17th it was 160, and markedly irregular; and on the following day it was too rapid to count. The whole heart, eleven hours after death, was flabby and soft.

Typhus Fever.—In two patients, who were seen respectively on the 6th and 7th day of the disease, the pulse was 80 and 96 in the minute; in the former it rose on the following day to 120. During the second week it ranged, with the exceptions about to be described, from 100 to 150; and, with those exceptions, in one case only was it as low as 100, and that was seen on the 8th day of the disease—its usual range being from 108 to 120.

Omitting for the present six cases, in which the pulse was at some period of the disease very irregular in force and frequency, and even sometimes intermitting, the cases that recovered so far as the fever was concerned, and those cases that were only seen once, there remain twenty-four cases of which I have notes of the pulse, taken on separate days, the number of days varying from two to nine. In seventeen of these cases it either kept up at the rate it was beating when first observed, or rose till the patient's death. In three of the seven cases which deviated from this rule there was a slight

effusion of blood into the cavity of the arachnoid, coincident
with a fall in the pulse of six, of eight, and of forty beats in
the minute.[1]

In two there was an unusual amount of congestion of the
meninges and substance of the brain, with an effusion of
serosity on the convex surfaces of the brain; and in one of
these two the fornix was distinctly softened. In the sixth
case the pulse, when the patient was first seen, was 90;
during the night he had an attack of convulsions, and on the
next morning it had risen to 96; but on the following day it
had again fallen to 90: so that it is probable that the rise in
the pulse on the second day was owing to the effect of the
muscular exertion during the convulsions not having passed
off at the time I saw him. The seventh—the only real exception to the rule—was an old woman seventy years of age,
seen for the first time on the 6th day of the disease, when her
pulse was 80; on the following (the 7th) day it was 120; and
on the 8th—i.e. during the last twenty-four hours of life—it
fell to 110.

The pulse in six cases was irregular, or irregular and
intermitting, when the first notes of its state were taken. In
two of these cases it was respectively 80 and 90, and very
irregular; in both cases it rose the following day about 20
beats, finally attained a rate of 140 to 160, and became from
the time of its sudden rise regular in force and frequency.
In another case it was, when the patient was first seen, 100—
irregular and intermitting: on the next day it rose to 120,
and was then regular, and free from intermissions. In a
fourth case, admitted on the 8th day, the pulse rose during
the four following days from 96 to 108, and continued regular
in force and frequency; on the 13th day it rose to 120, and
became irregular; it was intermitting on the 15th day; and
the patient died on the 17th day of the disease. In the
remaining two cases the irregularity of the pulse was unin-
fluenced by the rise or fall in the rapidity of the heart's
beats; one of the two had hypertrophy and dilatation of the

[1] In two of the cases in which the pulse continued to rise till the patient's
death there was meningeal apoplexy; in one of the two it is probable that
the effusion of blood took place some days before death, in the other after the
last note of her pulse was taken.

heart, with some amount of aortic and mitral valvular disease; the heart of the other was loaded with fat, though in general appearance healthy. Of the three cases in which the rise in the pulse was accompanied by a change from irregular to regular, the hearts of two were perfectly healthy; that of the third was somewhat hypertrophied, and in it the mitral valve was very slightly diseased; the heart of the patient whose pulse became irregular as it rose in frequency was by some accident not examined.

Of the patients who were convalescent before the disease began which caused their death, the pulse in one was 120 on the 8th day, and fell by the 14th to 76; in another it was 120 on the 10th day, and by the 14th it had fallen to 84; while in a third, a very mild case, it reached its maximum, 96, on the 9th day, and by the 12th day was only 84.

From the earliest period of the disease that any of the forty-three patients came under my observation, the pulse was decidedly soft, gradually became weak, then very weak, and in many cases, during the last few days of life, imperceptible. Generally small, it was occasionally full, but still retained its extreme softness.

COUGH AND PHYSICAL CHEST SIGNS.[1]

Typhoid Fever.—Twelve of the twenty-three patients whose cases I am analysing had cough. Sonorous rale was heard more or less extensively in the chests of eleven of the twelve; in the majority, mixed with a little mucous rhonchus; two expectorated a little colourless mucus. These rales were present when ten of the eleven were first examined on the 5th, 7th, 13th, 13th, 14th, 14th, 14th, 14th, 16th, and 28th day. In one case there was no sonorous rale till the 12th day, the patient being first seen on the 6th day.

Typhus Fever.—Twenty-one of the forty-three patients labouring under typhus fever had cough, generally slight in amount, and accompanied by little expectoration. Sonorous

---

[1] I have, of course, omitted the physical signs of pneumonia, pleurisy, etc., as the different proportion in which they occurred in the two diseases we are considering will be *demonstrated* by the lesions found after death. I need scarcely remind the reader that I am here speaking only of cases that proved fatal, and were examined after death.

rale was present in seven of these cases; three had mucous rale more or less abundant, without sonorous; and in nine there was during life some want of resonance of the most depending part of the chest, *i.e.* the portion corresponding to the most depending portion of the lung, the patient being in the recumbent position, and on his back; this region does not, it will be observed, include the extreme base, the root or apex of the inferior lobe; the respiratory murmur at the same point was feeble and coarse, seemed muffled or veiled, and was accompanied with either a few mucous clicks or submucous rale. After death these physical signs were found to be accompanied by an intensely congested condition of the corresponding pulmonary tissue, occasionally passing into absolute consolidation. Doubtless the same physical signs were present in many other cases, but from the state of the patients very many were unable to be raised in bed sufficiently for the posterior parts of their chest to be examined.

SLOUGHING.

Typhoid Fever.—Sloughs formed over the sacrum in two cases; in one toward the termination of the second, and in the other at the end of the fourth week. In a third case, the left lower extremity, as high as the knee, sloughed. That it was not owing to pressure, was proved by the discoloration first showing itself on the dorsum of the foot, and on the anterior as soon as on the posterior part of the ankle. The discoloration commenced on the 24th day of the disease.

Typhus Fever.—An oval portion sloughed out of the corner of both eyes in one patient, and of one eye in another; in the latter case there had been opacity of the cornea for some years before the patient's admission into the hospital.

In one case, on the 11th day, the dorsum and ankle of either foot assumed a purplish hue, and appeared mottled, exactly resembling the corresponding part in the case of typhoid fever, in which the lower extremities eventually sloughed; this patient died the day after the discoloration showed itself.

In three cases sloughs formed over the lower part of the back; in one of these a second slough formed on the shoulder, and in another on the occiput, shoulder, malleoli, trochanters-condyles of the femur, angles of ribs, and in fact in the progress of the case, on every part exposed to the slightest pressure. The sloughs in these cases began to form on from the 13th to the 16th day of the disease.

ERYSIPELAS.

Typhoid Fever.—Erysipelas occurred in seven of the twenty-three cases. In four of the seven it was very trifling in amount and extent, in none spreading beyond the upper lip and nose. In a fifth case it was by no means severe, and was limited to one side of the head. In these five cases it commenced respectively from the 12th to the 34th day of the disease. In two others it made its appearance after the fifth week, dating from the outset of the fever. In these two cases it affected both the head and face, and caused the death of the patients.

Typhus Fever.—In two cases only was erysipelas a complication. In both it was very severe, and confined to the head and face; in one of the two it commenced on the 18th day of the disease; in the other at an uncertain date, but certainly near the termination of the fever.

Of the nine cases of erysipelas above referred to, seven were females.

THE PATHOLOGICAL LESIONS AND CADAVERIC CHANGES NOTED ON EXAMINATION AFTER DEATH OF THE BODIES OF THE SIXTY-SIX PATIENTS WHOSE SYMPTOMS HAVE BEEN ANALYSED.

My object being to analyse the cases of typhoid and typhus fevers with reference to each other, *i.e.* for the special purpose of comparison, and not with the intention of determining the symptoms and appearances found after death from the two diseases, I have thought it useless to include in this analysis the deviations from normal structure noted in the cases of typhoid fever which proved fatal after the thirty-fifth day, and in those of typhus fever which proved fatal after the twenty-ninth day, except so far as relates to traces of ulceration of the intestinal mucous membrane, and of the larynx, pharynx, œsophagus, and stomach, and the remains of blood in the cavity of the arachnoid. The same purpose has rendered unnecessary, that which would be very necessary if my object had been to determine the symptoms and the lesions of the two affections positively, and not comparatively—viz., a description of a third set of fatal cases, taken indiscriminately of other acute diseases. Though I may occasionally be tempted to trace the relations between the symptoms and appearances discovered after death, it would extend my paper far beyond the limits assigned to it, if I should do so in many instances. No such attempt is necessary for my special purpose, *i.e.* the proof of the non-identity of the two fevers.

CADAVERIC RIGIDITY.

Typhoid Fever.—Sixteen bodies of the twenty-three patients who died of typhoid fever were examined with reference to the presence and amount of cadaveric rigidity. The condition of seven of the sixteen was noted within twenty-four hours, six between twenty-four and thirty-six. one forty-two and a half, one fifty, and one fifty-eight, hours after death.

In one of the sixteen, examined twenty-two and a half hours after death, there was no rigor-mortis, and in another, examined thirty hours after the fatal termination, it was only moderately well marked; in all of the remaining fourteen it was well marked at the times, respectively, at which they were examined.

Typhus Fever.—The bodies of thirty-four of the forty-three patients were examined with reference to this point; fourteen of them within twenty-four hours after death. In six of these fourteen the cadaveric rigidity was well marked throughout the body; in five it had in a great measure disappeared from the upper extremities; in one from the lower; in one it had entirely disappeared from the whole body; and in one it was little marked. In thirteen cases the body was examined between twenty-four and thirty-six hours after death. In one of these thirteen only was the rigor-mortis well marked in the upper and lower extremities; in four it had disappeared from the upper limbs; in three it was moderate in the legs and arms; and in five it was but little marked in either of the extremities. Of seven other bodies examined, with respect to the point we are considering, more than thirty-six hours after death, it was well marked in one forty-eight hours after death; it was moderately well marked in another forty-two hours, and had disappeared from a third forty-two hours, and nearly so from a fourth forty hours, after death;—while it was present in the lower extremities, examined in the remaining three of the seven, respectively, thirty-eight, forty-five, and fifty-two hours after the termination of life.

Thus, cadaveric rigidity was well marked in all the extremities of six of the seven bodies of the patients who died from typhoid fever and were examined during the first twenty-four hours after death with reference to the point in question; while it was well marked in all the limbs in six only out of fourteen dead from typhus fever examined during the same period; or if we take the whole of the cases, it was more or less absent in two of the sixteen bodies of the patients who died of typhoid fever, i.e. one-eighth of them, or in the proportion of 12·5 per cent.; while it had more or less disappeared, during the same period, from twenty-six of the thirty-four cases of typhus fever, i.e. from more than three-fourths of them, or in the proportion of 79·4 per cent. I was not aware of this remarkable difference having existed, till I made this analysis, or many points of interest connected with it might have been made out, but then I have the satisfaction of knowing, although I have ascertained less on the point than I might have otherwise done, that in what I observed I could have been biassed by no pre-conceived opinion on the subject. Anxious to ascertain the real cause of the difference, I have examined the two groups, i.e. those of typhoid and typhus fever, with reference to the state of the weather at the time the subjects lay in the dead-house, the age and previous state of health of the patients, the local complications, and the duration of the disease in the separate cases included under each group. The result of my investigations on these points is, that none of these circumstances was the cause of the difference observed in the duration of the cadaveric rigidity, so that it could only have been due to some peculiar state of the system, induced by the disease itself. The only one of the fifteen cases of typhoid fever in which there was no cadaveric rigidity was that in which the coma and prostration preceding death for some days was the most extreme.

As the subjects were removed from the shell to the dead-house table by the arms and legs, it is evident that force was applied to the knees in such a mode as to prevent their flexure, while it was applied to the arms so as to make them bend, and this probably was the cause of the cadaveric rigidity being less marked in the latter than in the former limbs in so many cases, but then the same mode of removing the body from the shell was used in the cases of typhus and typhoid fevers, and therefore, if the cadaveric rigidity had not disappeared spontaneously from the upper extremities in the former, it was overcome with a much less amount of force than in the latter.

SPOTS.

Typhoid Fever.—In one case only was there a trace after death of any spot marked during life. It was a very faintly marked, brownish point, and would undoubtedly have escaped notice if the rose-spot which caused it had not, during life, been encircled with an ink-mark. It could by no possibility have been confounded with the spots about to be described under the head of typhus fever. It was limited to the surface, and, on section, was seen not to extend to the cutis.

Typhus Fever.—On the surface of the trunk and extremities, small spots of a purple colour were detected in twenty-seven cases; in eleven of the forty-three cases of typhus fever I am analysing, the spots had disappeared before death; no note was made of their presence or absence in the remaining five cases.

The spots noted during life as becoming paler on pressure, were after death of a faint brownish purple hue. Those marked as unaffected by pressure during life retained generally the appearance they presented before death, and in some instances the ink-marks made during life indicating that a particular spot had passed through all the *three stages* described in a former part of this paper, under the head

' mulberry rash,' were still visible, the spot after death presenting the character of the third stage, *i.e.* a non-elevated purple spot, with well-defined border, unaffected by pressure.

As during life, so after death, the spots situated on the most depending parts of the body, the subject being on its back, were the darkest in hue, and were often well marked when those on the anterior surface were scarcely visible. That this difference in hue was dependent on position, was in some measure proved by the fact, that the intensity of the hue gradually increased down the sides of the trunk, *i.e.* passing from before backwards.

A piece of skin being removed from the subject, the following appearances were observed with the aid of a lens,—a faint brownish red or purple hue of the spots marked, as only fading on pressure during life, limited to the surface of the cutis. The purple colour of the well-defined spots, unchanged by pressure during life, affected the whole thickness of the cutis, and even extended into the subcutaneous tissue; a few minute vessels, still loaded with blood, converged towards the discoloured spot, but none were discernible in the spots themselves; their colour appeared to be due to infiltration of the tissue by a solution of hematin. The hue of these spots was even darker below the epidermis than on the surface.

That the spots observed during life were the same as those noted to be present after death, was proved by the ink-marks remaining which had, before death, been placed around several of them for the purpose of securing attention to the same spots throughout their varying changes. The absolute identity of the spots was thus demonstrated.

As no spot was to be seen, with the one exception previously referred to, within the circle made during life around the rose-spots of typhoid fever, it was indisputably proved that those spots were not permanent. As no patient affected with typhus fever died while the mulberry rash was in its first stage, I am unable to say whether, in that stage, *i.e.* while the spots constituting it disappeared on pressure, they would have been visible after death. I should suppose not, *a priori.*

Miliary Vesicles.—As I stated while analysing the symptoms, miliary vesicles were detected in four of the cases of typhoid fever after death, and in three of the cases of typhus. The difference in the proportion being, as I then pointed out, due to the *age* of the patients rather than to the *disease.*

VERGETURE OR DISCOLORATION OF THE POSTERIOR SURFACE OF THE TRUNK AND EXTREMITIES.

Of the difference on this point my notes enable me to say nothing positive, because I failed to record its varying inten-sity. To a greater or less extent it was present in all the cases of both groups of which notes on the point were made. My impression—but how fallacious impressions are, none can be more deeply sensible than myself—is, that it was much deeper in hue, and extended far higher up the sides of the trunk, the subject being on its back, in those dead from typhus than in those dead from typhoid fever.

GREEN OR PURPLE DISCOLORATION OF THE CUTIS INDICATING THE COURSE OF THE LARGER VEINS.

Typhoid Fever.—This cadaveric change was not present in a single instance.

Typhus Fever.—Excluding five cases that survived more than twenty-nine days, discoloration in the course of the veins was observed in six, or in nearly one-sixth of the remaining thirty-eight cases.

GREEN DISCOLORATION OF THE WALLS OF THE ABDOMEN AND THORAX.

Typhoid Fever.—Omitting four cases that survived beyond the thirty-fifth day of the disease, two cases of which no notes on the point were made, there remain eighteen of the twenty-three cases of typhoid fever.—In three or one-sixth of the eighteen cases the abdominal walls were more or less discoloured, the subjects being examined, respectively, twenty-four, twenty-six, and thirty-six hours after death.

Typhus Fever.—Of the thirty-eight of the forty-three cases available for analysis, with reference to this point, the abdominal parietes were discoloured in ten, or more than a fourth. These subjects were examined, respectively, thirty-eight, twenty-five and a half, forty-two, twenty-six, fifty-two, twenty-four, twenty-seven and a quarter, forty, twenty-seven, thirty-five and a half, hours after death.

That the discoloration was due to some cause acting from within, was proved by those parts which were protected from the action of—say a gas generated within—retaining their natural hue; when the liver projected below the ribs, that portion of the abdominal wall with which it lay in contact, preserved its natural colour, and in one instance, when the bladder was distended, its position was clearly marked out by the green hue of the abdominal parietes around. The inter-costal spaces were always affected before the skin covering the ribs, and the cutis over the larynx before the sides of the neck; the skin around the mouth before the other parts of the face. In one case in which there was gangrene of the lung, the subject, æt. twelve, being examined twenty-six hours after death, green discoloration of the intercostal spaces was well marked, while the skin over the ribs retained its normal appearance.

EMACIATION.

Typhoid Fever.—In eight, or nearly one-half of the eighteen cases, there was marked emaciation; in five of the eight, extreme emaciation; in five, no emaciation; of five cases no note was made.

Typhus Fever.—In seven, or less than one-fifth of the thirty-eight cases, there was more or less emaciation; in three of the eight only was it extreme; in seventeen cases there was no emaciation; of thirteen cases no note on this point was made.

MUSCLES.

Typhoid Fever.—In one case only were the muscles noted to be particularly dark in hue.

Typhus.—In six, or about one-sixth of the thirty-eight cases, the muscles were noted to be of an unusually dark colour. In two cases there was a considerable quantity of dark loosely coagulated blood in the substance, and anterior and posterior to, but within, the sheath of the rectus abdominis; in both instances it was situated between the umbilicus and pubes, in one of the two in both recti, in one in the left rectus only; the clot in the former case extended for about six inches in length, in the latter two only. The muscular substance in both was softened at the part.

HEAD.

Typhoid Fever.—Fifteen only of the twenty-three cases of typhoid fever are available for analysis, the remaining eight either lived more than thirty-five days, or I was unable to examine the head.

The consistence of the brain generally, in the fifteen cases, was normal; there was no trace of softening or abnormal induration in any portion of the cerebral substance. Seven of these fifteen brains were examined more than twenty-four hours, one forty-four and a half hours, and one as late as fifty-eight hours, after death. The two latter, however, were examined in the month of January, the thermometer, during the time the second case lay in the dead-house, standing below 32° F.

In one case there was no trace of the commissura mollis: the subject—a man thirty years of age—was examined thirty hours after death, in the month of October, the weather at the time being wet and cold. In five of the fifteen the supra cortical layer of white matter was more or less marked.[1]

Congestion of the cerebral substance.—Fifteen of the twenty-three cases of typhoid fever were examined with reference to this condition of the brain, and in two of the fifteen—*i.e.* less than one-seventh, or in the proportion of 13·4 per cent., the red points were more numerous than natural.

Membranes.—The dura mater retained its normal appearance in every one of the fifteen cases. In one case only was there marked congestion of the pia mater, and in only four others slight increased congestion of the larger vessels of the

[1] See Baillarger, *Séances de l'Académie de Médecine*, June 21, 1840.

pia mater. In the remaining ten cases the membranes were normal, or paler than natural, so that the non-congested were to the congested in the proportion of two to one, and to the intensely congested, fourteen to one. In nine only of the fifteen cases was any note made of the facility with which the membranes could be stripped from the convolutions of the brain, and in one case only was it noted that they were able to be removed with abnormal facility, and in larger portions than natural.

Fluid contained within the Cranial Cavity.—The quantity of fluid found after death within the cavity of the arachnoid on the lower surface, and at the base of the brain, was noted in seven of the fifteen cases available for analysis; in eight cases no note was made on this point. The amount varied from half a drachm to an ounce, the average quantity being about half an ounce. *In all the cases it was colourless and transparent.*

Fluid of a similar character was noted to be present in the lateral ventricles in thirteen cases; the quantity varied from half a drachm to an ounce, the average quantity being about two or three drachms. Immediately beneath the arachnoid, or infiltrating the meshes of the pia mater, there was some effusion of colourless serosity in nine cases; in six others no note on the point was made, probably from there having been in these cases no deviation from health. In one case only was it noted to be considerable; in the other eight it was described as ' a little,' ' very little,' ' very trifling.'

Choroid Plexus.—There was no congestion of the vessels of the choroid plexus in any of the cases examined with reference to the fact.

Typhus Fever.—Omitting the cases in which no examination of the head was made after death, and those which survived beyond the twenty-ninth day of the disease, there remain thirty-six of the forty-three cases for analysis. In four of these thirty-six the consistence of the brain was slightly diminished; in one of the four the softening had, in the septum lucidum and fornix, attained a considerable degree; in a fifth case there was slight softening of the fornix, the remainder of the brain having a normal consistence; while in a sixth case there was softening of the septum lucidum only.   The first four subjects were examined respectively thirty-six, forty-eight, forty, and twenty hours after death, the last being the case in which there was considerable softening of the fornix and septum lucidum; the examination of the head in the fifth case was made fourteen, and in the sixth twenty-two and a half hours after the death of the patients.   In a seventh case, examined thirty-eight hours after the fatal termination, there was decided softening of the left half of the cerebellum.   With these seven exceptions, the brain retained its normal consistence.   In two cases, although carefully sought for, there was no trace of the commissura mollis; had this absence been only apparent— i.e. due to softening—the true nature of the case would have been manifested by an examination of the ventricular surface of the thalami optici; the serous membrane covering which would in such case have been wanting at the point where the cord of nervous matter emerges from the thalami.   In one case there was an aperture in the septum lucidum, not formed by softening or handling; the edges of the perforation were firm and smooth, the serous membrane lining the two lateral ventricles being apparently continuous over its edges.   The supracortical layer—i.e. a film of white matter spread over the outer surface of the grey matter—was well marked in twelve cases, in two others imperfectly; no note with reference to the point was made in the remainder.   For reasons into which I cannot at present enter, I believe this layer of white matter not to have been due to decolorisation of a portion of the grey by maceration.[1]

Congestion of the Cerebral Substance.—In fifteen of the thirty-six cases—i.e. rather less than one-half, or in the proportion of 41·8 per cent.—the red points scattered over the cut surface of the brain were more numerous than natural.

Membranes.—In ten cases there was marked congestion of the dura mater; in five it was thickened and opaque— three of the five were more than fifty years of age.

In twenty-one of the thirty-six cases the larger vessels of the pia mater were more or less distended with blood.   In eight of these twenty-one cases the smaller vessels were also

---

[1] See Baillarger, *op. cit.*

congested ; and in one case, in which the larger vessels were not abnormally congested, the smaller were minutely injected. In seven of the twenty-one cases the congestion was trifling in amount. In nine cases the vessels of the pia mater appeared to be in a normal condition—at any rate there was in these nine no abnormal congestion. In four other cases there could have been no great deviation from a healthy state, as no note of their condition was made, although other points respecting the condition of the brain and its membranes were recorded. So that, if we consider the vessels of the pia mater to be normally injected in these four cases, the congested still bear to the non-congested the proportion of 160 to 100.

In seven of the thirty-six, or in one-fifth of the cases examined, there was intense congestion of the pia mater, while, as was before shown in the cases of typhoid fever, the moderately-congested bore to the non-congested the proportion of 1 to 2, and there was only one case in which the pia mater was intensely congested of the fifteen examined.

In eleven cases only was the facility with which the membranes separated from the surface of the convolutions noted, and in nine of the eleven they did so with abnormal facility, and in such large portions that my notes state that the membranes peeled off *en masse*. No portion of the cerebral substance was in any case removed with the membranes; the facility, therefore, with which they separated from the cortical substance was not owing to softening of the grey matter.

I deeply regret that this particular was not more frequently noted, as, when well marked, it is one of the most characteristic appearances found after death from typhus fever, but by no means the anatomical character, as in one of these eleven they were removed with difficulty, and in another case with only slightly increased facility. The quantity of fluid found after death on the convex surface, and at the base of the brain within the cavity of the arachnoid, was noted in twenty-five cases. In ten others, probably for the reason before assigned, no note was made. The quantity of fluid varied from about two drachms to two ounces; the average quantity being one ounce. In three cases it was slightly yellowish; in the others (excepting the cases of hemorrhage into the cavity of the arachnoid) it was transparent and colourless.

The lateral ventricles contained from a few drops to one ounce of transparent colourless fluid; the average quantity was from about two to three drachms.[1]

More or less serosity was infiltrated into the meshes of the pia mater, or effused beneath the arachnoid, in twenty-three cases. No note was made on the point in the remaining cases, probably for the reason before assigned—*i.e.* that in these there was little or no deviation from health.

The quantity of serosity was decidedly greater in a large majority of the cases of typhus fever than in the cases of typhoid fever; the amount of the fluid having been in the former described by the terms ' much,' ' considerable,' and in two only of the twenty-three by the expression ' very little.'

Choroid Plexus.—In four cases the vessels of the choroid plexus were noted to be abnormally distended with blood.

HEMORRHAGE INTO THE CAVITY OF THE ARACHNOID.

Typhoid Fever.—In nineteen of the twenty-three cases the head was examined after death; and in none of these was there the slightest trace of blood in the cavity of the arachnoid.

Typhus Fever.—In thirty-nine cases the head was opened, and in five of them coagula of various sizes were found within the cavity of the arachnoid. In every case the coagulum was in the form of a delicate red film, varying in thickness, and consequently in hue, in different cases and in different parts of the same clot. It was almost colourless where thinnest, bright red where a little thicker, and deep purple at the thickest parts. It was in every case situated on the

---

[1] I think it right to state that the amount of fluid was not *measured* in these cases; but as the quantities were estimated at the time the examination of the head was made by the same observer, it is probable that the comparative amounts are correct, although the absolute quantities are not available for accurate calculation. The fluid ought to have been removed by a pipette and measured, as it was by Dr. John Reid, in his admirable researches into the pathological appearance found after death in fever. But as my guessed quantities differ but little from those obtained by accurate measurement by that philosophic observer and reasoner, I trust they are not far from the truth.

convex surface of the brain, and in one stretched from the anterior lobe to the tentorium, and from the median fissure to a point corresponding to a line drawn transversely, just above the external auditory foramen. In one case it consisted of two or three delicate fibrinous films only. When the dura mater was reflected, part of the clot adhered to the layer of arachnoid lining that membrane, and part to the layer of arachnoid covering the pia mater. In three of the five cases the clot was double—*i.e.* existed on both hemispheres of the brain. In two cases it was confined to the right side.

In one of the five it was accompanied by effusion of blood into the substance of the rectus abdominis. The substance of the brain was firm in four of the five, and apparently healthy in all. The vessels of the cerebral substance and its meninges were not particularly congested; the blood in the vessels of the pia mater was fluid, but could not be pressed out of them into the cavity of the arachnoid. No aperture could be found from which the blood had escaped—the sinuses were perfectly healthy: the source of the hemorrhage could not, consequently, be discovered.

PHARYNX AND LARYNX.

I have conjoined the appearances found after death in these two organs, because both were in numerous instances diseased in the same subject; and because the relation which the pharyngeal bears to the laryngeal affection is important in a practical as well as in a theoretically pathological view.

The term inflammation has been used, because the appearances found after death, and the signs and symptoms observed during life, so closely resemble, if they are not identical with, those described by that term, that I cannot follow Rokitansky, and call these phenomena 'diffused congestive typhus processes,' especially as that author offers no proof that these local changes are peculiar to typhoid fever.

Typhoid Fever.—The larynx and pharynx were examined in fifteen of the twenty-three cases—they were both healthy in six, *i.e.* more than one-third, or exactly in the proportion of 40 per cent.

Ulceration of the pharynx was found in four cases; in one of the four there was an ulcer seated on the posterior aspect of the velum pendulum palati and uvula, by which the mucous membrane covering the latter and a small part of the former, was completely destroyed; the breadth of this ulcer was four lines; its edges were bright red, and not elevated; its floor, formed of submucous cellular tissue, was dusky red; the ulceration was quite superficial. In the same case there was a similar but smaller ulcer on the hard palate, and the arytæno-epiglottidean folds were considerably thickened, the chordæ vocales swollen, the mucous membrane of the larynx generally congested, and covered with mucopurulent fluid. Erysipelas, trifling in extent, had affected this patient a few days before death. In another of the four cases there were two or three small ulcers on the posterior wall of the pharynx. In the third an oval ulcer, half an inch in width, partially divided into two by a strip of apparently healthy mucous membrane, was found in the pharynx, just at its junction with the œsophagus; the floor of this ulcer was formed by the submucous cellular tissues of a yellowish colour, its edges, like the mucous membrane of the pharynx generally, were very pale; and there was in the same subject a second small superficial ulcer, seated a little below the one just described. In the fourth case four ulcers were seated on the posterior wall of the pharynx; one of the four ulcers was three-quarters of an inch in width, irregular in shape, its edges slightly elevated, sharp, and of a dark purple colour, its floor formed of the congested naked fibres of the middle constrictor of the pharynx: two or three similar, but much smaller ulcers, were seated around the larger one; the whole mucous membrane of the pharynx was dusky red. In the three latter cases the mucous membrane of the larynx was pale, and healthy in aspect; in three of the four cases, therefore, the larynx was healthy. In a fifth case there was ulceration and enlargement of both tonsils—increased vascularity of the pharynx, and redness of the upper and under surface of the epiglottis. In two cases there was distinct thickening (from submucous effusion of serosity) of the arytæno-epiglottidean folds and epiglottis; in one of the two there was also effusion of serosity beneath the whole mucous membrane of the pharynx and larynx—in both the serosity was colourless and transparent, and the mucous membrane itself of the larynx and pharynx pale. Both patients were suffering from erysipelas of the head and face at the time of their death.

In one case the pharynx was dusky violet, the upper and under surface of the epiglottis of a bright scarlet colour from minute injection; and there was a small ulcer on the corresponding parts of either chorda vocalis. The larynx appeared healthy in another case, in which there were numerous collections of a purulent-looking fluid, varying in size from a pin-head to a small sweet-pea beneath, and elevating the mucous membrane of the pharynx, that membrane itself being pale. This patient suffered from erysipelas a few days before his death.

The conditions of the larynx and pharynx discovered after death, in the fifteen cases, may be thus summed up:—

No vestige of old disease in any of the cases.

Both organs healthy in six, or, if the two cases be added in which the disease of the pharynx in the one, and of the larynx in the other, supervened after the termination of the fever, in eight cases, i.e. in the proportion of 53 per cent.

Ulceration of the pharynx in one-third of the cases.

Ulceration of the larynx in one case.

Signs of inflammation of the pharynx in six cases; but in two of these the inflammation set in after the termination of the fever. As two of the cases of ulceration of the pharynx were unattended by any other signs of inflammation of that organ, the pharynx was diseased during the progress of the fever in eight cases.

Signs of inflammation of the larynx in five cases.

Larynx and pharynx diseased in the same subject (excluding one case in which erysipelatous inflammation had set in after the fever had terminated) in three cases, that is, in one-fifth of the cases in which the organ was examined.

Larynx healthy, pharynx diseased, in three cases, or one-fifth of the whole examined.

Larynx diseased, pharynx healthy, in one case; but in this case it was doubtful whether the disease was, during life, confined to the larynx, although no morbid appearance could be discovered in the pharynx after death.

E

From this analysis, I think it may fairly be concluded, that in these cases the laryngeal was secondary to the pharyngeal affection, and that *in typhoid fever laryngitis independent of pharyngitis is extremely infrequent.*

Typhus Fever.—The larynx and pharynx were both examined after death in twenty-six of the forty-three cases of typhus fever I am here analysing.

Both organs were healthy in sixteen of the twenty-six cases. In one other case they were both healthy, with the exception of a little blood effused beneath the mucous membrane of the pharynx. In the remaining nine of the twenty-six cases, there were unequivocal traces of disease. The larynx and pharynx were deep purple, and covered with slimy mucus in one case. In four there were unequivocal traces of inflammation in both organs; thus, in one of the four the mucous membrane of the pharynx was deep red, of the larynx vivid scarlet, the redness on minute inspection being found to be punctiform; in another of the four the lining membrane of the pharynx was of a dirty yellowish colour, and so soft that it was removeable by the gentlest scraping; the chordæ vocales swollen, the rima glottidis a mere chink, the mucous membrane of the larynx generally vividly injected and covered with muco-purulent fluid, whilst on the chordae vocales, and on the mucous membrane lining the larynx above the chords, were numerous shreds of white opaque lymph-like matter, readily removeable. In the third case, the lining membrane of the pharynx was covered with thick mucus, felt rough, apparently from enlargement of its follicles, and was of a dull purple colour; there was a small ulcer on either chorda vocalis, but no other trace of inflammatory action within the larynx. The pharynx in the fourth case was studded with small yellowish spots, from which, on section of the mucous membrane covering them, a drop of purulent-looking fluid exuded. The lining membrane of the larynx in the same subject was dusky red, the chordæ vocales and arytæno-epiglottidean folds distinctly thickened from effusion of serosity into the submucous cellular tissue.

Old disease of the parts was present in two cases, the subjects being aged respectively fifty-six and forty-five; in one of the two the pharynx was congested; the mucous membrane of the larynx, covered with dirty, frothy mucus, was opaque and somewhat greenish in hue; the under surface of the epiglottis was irregularly thickened, so that it presented a mammillated appearance; just below the left chorda vocalis was a round aperture leading to a small cavity containing some sloughy matter; the base of the arytænoid cartilage, ossified and necrosed, was exposed. The other of the two cases terminated fatally on the 17th day of the disease. No history of the patient prior to admission could be obtained; after death, there was an old cicatrix on the posterior wall of the pharynx, and a small superficial ulcer on the same part; the mucous membrane of the pharynx and upper surface of the epiglottis was of a deep grey colour. Taking into account the cicatrix, the colour of the mucous membrane, and the duration of the fever, we cannot but conclude that the superficial ulcer was the consequence of chronic inflammation of the pharynx, which had existed prior to the attack of typhus. In one case in which the mucous membranes of the larynx and pharynx were pale and otherwise healthy, there was spread over the former some purulent fluid.

In one case only was there an ulcer in the pharynx, the result of recently established diseased action. It was small and superficial, and seated at the base of the left anterior pillar of the fauces. The mucous membrane of the pharynx was in this case of a deep red colour, and covered with finely granular, yellowish lymph. Similar granules of lymph covered both surfaces of the epiglottis. When the lymph was removed from the latter, the mucous membrane covering it was seen to be vivid scarlet; the lining membrane of the larynx generally was of a pale rose-red, the chordæ vocales slightly thickened. The subject of these serious lesions was attacked with phlebitis after he had completely recovered from a mild attack of typhus fever, and had even left his bed; it was during the second attack that hoarseness supervened. There had been no pharyngeal symptoms during the progress of the fever.

To sum up:—Of twenty-six cases in which the larynx and pharynx were examined after death, they were

Both healthy in seventeen cases, i.e. in the proportion of 65·4 per cent.; or if the two cases be added in which the disease was evidently of old standing, and the one in which it supervened after the patient had recovered from the fever, twenty cases, *i.e.* in the proportion of 77 per cent., passed through the disease without any affection of these organs.

In five cases there were signs of inflammation of both larynx and pharynx, *i.e.* in about one-fifth of the cases. In one of the five there was ulceration of the larynx.

Inflammation of the larynx, the pharynx being free from lesion, in one case.

In no instance was the pharynx diseased and the larynx healthy, but in two of the five in which both were inflamed, the lesion of the pharynx was much more profound than that of the larynx.

Ulceration of the pharynx as a consequence of the fever was not detected in a single instance.

Thus it may be stated that if the laryngeal affection in typhus fever be not invariably preceded by pharyngeal disease, it is almost always so. The difference between the two diseases as exhibited by the great tendency to pharyngeal ulceration, in the cases of typhoid fever (ulceration of the pharynx occurred in one-third of the cases) and by the total absence of any such lesion in the cases of typhus fever, is remarkably striking.

The relation which existed between the laryngeal and pharyngeal affection and erysipelas was undoubtedly intimate.

ŒSOPHAGUS.

Typhoid Fever.—The œsophagus was examined in seventeen of the twenty-three cases. In sixteen it was healthy.[1] In one it was extensively ulcerated. The ulcerations, several in number, extended five and a half inches upwards from just above the cardiac orifice of the stomach. The circular muscular fibres of the œsophagus 'were at places exposed.

---

[1] There is in the normal condition of the parts a marked difference in hue between the colour of the mucous membrane of the pharynx and œsophagus. The somewhat purplish colour of the former generally ceases abruptly on a line corresponding to the upper border of the larynx. I mention this because I have occasionally observed this appearance described by those unaccustomed to examine these organs as a morbid appearance.

One of the ulcers was three inches in length, and half an inch in breadth. All were longer than they were broad. The edges of the majority were slightly elevated. The mucous membrane between was here and there finely injected.

Typhus Fever.—The œsophagus was examined in twenty-four of the forty-three cases. It was healthy in all.

Covering the œsophagus is frequently observed a thin layer of opaque white curdy matter. Microscopic examination has demonstrated to me that this layer is composed of epithelium. Whether it separates more readily in the one disease than in the other is worthy of investigation, especially with reference to a condition observed in the kidney tubes. My notes do not enable me to determine the comparative frequency of this probably cadaveric change in the two diseases I am here considering.

STOMACH.

Typhoid Fever.—Excluding the cases in which the stomach was not examined, and those which survived the thirty-fifth day of illness, there remain fifteen cases for analysis with reference to the condition of the stomach generally, and twenty with respect to the presence or absence of ulceration of that organ.

The cases that proved fatal after the 35th day are available so far as concerns ulceration of the organ, because unequivocal traces of that lesion are left in the form of cicatrices for some time after the healing process is completed.

If any appearance of healed ulcers in the stomach had been discovered in the cases that proved fatal after the termination of the fever, then a question might have been raised as to whether the cicatrices had existed prior to the commencement of the fever. But no trace of pre-existing ulceration was detected, therefore these cases may be admitted as unimpeachable evidence.

Colour.—No note of the colour was made in four cases. In these four it must have been healthy, or nearly so. In six cases it was pale. In one there was scattered over the whole mucous membrane some bright red lines and patches.

In another there was punctiform redness, and softening of
the mucous membrane to the extent of three inches, commencing from the pylorus, and stretching towards the
cardiac extremity; it was in the same case mammillated to
near the cardiac extremity, *i.e.* commencing at the pylorus.
The mucous membrane retained in this case its normal
consistence at the cardiac extremity. There were a few rugæ.

In two cases the mucous membrane was somewhat grey.
In one of these cases the posterior portion of the great cul-
de-sac was speckled with deep red, the mucous membrane of
the cardiac extremity was rather soft, the remainder of the
organ normal in consistence and thickness. In the other of
these two cases the mucous membrane was rugose and mammillated—with the exception of the great cul-de-sac—
generally softened, the softening especially affecting the
pyloric half. In two other cases there was marked increase
in the vascularity of the cardiac extremity of the stomach.

Ulceration.—In one case only was there recent ulceration.
In this case the mucous membrane of the stomach was pale
and smooth, its consistence and thickness normal. Scattered
over the anterior and posterior wall and greater curvature
were numerous minute ulcers, varying in size from a pin
point to a line in diameter; their edges and floors were pale;
the former rounded, the latter formed of submucous cellular
tissue.

In no case was there any trace of old ulceration, or of
chronic inflammation [1] of the organ.

Softening.—In ten cases the mucous membrane retained
its normal consistence. In two it was slightly softened at the
cardiac extremity; in three near the pylorus; in one of
these three there were numerous red spots on the posterior
wall of the stomach, varying in size from a mere point to a
pin-head. The softening in this case was limited to the red
spots and their immediate vicinity, and in another of the
three cases the softening of the pyloric portion of the
stomach was accompanied by punctiform redness.

[1] I do not include mammillation of the mucous membrane of the stomach
under the term of chronic inflammation of that organ. The true signification of this condition of the membrane, it appears to me, has yet to be determined.

In no instance was any softening approaching perforation observed. In no instance was the mucous membrane firmer than natural; in no instance softened throughout the organ.

Thickness.—In one case the mucous membrane was noted to be generally somewhat thickened. In six cases it was recorded to be of normal thickness.

Mammillation.—In two cases there was no mammillation; in one nearly the whole membrane was in that state; in two cases it existed from the pylorus to near the cardiac extremity; in three it was limited to the vicinity of the pylorus; while in five of the fifteen cases no note of this particular was made.

Typhus Fever.—Omitting the cases of which no notes were made with respect to the condition of the stomach, and those which survived the 4th week of the disease, there remain for analysis generally thirty-seven cases, and with respect to ulceration forty-two.

Colour.—The stomach was noted to be pale or healthy in colour in twenty-three of the thirty-seven cases. It was of an uniform dusky grey hue in two cases. There was punctiform redness along the greater curvature, and anterior and posterior surfaces of the mucous membrane adjoining, in one case, minute hemorrhagic spots in the cardiac extremity in two cases; some redness of the great cul-de-sac in one case. The mucous membrane in the four last-mentioned cases retained its normal colour in the other parts of the organ.

There were signs of chronic inflammation of the mucous membrane of the stomach in seven cases, *i.e.* it was grey, speckled, thickened, altered in consistence, or covered with tough mucus, and in four of the seven there were unequivocal cicatrices.

Ulceration.—In one case the mucous membrane of the whole stomach was remarkably rugose, mammillated from pylorus to cardia, and of a dull roseate hue; in the great cul-de-sac the redness was remarkably vivid, and on minute inspection was found to be punctiform. Three inches from the pylorus, scattered over a space about an inch and a half in circumference, and seated on the posterior wall of the stomach, were nine ulcers, varying in size from a pin-point to No. 4 shot; their edges were well defined and not discoloured; there was no softening of the mucous membrane; on the contrary, it was noted as rather tough.

In no other case was there evidence of recent ulceration, for it so happened, as has been before remarked, that the old cicatrices were observed only in those cases which proved fatal during the progress of the fever. The ages respectively of the subjects in which the cicatrices were noted were 33, 40, 42, 56, and 61 years.

Mammillation.—The presence or absence of this condition of the mucous membrane was recorded in fourteen cases only. In one, the case before referred to, it was general. In six, it was limited to the vicinity of the pylorus. In seven cases there was no mammillation.

Consistence.—The mucous membrane was noted to be of normal, or nearly normal, consistence, in twenty-two cases. It was generally rather firmer than natural in four. In one of these four there were recent ulcers; in two others cicatrices of old ulcers; in one case,—in which the mucous membrane was of a reddish hue posteriorly, of a darker red anteriorly, and of a vermilion tint along the great curvature, the redness being punctiform and capillary,—the consistence, which was generally natural, was, at the reddest parts, slightly increased; the same parts were also thicker than natural. No note was made with respect to the consistence of the mucous membrane in one case. In four, it was generally softer than natural; in one of these four, the cardiac extremity was disproportionately soft. In four cases there was such extreme softening of the great cul-de-sac, that it ruptured in the removal or in the washing of the organ. The ages of these four subjects were 33, 49, 50, and 50. Two of these cases terminated respectively on the 12th and 16th day of disease; the other two during the course of the fever, but the exact date was never ascertained.[1] In no case was the mucous membrane in the vicinity of the pylorus softer than that covering the cardiac extremity.

---

[1] I shall reserve, till another opportunity, the minute analysis of these cases of perforation; the number is too few to lead to any satisfactory conclusion; and I have accounts of others, which may be added to these, though not admissible in this place, because they do not come within the limits I have laid down for the cases here analysed.

Thickness.—In three cases the mucous membrane was noted to be generally increased in thickness. In one case (before referred to) it was partially thickened; in twenty-one cases it was noted to possess its normal thickness.

DUODENUM.

Typhoid Fever.—Excluding eight cases, which either survived the fever, or were not examined with reference to the condition of the duodenum, there remain for analysis fifteen cases. There was no marked deviation of the duodenum from health, in ten of the fifteen. In one its mucous membrane was finely injected, and in another it was reddish-grey; in both of these cases there was redness and softening of the pyloric portion of the stomach. In one case there was vivid redness of the upper part of the duodenum, the stomach being perfectly healthy in appearance. In two cases the mucous membrane of the duodenum was pale grey; in one of the two the stomach was greyish, and in the other there was considerable redness, in patches and lines, of the latter organ. In no case was there any trace of ulceration.

Typhus Fever.—Six cases being omitted as not available for analysis, except in so far as traces of ulceration of the organ are concerned, there remain for examination thirty-seven of the forty-three cases here considered.

In twenty-eight the mucous membrane appeared perfectly healthy. In two it was stained yellow, and slightly softened; in one of these two the mucous membrane of the stomach was in the same state. In one case, the mucous membrane of the duodenum was vividly injected; in five others it was of a grey colour. In one of these five Brunner's glands were remarkably prominent. Signs of chronic inflammation of the mucous membrane of the stomach existed in four of the six cases last referred to, old cicatrices having been noted in that organ in four of them; and in the other two of the six the mucous membrane of the stomach was pale grey, though otherwise healthy in appearance.[1]

[1] As some persons have spoken of the solitary glands at the lower part of the ileum as Brunner's glands, I think it well to state that I intend, here and elsewhere, to limit the term to those glands described by Brunner as existing in the duodenum. They are well known to be very different in structure and situation from the solitary and agminated glands found in the ileum.

In one case there were some hemorrhagic spots beneath the mucous membrane, on the edges of the valvulæ conniventes, the intervening membrane being pale and healthy.

In no case was there recent ulceration, and in no case traces, in the form of cicatrices, of healed ulcers.

From this analysis, I think the conclusions may legitimately be deduced, that the duodenum is rarely affected in fever, and that it is not common for it to be the seat of chronic inflammation, unless in conjunction with, and probably secondarily to, the same affection of the mucous membrane of the stomach.

JEJUNUM AND ILEUM.

Typhoid Fever.—Seventeen cases proved fatal before the thirty-fifth day of the disease; only these seventeen, therefore, can be examined with reference to the colour and consistence of the mucous membrane; but all the twenty-three are evidence with respect to the presence or absence of ulceration.

Colour.—The mucous membrane generally was pale or healthy in eleven of the seventeen cases. The whole membrane was finely injected in one case; in another there was ramiform injection in patches; in two others the lower part of the ileum, in one two feet, in the other five inches, upward from the ileo-cœcal valve, was finely injected; in this latter case the jejunum was, like the duodenum, greyish, while the upper part of the ileum was pale. In another case the jejunum and upper part of the ileum was ash-grey, the lower part of the ileum pale. In one case two feet of the ileum were of a grey colour; this case proved fatal on the 25th day of the disease.

Consistence.—Notes on this point were made in fourteen cases only; in eleven of the fourteen it was natural, in three softer than normal. In one of the three cases the softening was confined to the lower two feet of the ileum; in the other it was general, but slight in amount; in all three the mucous membrane was pale and of normal thickness.

Agminated Glands or Peyer's Patches.—These organs,

the functions of which are entirely unknown, but whose structure Boehm has so well described, were ulcerated in the twenty-three cases I am here considering; and as the proof that the lesions of these patches observed in England are the same as those observed in France is of importance for establishing the identity of the cases I have here called typhoid fever with those described by Louis and Chomel under the same name, I must enter a little fully into the description of the changes these patches had undergone in the twenty-three cases here analysed.

(a) In one of the cases which proved fatal on the *twelfth day, i.e. the earliest* period of the disease at which either of the twenty-three patients died, the following lesions were noted to exist in the ileum. About seven feet above the cœcum, the solitary glands were very distinct, in the form of raised opaque white spots. Six feet above the ileo-cæcal valve was one of Peyer's patches, the *inferior portion* of which was thickened, and of a pinkish hue; from thence downward every patch was thickened; the amount of the thickness and the superficial extent to which each patch was affected, increased as they approached the ileo-cæcal valve. On one patch, situated about three feet from that valve, the mucous membrane was destroyed at several spots, by as many minute ulcers, each about the size of a pin's head; from this point downward every patch was more or less ulcerated, thickened, and distinctly, and in some places considerably, raised above the level of the surrounding mucous membrane. The lowest elliptical patch was three inches in length, thicker than any above it, covered with thick rugose mucous membrane. On it were several ulcers, the largest irregular in shape, about three lines in diameter, the smallest not bigger than a pin's head. The floors of the ulcers were formed of submucous cellular tissue of a deep yellow colour. The mucous membrane on the diseased patches was of a pale purplish colour, and softened; the minute pits observable naturally on the patches, were much more apparent than in the healthy state. The thickening of the patches appeared due to an increase in the thickness of the mucous membrane, and of the submucous cellular tissue, and not to any deposit in the latter. The size and thickness of the solitary glands increased as they

approached the ileo-cæcal valve; near this part some were as
large as split peas. On the apices of several was a small
opaque yellow spot, and on others a minute black point. The
mucous membrane between the glands at the lower eighteen
inches of the ileum was highly vascular; but neither softened
nor altered from its normal thickness. The peritoneum immediately over the diseased patches was of a palish purple
colour, finely injected, the vessels   running.   in two directions,
longitudinally and transversely, *i.e.* crossing each other at
right angles.

(*b*) The following is the description of the condition of the
last three-and-a-half yards of the ileum in a man who died
of hemorrhage from the intestines on the *twenty-fifth day* of
the disease.

About three-and-a-half yards above the ileo-cæcal valve
was one of Peyer's patches, opaque and thickened at intervals;
the opacity and the thickening were seen, on section through
the substance of the patch, to be due to a white deposit,
seated in the submucous tissue. The mucous membrane
covering the patch was pale, and of normal consistence. On
the next patch were two thickened spots, each three-eighths
of an inch in diameter. The deposit in the submucous tissue
which caused the thickening was of a pink colour; the
mucous membrane covering this patch was pale and softened.

Every patch from the last described, to about half a yard
above the ileo-cæcal valve, was more or less thickened. The
thickening did not, in the majority of cases, affect the whole
gland, but was found in spots only; the portion of the patch
between the spots appeared tolerably healthy. Where, however, the whole gland was slightly thickened, then some spots
were much thicker than the general mass of the patch; the
parts most affected measured about a line and a half in thickness, and had a pink colour; the thickening being evidently
due to a pale friable deposit in the submucous cellular tissue.
The mucous membrane covering the whole gland was softer
than that adjacent to it; and that over the pink and thickest
spots, softer than that over the pale and thinner portion of
the patch. The solitary glands, at this part of the intestine,
were, generally, scarcely visible; but here and there were a
few opaque, and slightly elevated, and two were as large as

split peas. The mucous membrane over the two was slightly softened, and decidedly softer at their apices than at their bases. The submucous tissue was of deep red at these spots. About half a yard above the ileo-cæcal valve was a Peyer's patch, much more thickened than those above described. The mucous membrane covering it was of pulpy softness. At its superior part was a round spot with red edges, the centre of which was occupied by an opaque yellow struc- tureless mass, readily detached ; by its removal, a thin layer of submucous cellular tissue was exposed. On the lower part of the patch was a spot about one inch in diameter, thicker than the other parts of the gland, of a red colour, its centre occupied by an ulcer three lines in diameter. The floor of this ulcer was formed of the transverse muscular fibres of the intestine ; to its edges, which were jagged, and overlapped the floor, were attached threads of tough, opaque, deep yellow, sloughy-looking matter, similar to that observed at the upper part of the patch, and described above as structureless, i.e. to the unassisted eye. Passing downwards there was, a little nearer to the cæcum, another patch of a deep grey colour, having on it an ulcer resembling the one last described, but larger and deeper ; attached to its edges were, as in the last, opaque yellow sloughs. Water thrown into the superior mesenteric artery welled forth freely from the edges of this ulcer ; doubtless from it, therefore, the hemorrhage of which the patient died proceeded.

Every patch from this point to the ileo-cæcal valve was more or less destroyed by ulcers resembling the last described. The solitary glands in this part of the ileum were larger than those in the upper portion.

(c) The patient whose intestine presented the appearances I am now about to describe, died on *the forty-sixth day* of illness, from perforation. The appearances illustrate well the process of healing of the ulcers, and also the chronic, atonic ulcers, which often continue long after the fever has run its course, and frequently prove fatal by perforation. I cannot refrain from pointing out to the reader the importance of the knowledge of the existence of these atonic ulcers in a practical point of view, as influencing, that is, the treatment and the prognosis. The lower part of the jejunum and the upper part of the ileum, in this case, had a peculiar opaque appearance; their consistence and thickness were normal. About three feet above the ileo-cæceal valve, at the inferior portion of one of Peyer's patches, was a grey spot, half-an-inch in diameter; the centre of this spot was pale, smooth, shining, and slightly depressed below the level of the surrounding tissue. There was no puckering around it. This mode of healing of typhoid ulceration of the gut explains the fact, that diminution of the calibre of the intestine never follows the healing of this form of ulcer, as pointed out by Rokitansky. It appeared to be the remains of an ulcer. From this spot downwards, to about eight inches above the cæcum, every patch was more or less diseased, i.e. of a deep grey colour; and on every one were healed, or apparently healing, ulcers. In neither of these healing ulcers was there any free fringe of mucous membrane. Between the patches were some small round superficial ulcers, the floors of which were pale, the edges grey, but not elevated. Nine inches from the ileo-cæcal valve, all the coats of the intestine were perforated, and an aperture from the interior of the bowel into the peritoneal cavity was formed, three-eighths of an inch in diameter. The edges of the aperture were well defined; the mucous membrane around it pale, and slightly softened. Through this opening the contents of the bowel had escaped before death.

The whole of the coats of the gut had been perforated, during life, through the next Peyer's patch, but the fæcal matter had been prevented from escaping through the aperture, in consequence of the peritoneal surface around the orifice having adhered, by dense false membrane, to the fundus of the uterus. The edges of the opening, like the remainder of the patch, were grey, and not thickened. On the same patch were two ulcers, the size of the aperture last described; their floors were pale, and formed by the transverse muscular fibres of the gut; their edges scarcely, if at all, elevated, and, like the whole patch, deep grey. On the patch, immediately above the valve, were several small superficial ulcers, and some smooth, pale, shining, and slightly depressed spots, apparently healed ulcers. Between the three last described patches were many small round grey spots. On these there were no traces of previous ulceration; they appeared to have undergone resolution without proceeding to the stage of ulceration. They were scarcely thickened, and the grey colour assumed a deeper tint when the surface of the mucous membrane was removed by gentle friction. This latter is a very important fact with reference to the question, whether the change of colour was cadaveric, or the result of diseased action. The whole mucous membrane of the lower portion of the ileum was pale, rather soft, somewhat opaque, but of normal thickness.

(d) In the following account of the appearances found in the ileum after death, on the 28th day of the disease, are detailed the conditions which precede one mode of perforation, viz. that by *rupture* of the peritoneal coat. The upper part of the ileum was of a pale ash grey, normal in consistence and thickness. About four and a half feet above the ileo-cæcal valve was one of Peyer's patches, slightly thickened, the mucous membrane covering it softened, and very vascular. The next patch was similarly affected. On the next, *i.e.* descending towards the valve, was a large ulcer, by which the coats of the intestine had been so much thinned that an aperture was formed in washing them. From this point downward every agminated gland was more or less destroyed by ulceration. On the floors of some of the ulcers were large sloughs of a yellow colour, soft, but moderately tough; around the edges of others were small masses of pale yellowish deposit, friable, and of cheesy consistence. The floors of the ulcers generally were formed by transverse muscular fibres. From the centre of some of them, however, the muscular fibres had disappeared, *and a delicate layer of peritoneum only separated the contents of the intestine from the abdominal cavity.* The edges of the ulcers were elevated, and of a grey or slate colour. The mucous membrane, between the agminated glands, was rather pale, and slightly softer than natural. The peritoneum covering the ulcerated patches was more vascular than elsewhere; and on that membrane, corresponding to the floor of some of the ulcers, were some shreds of recent lymph.

I have detailed in the above four cases two forms of thickening of the agminated glands. One, in which the thickening depended on the deposit of a pale whitish friable matter, of cheesy consistence, *in the substance* of the submucous cellular tissue—the *plaques dures* of Louis; and another, in which the thickening was due to swelling of the mucous and submucous tissues,—the *plaques molles* of the same author.   Ulceration follows both forms of thickening.

These cases further illustrate the following facts :—

1st, That ulceration of the solitary and agminated glands may commence in two modes ; on the one hand, by softening of the mucous membrane, abrasion of the extremely softened superficial tissue, and then enlargement of the breach of continuity thus formed, in depth and extent, by simple ulceration ; on the other, by sloughing of a portion of the submucous tissue containing the before-described deposit, and of the mucous membrane over it, and then extension of the ulcer in breadth and width, by the separation of minute sloughs from the edges of the breach of continuity, left after the separation of the slough first formed.

2nd, That when the whole of the deposit has sloughed out, no fresh deposit is formed ; and that, consequently, as the whole of that deposit is seated in the submucous tissue, destruction of the muscular fibres of the intestine must be the result of simple ulceration.

3rd, That resolution of the disease affecting the patches may in some cases occur before ulceration has taken place.

4th, That ulcers of considerable size may heal.

5th, That no contraction follows, within a short period, the healing of the ulcers.

6th, That ulcers, dependent for their origin on the presence in the system of the fever-poison, may, after the fever has run its course, continue to spread, retard recovery, and even cause death by perforation.

7th, That while some of the ulcers are undergoing the healing process, others may be spreading ; or, as Rokitansky says, may pass into the state of atonic ulcers.

These atonic or simple ulcers left after the termination of the fever, are a frequent cause of lengthened duration of illness in cases of typhoid fever.

Four cases only of twenty-three offered examples of the *plaques dures.*

In no case that proved fatal after the 30th day was any of the whitish deposit discovered in the submucous cellular tissue; and this agrees with the experience of Louis, for the thirteen examples of the *plaques dures* detailed in his great work on Typhoid Fever proved fatal before the 30th day of the disease. I doubt, however, if it be correct to regard all the cases which proved fatal at a later period as examples of the *plaques molles*, because it is probable that the deposit constituting the *plaques dures* takes place at an early period of the disease.—(I have seen it very extensive in the intestine of a girl who died four days after she had been engaged at the wash-tub, at which time she felt quite well. I am indebted for the history of the case to my friend Mr. Sankey. I saw the girl the last day of life, and was present at the examination after death.)—And it is further probable, that before the 30th day the whole of this foreign matter, incapable of more than the lowest cell-development, would be thrown off by sloughing.

This view of the matter receives confirmation from the condition of the mesenteric glands in many cases.

From these organs the typhous matter, as it has been called, is not thrown off, as from the agminated glands, by sloughing. In them, accordingly, we find this deposit long after the thirtieth day. In one of the cases above described, which proved fatal on the 28th day of the fever, had the patient survived another day or two, the few pieces of yellowish cheesy matter which still adhered to the sides of the ulcers would have been thrown off, and there would have remained no proof that the case had been an example of the *plaques dures*.

The ulcers, as a general rule, increased in superficial extent as they approached the ileo-cæcal valve. When one portion of a patch was thicker than another, the portion of the patch next the ileo-cæcal valve was usually the thicker.

Healing ulcers were found in every case that proved fatal after the 30th day, and also in one case that *probably* had been ill only twenty days when the fatal termination took place. No effort at separation was discovered in the other cases that proved fatal before the 30th day. This fact affords additional ground for believing that the attempt I made to fix the duration of the disease from the duration of the eruption, at the commencement of this paper, was successful.

F

Perforation.—Three patients, or rather less than one-eighth of the patients whose cases are here analysed, died from perforation of the intestine, respectively on the 17th, 31st, and 42d day of disease. The perforation in all three took place through the floor of an ulcer seated on one of the agminated glands. In two of the three, perforation occurred in the lower nine inches of the ileum ; in one, three feet above the ileo-cæcal valve. In two of the three the coats of the intestine were destroyed through their whole thickness at another spot from that at which the perforation which proved fatal took place; but the contents of the bowels had been prevented escaping through the aperture first formed, by adhesions, in the one case, to the fundus of the uterus, and in the other, to a fold of the intestine. It will be observed, that in one of the three cases certainly the fatal perforation took place after the termination of the fever.

This fact, as I have before stated, is of the highest practical importance. It is not to be supposed that a case continues to be typhoid fever so long as ulceration, even active ulceration, of the agminated glands exists. The fever, the true fever, runs its course, but having excited, during that course, ulceration or inflammation of any organ or set of organs, that ulceration, or that inflammation, continues to its termination irrespective of the duration of the specific disease. This appears to me to be the key to much of the difficulty surrounding the study of the duration of continued fevers.

Solitary Glands.—These bodies were visible in six cases, enlarged slightly in three, ulcerated in six ; no note of their condition was made in eight cases, so that in these eight they could have deviated little, if at all, from the healthy appearance, *i.e.* could have been scarcely, or not at all, visible. Four of these eight cases survived the fever. They were generally more diseased in the vicinity of the cæcum than higher up the intestine.

When ulcerated, the breach in the continuity of the mucous membrane over them appeared to take place, either by the formation of minute sloughs on their apices, which, when thrown off, left small ulcers, or by softening of the mucous membrane covering their most prominent part.

Typhus Fever.—Colour.—The mucous membrane of the jejunum and ileum was healthy in colour in 34 of the 39 cases of which notes on this point were made; in four, however, of the thirty-four there was some ramiform injection of the larger vessels at intervals, apparently due to position.

In two cases hemorrhagic spots existed beneath the mucous membrane. In one of the two, these spots, about twenty in number, were scattered over the upper eighteen inches of the jejunum; their size varied from a small pin's head to a line and a half in diameter; the largest were of a deep purple colour, the smaller red. All were hard to the touch, and distinctly elevated. When firmly pressed, their contents, which were fluid, spread irregularly beneath the surrounding mucous membrane. Apparently entering into several of these spots, small vessels, filled with fluid blood, could be traced. The intervening mucous membrane was pale and of normal consistence. In the other of these two cases, the mucous membrane of the ileum, from four feet above the ileo-cæcal valve to nine inches from the same spot, was finely injected. Some of the larger veins were filled with dark blood, and in their vicinity were small spots of ecchymosis. The mucous membrane itself was rather thin and soft. In one case the jejunum was finely injected, while the ileum was pale; in another, both divisions of the intestine were deep grey; and in another case, the fine injection was limited to the lower part of the ileum.

Consistence.—In twenty-nine cases the mucous membrane was of normal consistence, or nearly so; in six, it was generally slightly softened; in one case before referred to, the softening was confined to the lower part of the ileum, the same part being finely injected. The upper part of the jejunum was rather soft in a case in which the mucous membrane of the ileum was normal in consistence. In one case only was there any notable thinning of the mucous membrane, and in that case it was conjoined with softening and redness.

Peyer's Patches, or the Agminated Glands.—With three exceptions, these organs were perfectly healthy, *i.e.* neither elevated, reddened, softened, nor ulcerated. In fourteen cases they were scarcely visible; in sixteen they were noted to be visible, and normal in appearance. I have not considered that appearance, likened by French pathologists to the newly shaven beard, as a deviation from health. This condition was observed in four of the above cases. In the other ten instances, the whole intestinal canal was carefully examined, and recorded as *perfectly healthy*, but no note was made as to whether the patches were visible.

The following are the particulars of the appearances presented by the three cases in which the patches deviated from their normal condition. In one case, the patient, a child æt. ten years, died on the forty-fourth day of illness, and the thirty-first of her residence in the hospital. There was found, after death, extensive tubercular deposit in both lungs, and a large gangrenous abscess in the left. About eighteen inches from the commencement of the jejunum was a Peyer's patch, beneath the mucous membrane of which, *in distinct points*, was some yellow opaque matter; the tissue of the gland between these *points* was healthy in all particulars. The next three or four patches resembled the last described. Then followed six perfectly healthy; then one resembling the first; after which every patch was normal in all respects. The mesenteric glands were enlarged, especially about the centre of the mesentery. On section, some of them were found studded with yellowish white masses, about the size of pins' heads.

This was evidently a case of tubercular disease of the agminated and mesenteric glands. These organs bore *no* resemblance to the same parts taken from a patient who had died at the same period, after recovering from typhoid fever. The situation of the diseased patches and mesenteric glands, the form and nature of the foreign matter deposited in them, and finally, the fact of the whitish matter of the *plaques dures*, with which alone it could by any possibility have been confounded, never having been seen in the agminated glands after the 30th day, while this patient died on the 44th day of the illness,—all unequivocally prove that this was not a case of typhoid fever; while the general appearance, and the situation of the deposit, and the existence of tubercle in the lung, as undoubtedly prove that it was an example of abdominal tubercular disease.

In the second case, which proved fatal during the fourth

week of the disease, the lower eighteen inches of the ileum were intensely congested—the large veins distended with dark blood—the mucous membrane of a dusky vermilion hue, the bodies of Peyer's patches slightly thickened, and of a deeper red than the surrounding membrane. At the same part the mucous membrane was somewhat softened, but not more so on the patches than around them. Some of the mesenteric glands in this case were visible, but not enlarged; the mucous membrane of the cæcum, and ascending colon near to the cæcum, was highly vascular and softened—the under surface of the ileo-cæcal valve an uniform dusky purple red. This case, then, was one of dysentery, in which the inflammation extended somewhat higher up the ileum than usual, and involved the mucous membrane covering the elliptic patches, in common with that around them. The inflammatory action probably commenced at the under surface of the ileo-cæcal valve; at any rate, that spot deviated the most markedly from a healthy appearance. The third case was that of a woman aged thirty-nine years, who died on the 19th day of the disease. The mucous membrane of the jejunum and ileum was tinged with bile; the larger vessels were considerably congested. The thirteenth Peyer's patch, counting from the cæcum, was finely injected. The other patches were healthy, with the exception of the last and the last but one, on either of which was a very slightly thickened spot, of a greyish colour, about two lines in diameter, with a minute depression in the centre. The mesenteric glands were visible, but not enlarged; the mucous membrane over the patches was of normal consistence and thickness, the deviation from health was so trifling, that a friend present, well acquainted with the normal and diseased condition of these organs, considered them healthy; and I really cannot say, the thickening being so trifling, and the discoloration so pale, that there was any actual disease, but as I noted these appearances at the time, and there was a question whether there was a loss of mucous membrane at the minute depressed points, I have thought it well to give the particulars.

Thus, it may be said that recent disease of Peyer's patches was absent in every one of the forty-three cases of typhus fever.

Solitary Glands.—There was no deviation from the healthy condition of these organs in any of the cases of typhus fever.

LARGE INTESTINES.

Typhoid Fever.—The large intestines were not examined in three cases; four proved fatal after the 35th day of the day of the disease, so that so far as the colour and consistence of the mucous membrane are concerned, sixteen cases only are available for analysis.

The colour and consistence of the mucous membrane in ten of the sixteen were normal, or nearly so. In two of the ten there were ulcers on the mucous membrane of both cæcum and colon.

In two cases the mucous membrane of the large intestines was softened throughout; in one of the two it was pale throughout; in the other the ascending colon was deeply injected, the remainder of the gut being pale.

In one of the sixteen cases the mucous membrane of the cæcum was pale grey, and normal in consistence and thickness; the colon in the same subject being bright red, mottled with patches of grey : in another the lining membrane of the cæcum was slightly softened; the ascending colon, here and there, dull red and slightly softened, the transverse and descending colon being normal in consistence and thickness : the cæcum was pale in one case in which the ascending colon, just above the cæcum, was highly vascular, but from that part to its termination, pale. Its consistence in this case was normal. In the three last cases there were ulcers in either the cæcum or colon, or in both. In one case there was un-equivocal evidence of inflammation of the colon. The subject was a man æt. twenty-eight, who died on the 27th day of the disease; the mucous membrane of the colon immediately above the cæcum—which was pale and healthy in consistence and thickness—was minutely injected, and scattered over the same part were patches of a bright red colour. The mucous membrane at these deeply red parts looked rough-ened, the minute elevation being of a deeper hue than the floor on which they were seated; on the deepest-coloured spots were shreds of lymph-like matter, of a yellowish colour.

These patches of shreds had a transverse direction—*i.e.* ran round the intestine; and the shreds were capable of being removed without injury to the subjacent membrane. The mucous membrane itself was neither thickened nor softened, but was capable of being removed in larger and longer strips than usual, probably from softening of the submucous cellular tissue. At this part of the colon the solitary glands were not visible, but further on they were found without difficulty. They did not appear diseased in any way. There was no ulceration of the large intestines in this case.

Ulceration.—Twenty of the twenty-three cases may be considered with reference to this point—*i.e.* all those in which the large intestines were examined. In seven of the twenty, ulcers existed in the cæcum or colon, or in both. Generally round and small, they were occasionally oval, and of considerable size; in the latter case their long axis lay in the direction of the circular fibres of the intestine. Some-times their floors were formed of submucous cellular tissue, at others of muscular fibres, and in one instance by peri-toneum only. The following descriptions will show that their first development resembles, in all particulars, the origin of the ulcers observed in the small intestines in the cases here examined. A male, æt. 23, died on the 25th day of the disease; the colon was bright red, mottled with grey; scattered over its whole surface were numerous round spots about a line in diameter, elevated, some of them considerably, above the level of the surrounding membrane. Their centres were white and opaque, their bases grey. The white opaque central spot had, in some instances, separated at its circum-ference from the surrounding membrane, still, however, adhering to the submucous tissue; the line of separation was deep red. Again, at other places, this line had widened so as to form a complete furrow, the opaque white mass still adhering more or less firmly to the submucous cellular tissue; while in a third set of cases the opaque white mass had dis-appeared, and a small ulcer had been formed. The elevation of these spots was caused by an opaque white deposit in the submucous tissue. In the descending colon the deposit causing the elevation was greater in amount, and the round spots were larger and stood higher above the surrounding level, than in the parts of the colon near to the cæcum. In another male, æt. 28, who died on the 31st day of the disease, there were about twenty ulcers seated on the four inches of colon immediately adjacent to the cæcum; they were oval, and varied from one-fourth to one-and-a-half inch in length, the largest being one-half inch broad; their long diameter corresponded to the transverse fibres of the intestine. They were situated between the transverse folds of the gut. Their edges were undermined, grey and rounded; their floors formed of transverse muscular fibres; but in a few places there was little more than peritoneum to prevent the escape of the fæcal matter. There was no appearance of solitary glands in this case. In a third case, which proved fatal on the 46th day, the cæcum and ascending colon were thickly studded with ulcers, varying in diameter from one to four lines, the edges of which were scarcely elevated, their floors being formed by submucous cellular tissue, or transverse muscular fibres. In addition to these ulcers, there were interspersed among them numerous opaque white, smooth, shining spots, one or two lines in diameter, the borders of which were grey, the mucous membrane around being slate-coloured, and slightly puckered toward them.

It admits of question whether the ulceration in these cases had its origin in the solitary glands; and although, in the first case, the general appearance of the elevations studding the mucous membrane closely resembled enlarged solitary glands, yet I by no means feel confident that they were such in reality. The analogies of the *plaques molles* and *plaques dures* are clearly seen in the above cases, and the last case exhibits what was seen to be true with respect to ulcers in the small intestines,—viz., that while, after the fever had run its course, some of the ulcers might heal, yet that others might pass into the state of simple ulcers, and prolong the illness to an indefinite period.

Typhus Fever.—The large intestines were examined in thirty-seven cases before the termination of the 4th week of the disease. In twenty-eight of the thirty-seven the mucous membrane lining them was normal, or nearly so, in colour and consistence.

In one case the cæcum, in one the cæcum and colon

generally, and in one the cæcum and ascending colon, were congested. The congestion, though marked, was confined to the larger vessels, and was ramiform in character. In one case the cæeum and colon were pale, but slightly softened; and in one the softening was limited to the transverse arch.

In four cases only were unequivocal traces of inflammation of the mucous membrane of the large intestines present. A female, aged twenty-nine, died toward the end of the third or during the fourth week of the disease. The appearances found after death in the intestine have already been described. In another of the four cases, the patient, a woman, aged forty-seven, died on the 12th day of the disease. In the colon, just above the cæcum, were four large patches running transversely, of a deep red colour; the mucous membrane at this part was thickened, and decidedly softer than that around. Although it was in this case rather softer throughout the colon than usual, still it was not more so generally than might be considered within the range of health. With the exception of the patches, just described, the mucous membrane of the large intestine was pale. The third case also was that of a woman, æt. forty-three, who died on the 16th day of the disease. Scattered over the eighteen inches of colon next the cæcum, there were about twenty patches, varying from one-quarter to half-an-inch in diameter, irregular in shape, of a dull yellow colour, considerably elevated. The mucous membrane which immediately surrounded them was of a bright red colour, gradually fading as it receded into the natural hue of the intestinal mucous membrane. The yellow matter itself was readily removeable, friable, and finely granular. It appeared to be a deposit of lymph in and on the mucous membrane, a portion of the latter being carried away when the former was removed. In the transverse and descending colon were a few linear patches, resembling the yellow spots above described. Some of these ran transversely, others longitudinally; the latter appeared in some measure to correspond in course and situation to the longitudinal bands. The mucous membrane of the colon generally was rather soft, of normal thickness, and pale. The fourth case, in which there were signs of inflammation of the mucous membrane of the colon, was that of a male, æt. thirty. In the sigmoid flexure was a patch, about four inches in diameter, of vivid redness; the mucous membrane at the same part was decidedly softened. With these four exceptions, there was no trace of inflammation of the mucous membrane of the large intestines.

The frequency of dysentery as a complication of typhus fever, when patients are placed in unfavourable circumstances, ought to make us particularly careful in admitting such evidence (excepting M. Landouzy's [1]) as Gaultier de Claubrey has adduced in support of the opinion, that the typhus fever of camps and jails of old writers, and typhoid fever, are identical. For we see, even by the examples here brought forward, that lesions of a very serious nature may affect the intestinal mucous membrane in typhus fever; but, at the same time, we see also that these lesions are of a very different character from those occurring in typhoid fever. Therefore, to show that petechiæ, diarrhœa, and delirium,

---

[1] I may here briefly observe, that M. Landouzy appears to have had, in the prison at Rheims, cases both of typhus and of typhoid fevers. The presence of petechiæ by no means proves that a case is not typhoid fever. Petechiæ may occur in scarlet fever, small-pox, and in many other diseases (as all who have witnessed much of these affections will readily allow), when the patients are placed in unfavourable circumstances, and occasionally even under other conditions. There is no proof that the mulberry or true typhus rash was present in M. Landouzy's cases, or that true rose spots ever passed into petechiæ; nay, it is even within the range of probability that some of the so-called petechiæ were really flea-bites. Similar circumstances favour the spread of typhus and typhoid fevers. The poison of both appears subject to the same laws of development; therefore, where one exists there the other is likely to exist. The apparent discrepancies in the observations of the older writers on camp and jail fevers may probably be explained thus :— Their descriptions of the disease varied, because they had at least two diseases to describe, each capable of assuming a mild or a severe form. Now, the varied proportions in which these two diseases prevailed at different times, the presence of one disease only in the camp or jail, and variations in the severity of type, must have necessarily caused confusion in the accounts of camp and jail fever. The same confusion, from the same cause, exists in the descriptions of typhus fever by the writers of our own age, who have not drawn the distinction, which nature has, between typhus and typhoid fevers. The attempt to settle the question of the identity or non-identity of these diseases by a reference to old writers, appears as absurd as it would be for astronomers of the present day, with eyes in their heads, telescopes in their hands, and the heavens above them, to found their opinions respecting the movements of certain celestial bodies on the dicta of Ptolemy, or the observations of Copernicus.

were present during life in a number of cases, and that some lesion of the intestine was found after death in the same cases, is by no means to prove that these persons died of typhoid fever. The cases here analysed, like those recorded by previous writers, prove that neither typhoid nor typhus fever is gastro-enteritis.

MESENTERIC GLANDS.

Typhoid Fever.—These organs were more or less extensively and unequivocally diseased in all of the twenty-three cases I am considering. In every case they were larger than natural, and their volume increased as they approached nearer to the ileo-cæcal valve.

Their size varied from a pea to a pigeon's egg; their colour from pale rose to dark grey; their consistence from firm to soft and flabby, and soft and friable. The deep grey of these organs, with one exception, was limited to those cases which proved fatal after the 30th day. The four cases, also, in which they were recorded to be flabby, all proved fatal after the same date of the disease.

In three cases one or more glands were in a state of suppuration.[1] In two of the three the purulent-looking fluid, collected in a mass, was separated from the abdominal cavity only by a thin layer of peritoneum. In the third the purulent fluid occupied distinct points in the glands. Two of these three cases proved fatal, respectively on the 20th and 30th day, the third at least five weeks after the commencement of the disease.

In a fourth case, in which probably the suppurative process took place, the patient recovered, so far as the fever was concerned, and the glands were reduced at the time of death to a state in which they could no longer have exercised any injurious effect. This patient died of erysipelas, on the 86th day of illness.[2]

In four cases there was a deposit of opaque pale yellowish

[1] Though resembling in external characters true pus, this fluid differs considerably from that when seen by the aid of the microscope.

[2] For particulars of this very interesting case, I must refer the reader to the essay in a subsequent part of this volume (Case 33, p. 303).

friable matter in the substance of the mesenteric glands. This appeared to be exactly the same material as that seated in the submucous cellular tissue, corresponding to Peyer's patches; and microscopic examination demonstrated the identity of the minute structure of the two deposits. Three of the four cases in which this deposit was found proved fatal respectively on the 12th, 25th, and 46th days; the fourth at least five weeks after the commencement of illness, and three weeks after the admission of the patient into the hospital.

That the before referred to pseudo-suppuration sometimes occurs *around* this deposit, the annexed description of the appearances found after death in the mesentery of a man, aged thirty-three, who died on the 20th day of the disease, will, it appears to me, afford sufficient proof. The mesenteric glands were considerably enlarged. They varied in size from a pea to a walnut; just behind the cæcum was a mass, the size of a large pigeon's egg. Externally they were of a deep slate grey. On dissection, a considerable quantity of reddish purulent-looking fluid escaped from them. In the centre, and quite detached and loose, and bathed on all sides by this purulent-looking fluid, was a solid mass, in one of the largest glands about the size of a small walnut, of a delicate pink colour, finely granular externally and on section firm and friable. In some of the glands the disorganising process appeared to have proceeded further, the central solid pink mass being replaced by a semi-purulent clot. Microscopic examination demonstrated this mass to be made up chiefly of typhous matter, as it has been called.

The mesocolic glands were noted to be enlarged in five cases; in one the enlargement was limited to the vicinity of the colon adjacent to the cæcum, and these glands, which were dark-red and softened, contained some purulent-looking fluid.

In the case in which there was extensive ulceration at the lower part of the œsophagus, there was considerable enlargement of the corresponding *œsophageal lymphatic glands*.

In two cases the *lumbar glands* were enlarged.

Typhus Fever.—In one case, that of a child, æt. 10, in

whose lungs and agminated glands numerous tubercles were found, the mesenteric glands varied in size from a pea to a small bean, the largest corresponded to the middle of the small intestine. These glands contained some tubercular matter.[1] In the same case the mesocolic glands were dark grey and firm, and some of them were as large as peas. In another case, that of a child in whose lungs was found some tubercular deposit, the mesenteric glands were large and pale.

With these two exceptions, no deviation from a healthy structure was observed in the mesenteric or other lymphatic glands, in either of the forty-three subjects dead from typhus fever. So that patients labouring under typhus fever are exempt from acute disease of the lymphatic glands, at least to any appreciable extent. How much they differ in this respect from those affected with typhoid fever I need not here point out.

PERITONEUM.

Typhoid Fever.—In five of the twenty-three cases there were signs of peritonitis, *i.e.* increased vascularity, with effusion of turbid serosity and lymph, or recent adhesions. In four of the five cases the inflammation had extended over nearly the entire surface of the peritoneum. In three cases perforation of the coats of the gut appeared to have been the cause of the inflammation. In a fourth case the co-existence of perforation was a matter of doubt, as I was not permitted to complete the examination. In the fifth case the peritonitis depended for its origin on perforation of the peritoneum covering a gland in the process of recovery from a state of suppuration.[2]

Typhus Fever.—In no case was there any trace of recent peritonitis.

SPLEEN.

Typhoid Fever.—Weight.—Excluding the cases of the subjects under fifteen years of age, those which survived the

---

[1] See page 84.

[2] This case is given in detail in the subsequent paper on illustrative cases.

35th day of disease, and those the spleens of which were not
weighed, there remain only eleven cases for analysis.   The
average weight of the spleens in these eleven cases was
10 oz. 3 drms. avoirdupois ; neither of them weighed less
than 6 oz., two exactly 6 oz. each, and one as much as 14 oz. ;
the patients from whom the two former were obtained died
respectively on the 21st and 31st day of the disease ; the
last on the 27th.

The size of the organ was nearly in proportion to its
weight ; its vertical measurement varied from four and a half
to seven inches.

Consistence.[1]—The condition of the spleen with reference
to its consistence was recorded in fourteen cases that proved
fatal before the 35th day.   In four of these fourteen cases it
was decidedly softened, in one of the four pulpy ; these four
cases terminated respectively on the 23rd, 25th, 27th, and 28th
day of disease.   In the remaining ten cases the spleen was of
normal consistence ; these ten cases terminated respectively
from the 12th to the 34th day inclusive.

It is worthy of remark that seven of the fourteen cases
terminated fatally between the 20th and 31st days ; and that
it was in this group that the four cases of softening of the
spleen were found.   Now this is the period of the disease
in which M. Louis found the organ the most frequently
softened.

*Relation between Enlargement and Softening of the
Spleen.*—The four spleens which were decidedly softened
weighed respectively 11 oz., 13 oz., 13 oz. 4 drms., 14 oz.

Two of those which were as firm as in health weighed 11 oz.,
and 12 oz. 4 drms. ; the patients from whom these two were
removed, died on the 12th and 20th days of disease.   The
others weighed less than 10 oz. ; two of them only 6 oz., these
two died respectively on the 21st and 31st day of disease.

Typhus Fever.—The spleen was weighed in thirty-four of

[1] In examining the consistence of an organ, there is no certain standard
of comparison ; so that what one observer terms normal in consistence,
another may call softer than natural.   It is evident that the term of expression will vary according to each man's own idea of what the normal consistence of any given organ is.   I have endeavoured to restrict my application
of the term softening to those cases regarding which there could be no
difference of opinion.

the forty-three subjects aged more than fifteen years, who died before the termination of the fourth week of disease.

Its average weight was 7 oz. 5 drms.

In nine, or rather more than one-fourth, of these 34 cases, it weighed less than 6 oz. In one case, only 2 oz. 6 drms.

In seven, or rather more than one-fifth of the cases, its weight was greater than the average weight of the same organ in the case of typhoid fever. In two cases it weighed as much as 14 oz.

Its size was usually in proportion to its weight. Its vertical measurement varied from four to seven inches.

*Attempt to determine the co-existence of conditions which favoured enlargement of the spleen.—Sex.—*Of the above thirty-four cases, seventeen were males, and seventeen were females.

The average weight of the spleen in the seventeen males was 7 oz. 2 drms. Four of the seventeen spleens removed from the male subjects weighed less than 6 oz., two more than the average weight of the typhoid spleens, one as much as 14 oz., one as little as 2 oz. 6 drms.

If the male cases which proved fatal before the 21st day only be taken, the average weight of the spleen in them was 8 oz. 2 drms., one only weighing less than 6 oz., and two more than the average of the typhoid spleens.

The average age of these seventeen males was forty-six years eight months: the eldest was sixty-five, the youngest twenty-nine; eight of them were under fifty years of age.

The average weight of the spleen in the seventeen females was 8 oz. 4 drms., five of these seventeen spleens weighed less than 6 oz., and five more than the average weight of the typhoid spleens. The heaviest weighed 14 oz. 4 drms., the lightest 3 oz. 4 drms.

If the cases (female) which proved fatal before the 21st day only be taken into the calculation, then the average weight of the organ was 7 oz. 2 drms., five of the spleens weighing less than 6 oz., and three more than the average weight of the typhoid spleens.

The average age of these seventeen females was 43 years 9 months—the age of the eldest was 70, of the youngest 22 years—ten of the seventeen being under fifty years of age.

Thus it is evident that sex exerted no influence over the size and weight of the spleen in these thirty-four cases.

Age.—The spleens of thirteen subjects between the ages of 16 and 40 inclusive were examined before the termination of the 4th week from the commencement of the typhus fever. The average weight of the organ in these thirteen cases was 9 oz. 1 drm.—two of them weighing less than 6 oz.; six, or nearly one-half, more than 10 oz. 3 drms., *i.e.* the average weight of the spleen in those dead from typhoid fever.

The spleen was weighed in nineteen cases, the ages of which varied from 41 to 70 years inclusive. In these nineteen the average weight of the organ was only 6 oz. 6 drms.; six, or nearly one-third, weighed less than 6 oz.; one only weighed more than the average of the typhoid spleens.

Thus the age of the patients appears to have exerted an appreciable influence over the size attained by the spleen in the cases of typhus fever.

If, instead of taking the average of the spleen in these thirty-four cases, the weight of the organ in the subjects, whose ages corresponded with the ages of the cases of typhoid fever here analysed, *i.e.* were under 40 years, be considered, and these cases be still further limited to those which proved fatal before the termination of the 21st day of disease, then there will be nine cases for examination, and the weights of the spleens in these nine will nearly correspond with the weights of the same organ in the cases of typhoid fever,—thus the average weight of the organ in these nine cases was 10 oz. 4 drms., none weighing less than 6 oz., and six over the average of the weight of the same organ in the cases of typhoid fever.

But if the cases of the patients between 40 and 50 years of age, who died by the 21st day of the disease, only be considered—there were eight of them—the average weight of the spleen in these eight cases was 6 oz. 4 drms., and while four of the spleens weighed less than 6 oz., only one exceeded in weight the typhoid spleens.

The spleens of eight patients, whose ages exceeded 50 years, and who died before the 21st day of disease, were weighed. The average weight of the organ in these eight cases was 7 oz. 1 drm., one only weighing less than 6 oz., and none more than 9 oz.

Consistence.—The consistence of the spleen was notably diminished in thirteen cases. In these cases its consistence was characterised by the terms—pulpy, very soft, soft, rather soft.

In eighteen cases it retained its normal consistence. In these cases it was stated in my notes to be firm, healthy in consistence, or moderately, or tolerably firm, or not decidedly softened.

In the remaining twelve cases there was either old disease of the organ present, or the patients survived beyond the fourth week of the disease, or the consistence of the organ was not noted.

Influence of sex—season—local complications—cadaveric change—condition of the blood—age—and duration of the disease in determining the presence or absence of softening of the spleen.

Sex.—Nine of the eighteen subjects in which the spleen was of good consistence were males; nine females.

Six of the thirteen in which it was softened were males; seven females.

The proportion of males to females, in both instances, was, therefore, as nearly equal as was possible, so that sex exerted no influence in producing softening of the spleen.

Season.—Seven of the eighteen subjects, the spleens of which were of normal consistence, were examined during the six winter months, eleven during the six summer months:

Six of the thirteen subjects, in which the same organ was softened, were opened during the six winter months, seven during the six summer months. The latter, therefore, are in as nearly equal proportion as is possible, seeing the total is an odd number. Thus season, like sex, had no part in causing the change in the consistence of the spleen.

Local Complications of an Inflammatory Nature.—These appeared to exert little influence on the consistence or size of the spleen. Five of the eighteen cases in which that organ was firm, were uncomplicated, and four of the thirteen in which it was softened.

Was the Softening the effect of a Cadaveric Change?—Three of the cases in which the spleen was very soft, or soft, were examined respectively 8, 9, and 11 hours after death, and only three of the thirteen cases more than 30 hours after death, while eight of seventeen cases, in which the spleen was of normal, or nearly normal consistence, were examined more than 30 hours after death.

It appears highly probable that this change, then, was pathological and not cadaveric; for although the subjects, the spleens of which were so decidedly softened 8, 9, and 11 hours after the fatal termination, were examined in the months of July and September, yet the temperature was noted to be cool at the time the two former lay dead.

Relation between Softening of the Spleen and the Condition of the Blood.—Of six cases in which the blood was fluid, or in which there was merely a little soft black clot in the right side of the heart, two had the spleen soft, and four firm, and as there were eighteen of the latter to thirteen of the former, this condition of the blood could have exerted but little influence in producing the variations in the consistence of the spleen.

Age.—Of the thirteen subjects in which the spleen was noted to be of normal consistence or firm, there were—

Aged 30 years and under,   5 *i.e.* $\frac{5}{13}$, or in the proportion of 38·46 per cent.
... between 31 & 40 incl., 3 ... $\frac{3}{13}$, ...   23·07 per cent.
...   ...   41 & 50 ... 4 .. $\frac{4}{13}$, ...   30·77 per cent.
...   ...   51 & 62 ... 1 ... $\frac{1}{13}$, ...   7·68 per cent.

If to these be added the five subjects in which the organ was noted to be of tolerably firm, etc., in consistence, there will be—

Aged 30 years and under,   6 *i.e.* $\frac{6}{18}$, or in the proportion of 33·33 per cent.
... between 31 & 40 incl., 4 ... $\frac{4}{18}$, ...   22·22 per cent.
...   ...   41 & 50 ... 5 ... $\frac{5}{18}$,   ...   27·77 per cent.
...   ...   50 & 65 ... 3 ... $\frac{3}{18}$,   ...   16·66 per cent.

Of the thirteen subjects, the spleens of which were *decidedly* softened, there were—

Aged 30 years and under,   1 *i.e.* $\frac{1}{13}$, or in the proportion of 7·68 per cent.
... between 31 & 40 incl., 2 ... $\frac{2}{13}$, ...   15·38 per cent.
...   ...   41 & 50 ... 4 ... $\frac{4}{13}$, ...   30·77 per cent.
...   ...   51 & 62 ... 6 ... $\frac{6}{13}$, ...   46·15 per cent.

So that, of the spleens undoubtedly softened, rather more

than three-fourths belonged to subjects more than forty years of age, and nearly one-half to subjects more than fifty years of age; while of the spleens, the consistence of which was as firm as in health, decidedly less than half were removed from subjects more than forty years of age, and one only from a subject more than fifty years of age; and if to the latter group be added the five in which the consistence was so slightly diminished as not to be considered abnormally so, still less than half were removed from subjects the ages of which exceeded forty, and three only from subjects more than fifty, years of age.

Duration of the Disease.—Fifteen spleens of normal or nearly normal consistence, were removed from subjects, the duration of the disease in which was known.   Of these fifteen spleens there were,—

Belonging to subjects who had been ill a period not exceeding 14 days,   5
...   .   between 14 and 29 days, 10

Of ten spleens noted to be decidedly softer than natural, there were,—

Belonging to subjects who had been ill a period not exceeding 14 days, 7
...   .   between 14 and 17 days, 3

and not one of the four subjects in which this organ was noted to be *very* soft, had survived the 14th day of the disease.

Relation between the weight and consistence of the Spleen. —Twelve of the softened spleens were weighed, of these—

3 or one-fourth weighed less than 6 oz.
11 less than   ...   ...   9 oz.
1 weighed ...   .   11 oz. 4 drms.

Sixteen of the spleens of normal consistence were weighed, of these—

3 or rather less than one-fifth weighed less than 6 oz.
8 or one-half more than   ...   ...   9 oz.
2 as much as   ...   .   14 oz.

So that the smaller spleens appear to have been the softer.

From this rather lengthened analysis it is evident—

1. That the spleen was considerably enlarged in the cases of Typhoid and Typhus fevers here analysed.

2. That it is generally larger in the subjects dead from Typhoid than those dead from Typhus fever.

3. That if the cases of Typhus fever be limited to those, the

ages of which do not exceed forty years, then the relative difference in the weight of the spleen in the cases of Typhoid and
Typhus fevers, which prove fatal respectively before the 35th,
and the 28th day of the disease is considerably diminished.

4. That the average weight of the organ is exactly equal
in subjects dead from Typhoid and Typhus fevers, if the
cases of the latter disease only be considered, which prove
fatal before the 21st day of the disease, and which do not
exceed forty years of age, *i.e.* the age after which no case of
Typhoid fever (here analysed) proved fatal.

5. That after the age of forty, the spleen is much less
enlarged in Typhus fever than it is before that age. How
far this holds true with regard to Typhoid fever, the cases
here considered afford no means of determining.

6. That softening of the spleen in cases of Typhus fever
is much more frequent after the age of fifty, than before that
period of life.

7. That softening of the spleen both in Typhoid and
Typhus fevers, is much more frequent in those cases that
terminate unfavourably at an early period of either disease,
than in those which prove fatal at a later period.

8. That in no case of Typhoid fever (here analysed) was
the spleen found softened after the 28th day of the disease.

9. That softening of the spleen is much more frequent in
cases of Typhus fever before than after the 14th day of disease.

We may therefore conclude that the age of the patient,
and the duration of the disease, are the two circumstances
which exert the greatest influence in determining the presence
of softening and of enlargement of the spleen in Typhus and
Typhoid fevers.

LIVER.

Typhoid Fever.—Excluding eight cases, in which the liver
was not examined, or which proved fatal after the 35th day
of the disease, there remain fifteen for analysis.

Seven of the fifteen bodies were opened during the first 24
hours; eight between 24 and 58 hours after death: six during
the winter, nine during the summer months.

In eleven of the fifteen the consistence of the liver was
normal; six of these eleven cases were examined during the
first 24 hours after death, the remaining five between 24 and

44½ hours; five of the eleven were examined during winter months, six during the summer.

In four of the fifteen—*i.e.* about one-fourth—the liver was flabby; these four were examined respectively 11, 26, 32, and 58 hours after death, in the months of September, August, September, and January. The four cases proved fatal respectively on the 31st, ?th, 28th, and 30th days of disease.

In one of the four cases only was the organ noted to be of a doughy consistence, *i.e.* it received and retained the impression of the fingers with facility. This was the third of the four cases above-mentioned.

The colour was noted to be normal in thirteen cases; darker than usual in two cases—*i.e.* about one-seventh.

Typhus Fever.—Seven of the forty-three cases are ineligible for analysis.

Seventeen of the remaining thirty-six cases were opened during the first 24 hours after death; nineteen between 24 and 52 hours: sixteen were opened in the winter, twenty-five in the summer, months.

In fourteen of the thirty-six cases the liver retained its normal consistence; eight of these fourteen were examined within 24 hours, and five between 24 and 36 hours, after death: five during the winter, and nine during the summer, months.

In twenty-two, or three-fifths of the cases examined, the liver was flabby. Nine of the twenty-two were examined during the first 24 hours after death, thirteen between 24 and 52 hours after death: seven were examined during the winter, fifteen during the summer, months.

In seven of these twenty-two cases, *i.e.* in one-fifth of the whole number of cases examined—the liver was of doughy or putty-like consistence. Six of the seven were examined between 22 and 36 hours after death: three during the winter months, four during the summer. Five of these seven died on or before the 14th day of disease; two at an uncertain period of the disease, but on the 3rd and 6th days of their residence in the hospital, and therefore probably at an early period of the disease. While of twelve cases, the duration of which was known, and in which the liver was firm, or of normal consistence, eight—*i.e.* two-thirds—survived the 14th day of the disease.

The colour of the liver was normal in twenty-nine of the thirty-six cases; deeper than natural in seven—*i.e.* one-fifth.

The question examined above, it will be observed, is not that of the *absolute* cause of the softening of the liver in typhoid and typhus fevers, but that of the existence of external conditions, capable of accounting for the actual *difference* observed in the condition of the organ in the two diseases.

It will be seen, then, that about half the cases of either disease were examined during the first 24 hours after death, and, as near as possible, two-thirds of either disease during the summer months. The difference in the proportions of the cases in which marked alteration in the consistence of the organ occurred cannot, then, be attributed to any difference in the periods at which the cases of the two diseases were examined after death, nor to any difference in the temperature. Like the same change in other organs, as the kidneys and pancreas, it was probably the effect of the difference in the alterations in the solids induced by either disease, which difference was only manifested by the rapidity, etc., of the cadaveric changes.

GALL BLADDER.

Typhoid Fever.—Notes were taken of the **gall-bladder** and its contents in fourteen cases, which proved fatal before the 35th day of disease.

In two cases only was the bile distinctly green, and in both it was thin and limpid. In four cases it was greenish yellow; and in eight cases yellow or orange.

In one case, which proved fatal on the 46th day of the disease, two ulcers were found in the gall-bladder.

Typhus Fever.—The physical appearances of the bile were recorded in thirty-one cases.

In nine of them it was dark green; in nine greenish yellow; and in twelve yellow or orange.

In addition to this difference in hue, the bile was generally much thicker in typhus than in typhoid fever.

In no case of typhus was there any ulceration of the lining membrane of the gall bladder.

PANCREAS.

Typhoid Fever.—This organ was examined in thirteen of the twenty-three cases. In four it was flabby; in nine of normal consistence. In all it preserved its natural colour.

Typhus Fever.—In eight of thirty-four cases in which the pancreas was examined, that organ was flabby; in the remaining twenty-six it was normal in consistence. In eight cases it was deeper red than natural; in twenty-six it preserved its healthy hue.

KIDNEYS.

As the amount of blood in these organs could have caused but little change from their normal weight, and the cases I am here considering are limited in number, I shall not enter on that subject, although I have notes of the weight of the kidneys in sixty of the sixty-six cases here considered.

The microscopic examinations I shall also reserve for some other occasion. It is sufficient to say that such examinations exhibited a marked difference in the structure (after death) of the kidneys in the two diseases. In the one (typhus) the tubes were, in a much larger proportion of cases than in the other (typhoid fever), filled with detached epithelium scales. This separation I regard as cadaveric, and a part of that general tendency to the dissolution of tissue so eminently characteristic of typhus fever.

Typhoid Fever.—The kidneys were noted to be healthy in eight cases, congested in three, and pale in three. Of two others no note was made, so that they could have deviated but little in appearance from health.

Seven cases either survived the 35th day of disease, or those organs were not examined.

Consistence.—Excluding the above seven cases, the kidneys were noted to be flabby in one case, examined 47½ hours after death, in the month of October. In the other cases they were normal in consistence—at least they were recorded to be healthy.[1]

[1] In every case recorded as healthy the capsules were removed from the surface, and the kidney divided longitudinally.

In two cases there was slightly increased vascularity of the lining membrane of the pelvis of the kidney.

The *urinary bladder* was examined in nine cases which proved fatal before the termination of the fever. In one case only did it present any deviation from health. The following is a description of its appearance :—Scattered over the mucous membrane of the organ were numerous patches of deep red, and here and there patches of a dull yellow, slightly elevated, smooth on the surface, and surrounded by an areola of deep red. When the yellow matter was removed by the nail, a slightly abraded surface was exposed, as if the mucous membrane had been carried away with it.

Typhus Fever.—Both kidneys were congested in eight cases; the left kidney only in one case. In twenty-seven cases they were considered healthy in appearance.

Consistence.—In five cases they were recorded to be flabby, or soft and flabby in consistence. These five cases were examined respectively 16, 22, 27, 36, and 38 hours after death, and in the months of December, November, October, and May.

In thirty-one cases they were healthy.

In four cases the lining membrane of the pelvis was considered to be more injected than natural. In one of these cases it was studded with minute hemorrhagic points.

Seven cases either survived the fever, or were not examined.

The *urinary bladder* was examined in twelve cases, which proved fatal by the 28th day of the disease. In one there was found congestion of its posterior wall, with numerous minute hemorrhagic spots in the same situation. In another the mucous membrane generally was slightly more vascular than natural. While in a third case the anterior wall of the viscus was very finely injected.

In the remaining nine cases the organ was pale and healthy.[1]

PERICARDIUM.

Typhoid Fever.—In one case only was any deviation from

[1] Subsequent experience would lead me to suppose that I noted some kidneys as healthy which ought to have been regarded (comparatively) as softened.

the normal condition of the pericardium observed. In that case a few shreds of lymph were attached to the pericardium, covering the auricle. In every case the fluid retained the yellow hue proper to it, and its amount was considered natural.

Five of the cases were examined respectively 30, 32, 36, 44½, and 58 hours after death; three in the summer and two in the winter months.

Typhus Fever.—Excluding seven cases not available for analysis, there remain thirty-six for consideration.

In thirty-one cases no abnormal appearance was observed.

In five the serosity contained in the pericardium was of a more or less deep red colour. These five cases were examined respectively 16, 24, 24, 40, and 48 hours after death: four during the summer and one during the winter months. That the red hue was due to the transudation of the colouring matter of the blood, and not the consequence of effusion of blood, was proved by its containing no red corpuscles, by the number of epithelium scales diffused throughout it, by the deep red staining of the posterior wall of the auricles, and by a shade of discoloration bounding the edges of the veins coursing over the surface of the heart.

This cadaveric transudation of a solution of the colouring matter of the blood into the serosity contained in the pericardium, is another example of the greater tendency to decay impressed on the body by typhus than by typhoid fever; for it may be observed that the period that elapsed after death, before the above five cases were examined, was exceeded by that before which five of the cases of typhoid fever were opened. One of the former, in fact, was inspected in the month of December, only 16 hours after death. Three of these five patients were less than forty years of age; the one last referred to was only twenty-two, so that neither difference in age, nor external conditions, was the cause of the want of similarity between the two diseases with respect to the change under consideration.

HEART AND ITS CONTENTS.

Typhoid Fever.—Excluding those cases in which the chest was not examined, and those which survived more than 35 days from the outset of the disease, there remain for analysis fifteen cases.

In no case was there any recent endocardial disease; in one there was a congenital malformation, a communication between the right and left ventricles; and in another, slight thickening of the free edges of the mitral, and induration of the base of the aortic valves.

The substance of the heart was firm or healthy in consistence in five cases; soft and flabby, or flabby only, in five cases; the right ventricle flabby, the left normal, in one case; of four cases no note on this point was made.

Of the five hearts that were flabby, one was examined an uncertain period after death; the other four respectively, 11, 22½, 32, and 36 hours after the fatal termination. The body in which the right side was flabby, and the left firm was opened 27 hours after death; while the five subjects in which the substance of the heart was firm and normal in consistence, had been in the dead-house respectively 24, 30, 42½, 44½, and 58 hours.

The four hearts of which no note on the point here examined was recorded, were probably healthy in consistence, because other facts respecting them were noted. These four cases were examined within 20 hours after death.

The duration of the disease in the five in which the heart was flabby, was respectively 12, 21, 23, 25, and 28 days; in five cases in which it was firm, 20, 27, 30, 30, and 34 days; one case had lasted an uncertain time. In the four cases in which it was probably healthy, 17, 30, 32, and 33 days.

Thus four out of five cases in which the heart was flabby proved fatal by the 25th day of the disease, while only one out of nine of those in which it was firm, died so soon as the 25th day of disease. It will be remembered, that the only two cases of typhoid fever in which the cadaveric rigidity had entirely disappeared, proved fatal before the 25th day of disease. This seems to place the two series of facts in the same category.

Of six cases examined during the six winter months, the substance of the heart was flabby in only one; of eight examined during the summer months it was flabby in four.

Dusky-red Staining of the Lining Membrane of the Heart.

—No note with reference to this particular was made in seven of the cases; in five cases it was unstained; in one there was slight discoloration of the endocardium of the left auricle, and in two cases there was slight staining of the whole endocardium; so that in one-fifth only of the cases was the endocardium observed to be stained, and in these cases the description of the staining was qualified by the terms—'slightly,' 'slightly,' and 'a little.'

Condition of the Blood in the Heart.—Of fifteen cases eligible for analysis, no note was made in one. In four, examined respectively 58, 36, 22½, and 7 hours after death, the blood was fluid; in the last, however, it coagulated shortly after its escape from the body; and there was already formed a minute clot in the right ventricle.

There was a large clot, made up of a larger or smaller smooth, shining, yellow, fibrinous portion, from the substance of which much serosity could be pressed, and of a large, loose, dark crimson, almost black clot, joined to and lying beneath the former, in the right auricle and ventricle in ten cases; in all of these cases there was also a similar but smaller clot on the left side; and in seven of the ten cases, the fibrinous portion of the coagulum on either side of the heart was continuous with a clot in the pulmonary artery and aorta; and in several of these ten cases it was moulded at the lower portion to the shape of the upper surface of the sigmoid valves.

In four cases the blood was fluid in the venæ cavæ and pulmonary veins, while it was tolerably firmly, or decidedly firmly, coagulated in the right side of the heart.

In two of the three cases in which the blood was fluid in the heart, and did not coagulate after its escape from the body, the substance of the heart was flabby; in two other cases, in which a similar condition of that organ existed, the blood was firmly coagulated; and in five cases, in which it was firm, a firm coagulum was found in the right and left cavities of the organ.

Typhus Fever.—Eight cases either survived beyond the 29th day of the disease, or the chests were not examined.

Excluding six cases, the hearts of which were examined respectively 11, 20, 27¼, 36, 45½, and 48 hours after death, because no note with reference to their consistence was made, there remain for analysis twenty-nine cases; in fifteen of these the heart was flabby, in fourteen firm.

Of five hearts examined 20 hours or less after death, one only was flabby; of fourteen examined between 20 and 30 hours after death, four, or more than a fourth, were flabby; while the whole of those, *i.e.* nine, examined more than 30 hours after death, were in that condition. Since, as I have said, above two-thirds of the hearts examined more than 30 hours after death from typhoid fever, were firm or of natural consistence, and if, as is highly probable, those hearts of which no note was made were firm, then it will be seen that four-fifths of the hearts of the subjects dead from typhoid fever, which were examined more than thirty hours after death, were firm; while one-fourth only of the hearts of the subjects dead from typhus fever, which were examined more than 30 hours after death, were firm.

The day of the disease on which those cases proved fatal in which the heart was flabby, varied from the 9th to the 23rd day; a large majority of these patients died by the 16th day. The day of the disease on which those cases in which the heart was firm expired, varied from the 11th to the 22nd day; the large majority proved fatal by the 15th day, so that the duration of the disease could have had no material influence in producing the flabby condition of the heart. As I have shown above, the duration of the disease had a marked influence over the condition of the heart, with reference to the point we are considering, in the cases of typhoid fever.

Age had very little influence in modifying the consistence of the organ in typhus fever, for the average age of the group in which the heart was flabby, was 44; of that in which it was firm, 47; in the latter group there were six cases under 50 years of age; in the former, nine under the same age.

The external temperature, like the age of the patient, exerted little influence in modifying the consistence of the heart in the cases here considered; for of eleven hearts examined during the six winter months, four were flabby and seven firm; and of twenty-two inspected during the summer six months, nine were flabby and thirteen firm.

So that it seems probable that, in the cases of typhoid fever, the flabby condition of the heart was due to two causes,

—1st, a tendency imprinted on the muscular tissue by the disease when death occurred within 25 days from its outset; and, 2dly, the external temperature. Whereas in the cases of typhus fever here considered, although the latter cause might have had some influence, the principal, and by far the most active cause, must have been the impression produced on the heart by the disease itself. These opinions are still further strengthened by the fact, that so many cases of typhus fever prove fatal from the intensity of the general affection, and not from the supervention of local lesions, and that at all stages, even the most advanced, of the disease (*i.e.* excluding cases fatal after the 4th week). Now it is at the earlier periods of typhoid fever only that the state of the system at large produces death. Thus an explanation is afforded of the fact, that the duration of the disease had a marked influence in the production of the altered consistence of the heart in typhoid, and not in typhus, fever; the *difference* in the influence of the temperature of the two affections was probably more apparent than real, because the tendency to produce the flabby state of the heart in typhus fever was so great, that the influence of the weather could scarcely be observed.

Dusky-red Staining of the Lining Membrane of the Heart was observed in twelve cases. In eight of the twelve both sides of the heart were stained; but in four of the eight the right side was darker than the left, and in one only was the left side darker than the right; in three cases the staining was confined to the right side. There was no discoloration of the endocardium in twelve cases; no note was made in eleven cases; so that about one-third, or eleven out of thirty-six, had the lining membrane of the heart discoloured; or if we exclude from the calculation those of which no note on the point was made, one-half would be thus affected. On the other hand, of the cases of typhoid fever one-sixth only (or rather two-thirteenths), or if I omit from the calculation the cases of which no note on the point was made,—one-fourth only had the endocardium discoloured. It will be observed by the reader, that whichever calculation be used, the relative proportion is the same, and therefore, for the purpose for which these cases are here analysed, it is a matter of indifference which of the two be adopted.

In every case, save one, the substance of the heart was flabby at the same time that its lining membrane was stained. The subject which formed the exception—a man, æt. forty, who died about 28 days after the commencement of the disease—was examined in the month of November, 22 hours after death.

In every case, excepting two, in which the endocardium was noted to be unstained, the substance of the heart was firm ; these two cases were examined respectively 42 and 48 hours after death.

If the staining be viewed with reference to the date after death at which the cases were examined, the average number of hours which had elapsed from the hour of death till the subject was placed on the dead-house table, was, for the unstained, 24·7 hours—for the stained, 32·7 hours ; two-thirds of the latter group were examined more than 30 hours after death ; one-sixth only of the former more than 30 hours after the patients expired. So that the staining of the endocardium and the flabby condition of the heart depended apparently on the same causes.

Conditions of the Blood.—It was fluid in four cases ; fluid, but mixed with a few loose black clots, in four others ; these eight cases proved fatal on the 14th, 13th, 17th, 20th, 16th, 13th, 15th, and 17th days of the disease ; and were examined respectively 16, 27¼, 21½, 27, 22, 24, 45½, and 20 hours after death.

The blood was fluid in the left side only of the heart in six cases ; in two of these six there was a small dark coagulum ; in two a large, loose, soft, black, and small fibrinous clot ; in the fifth, a large, very loose, black clot, and much fluid blood ; and in the sixth, a large, soft, pale yellow and black clot in the right side of the heart.

In one other case, there was a small black clot in the right side of the heart, while the left was empty.

In two cases there was a large, loose, black clot in the right side ; in one of these two the left side of the organ was empty, and in the other it contained a small black clot.

A small fibrinous clot only was found in two instances on the right side of the heart, and in both these there was a small black coagulum found on the left.

A large fibrinous clot, with much fluid blood, occupied the right cavities of the heart in four cases, and in these four the blood was found in a similar condition on the left side, but in smaller quantity.

In three cases a large, loose, fibrinous clot, and much dark fluid blood, filled the right auricle and ventricle, and a small fibrinous clot lay in the left side.

In seven cases a large, loose, fibrinous, and black clot filled the right auricle and ventricle; in one of the two the left side of the heart was empty; in five it contained a small black, or black and fibrinous, coagulum.

In the remaining four of the cases of typhus fever in which the condition of the blood after death was noted, a firm, yellow, fibrinous and black coagulum filled both the right and left sides of the heart; two of these four cases proved fatal at an uncertain period, but before the 21st day of the disease; the other two respectively on the 16th and 17th day of the disease. The age of these patients was between 32 and 45 years. The two cases in which the coagulum was the densest and largest, were complicated with extensive lobar pneumonia, and one of the two with erysipelas.

The blood was fluid, or nearly so, in the aorta and pulmonary artery in nine cases, and in all these nine cases it was also fluid in the venæ cavæ and pulmonary veins; it was fluid in the veins in three other cases, in which its condition in the arteries was not noted.

In thirteen cases there was a clot of some size, fibrinous and black, in the pulmonary artery and aorta; in three of these thirteen cases it was fluid in the pulmonary veins and venæ cavæ; and in four others of the thirteen the latter contained loose black coagula.

In the same subjects the clot was firm and the heart flabby in three cases. The clot was firm, and the substance of the heart firm, in six cases.

The clot loose and the heart flabby in five cases; the clot loose, and the substance of the heart firm, in nine cases.

So that in these twenty-three cases there was no constant relation between the condition of the blood and that of the heart.

The fluid condition of the blood generally, was observed

in about equal proportion in the subjects dead from typhoid and typhus fevers, but with those exceptions there was a marked difference in the blood in the two diseases; it was far more profoundly diseased, *i.e.* it deviated far more from its healthy condition, in the cases of typhus, than in those of typhoid fever.

LUNGS.

Typhoid Fever.—Eight cases either survived the thirty-fifth day of illness, or I was not permitted to examine their chests after death.

The lungs in one of the remaining fifteen cases were healthy in all particulars; this case proved fatal on the 25th day of the disease, from hemorrhage from the intestines; there had been little or no heat of skin during life, and the pulse never exceeded 90; the general symptoms had been trifling. In another case there was only some mottled congestion of both lungs. Of this case I speak with hesitation —in truth, I think it ought probably to be arranged under the head of non-granular lobular consolidation, a condition with which, at the time I made the examination, I was but imperfectly acquainted, and which, consequently, I might have described by the term, 'mottled congestion.' In a third case, the only deviation from health was a considerable quantity of almost colourless frothy serosity in the apex of the right lung.

In all' of the remaining twelve cases, there was more or less extensive consolidation of the pulmonary tissue.

These twelve cases may be thus grouped:—

1st, Five cases of non-granular' lobular consolidation, distinctly circumscribed by interlobular septa. In one of the five, this condition was conjoined with granular lobular consolidation. In four of the five cases consolidated patches existed in both lungs. In neither of them, however, were both lungs equally affected. In the fifth case the left lung only was diseased.

2d, One case of non-granular consolidation, in separate patches, not bounded by interlobular septa; in this case portions of the pulmonary tissue, cut from the substance of•the lung adjacent to the consolidated portions, sunk in water, if slightly pressed before immersion. Both lungs were nearly equally affected.

3rd, Two cases of granular consolidation, in well-defined patches; whether these solidified portions were bounded by interlobular septa or not, was only imperfectly made out. In one of these cases the disease was limited to the left lung; in the other both lungs were affected; in the right, however, there was extensive lobar granular consolidation; in the left, lobular and lobar solidification.

4th, Two cases of granular consolidation, in distinct but not well-defined patches. In one of these two cases, the disease was double; in the other the right lung was affected with lobular, the left with lobar, consolidation.

5th, Two cases in which a state intermediate between the non-granular and the granular consolidation was exhibited. In one of the two the disease was double; in the other, limited to the left lung.

Physical Characters of Lobular Non-granular Consolidation.—Externally, a portion of lung in this condition has a mottled aspect, here and there are patches, varying in size from a single lobule to half or more of a lobe, of a deep bluish, chocolate, violet, or purplish slate colour, bounded by a well-defined augular margin, crossed,—if it includes more than one or two lobules,—and mapped out into smaller patches, by dull opaque whitish lines. On closer inspection, the outline, and the whitish lines intersecting the patches, are seen to be thickened interlobular septa. Scattered in the midst of the larger patches, are frequently to be found one or more comparatively healthy lobules, of a pale brightish pink colour, contrasting strongly with the hue of the surrounding tissue. Here and there, near the border of the large patches, may be seen, occasionally, lobules, the *centres* of which have assumed the dusky purplish tint; the *circumference* of the same lobules yet retaining their healthy colour. The dark patches feel solid and flabby; the pulmonary tissue, at these spots, has lost the resiliency of health. The pleura covering the lung either retains its natural appearance, or has a slightly milky aspect.

On section, the tissue corresponding to the dark patches is found to be of a deep purplish chocolate colour, gorged with non-aerated bloody-looking fluid; it breaks down with little or

H

no increased facility, nay, sometimes appears tougher, than in
health; has a uniform or nearly uniform section, i.e. there is
no appearance of granules, such as are seen in the consolidated
state of so-called vesicular pneumonia; sinks in water; and
like the patches seen externally, is bounded by interlobular
septa; but these divisions, between the consolidated and non-
consolidated tissues, are less marked, especially the most
superficial tier, so to speak, of lobules.[1]

A minute portion can be cut from the middle of a lobule
—the centre of which is dusky purple, and the circumference
brightish pink—which sinks in water; equally small pieces
of pulmonary tissue, taken from the circumference of the
same lobule, float.

The following account of the superior lobe of the right
lung of a girl, æt. fifteen, who died on the twelfth day of
disease, illustrates some points in the above description :—

Its posterior part had a mottled aspect; the darker portions being of a purplish slate and violet colour; the lighter
of a pinkish violet. The septa between the lobules was well
marked, white and opaque. The mottling was found, on close
inspection, to depend on the difference in colour of the
lobules. Some were dark throughout; the dark colour terminating abruptly at the interlobular septa. At places
several of these dark lobules were in contact, forming a deep-
coloured patch, crossed by the white septa. Some of the
lobules, here and there, were pale, but the centres of some of
those which were generally pale, were dark; the size of this
dusky central spot varied in different lobules, as if the non-
granular consolidation had commenced in the centre, and

---

[1] I have proved, by injecting the lung in this non-granular consolidated
state, common to all acute diseases of determinate duration, dependent for
their origin on a specific cause, and accompanied by febrile excitement, as
measles, scarlet fever, smallpox, typhoid and typhus fevers, that occasionally the centre of the lobule is really the point at which the diseased
action is first set up; but then it is doubtful how far this, in the cases
referred to, was dependent on an inflammatory condition of the bronchial
tubes, extending downwards to their termination in the vesicular tissue of
the lobules. The question can only be answered by an analysis of numerous cases, in which all the possible determining circumstances, i.e. the
co-existence of bronchial inflammation, etc., etc., are considered at full.
There was no trace in these cases of the bronchial fibrinous plugs, described
by some writers as invariably found in catarrhal pneumonia.

then spread till it involved the whole lobule. The pulmonary pleura had a slightly milky aspect. On section, the distinction between the lobules was well marked, and the difference in their colour almost as much so as on the surface. The paler lobules were crepitant, floated in water, and possessed their normal consistence. Some of the darker lobules contained a little air, others none; they sank in water, and broke down with facility under pressure. Parts of the middle and inferior lobes of the same lung were in a state of red, and parts of grey, hepatisation. The superior lobe of the opposite lung was natural in colour and consistence. The inferior lobe, natural in appearance anteriorly, was mottled *posteriorly*; the darker parts being non-crepitant, the bright red crepitant. The bronchial tubes of both lungs contained much frothy mucus; their lining membrane was bright red; its consistence and thickness were considered natural.

The following description of the lungs of a girl, æt. 16, offers an example of non-granular lobular consolidation, uncomplicated with the granular form. As in the last, the bronchial mucous membrane was the seat of increased vasenlarity; but the bronchial symptoms, during life, had not been prominent. The left lung weighed 16 oz.; was of a dark pinkish violet; externally scarcely darker posteriorly than anteriorly. Over the whole surface were scattered varioussized patches, of a deep purplish colour, from base to apex; the majority distinctly bounded by interlobular septa. The number of lobules in each patch varied from one to eight or ten; some of the darker lobules were situated near the anterior margin of the lung. On section, the darkest-coloured patches, seen externally, were saturated with bloody fluid, non-crepitant, sank in water, and had a uniform or nearly uniform section. The somewhat less dark-coloured patches contained much bloody fluid, but little air, yet floated in water. The whole lung, on section, was darker than natural, and the interlobular septa particularly distinct. It contained a considerable quantity of frothy serosity, but scarcely more posteriorly than anteriorly. The right lung in the same subject weighed 21¾ oz.; was gorged with reddish frothy serosity; felt rather more solid than natural, but every part floated in water. The bronchial mucous membrane in both lungs was intensely injected, of a dusky red colour; the redness being in streaks, punctæ, and patches. The bronchial tubes were filled with thin frothy mucus. In the case in which the non-granular consolidated portions of lung were not circumscribed, but passed imperceptibly into the crepitant tissue, the posterior part of the lung only was affected; and the still crepitant tissue was gorged with bloody serosity, and broke down with abnormal facility; both lungs were equally affected.

Granular Lobular Consolidation.—The physical appearances presented by the lobules thus affected, characteristic, as they are, of the second stage of pneumonia, are too well known to require description.

The following, offering an example of the well-defined lobular granular consolidation, was the condition of the superior lobe of the left lung of a man, æt. 28, who died on the 27th day of disease. In its substance were two or three masses, the size of filberts, firm to touch; on section, of a deep red colour, friable, distinctly granular, readily breaking down under pressure; the line of demarcation between the crepitant and consolidated tissue was well marked and defined. The inferior lobe of the same lung presented the following appearance:— A small portion overlapping the heart was pale and crepitant, the most inferior and posterior portion of the same lobe felt solid; contained no air; was very friable; had a granular fracture; of a pale red colour; sank in water; and, on pressure, gave exit to an opaque bloody muco-purulent fluid. The intermediate portion of this lobe was *non*-granular; of a deep purple colour; sank in water; contained no air; on pressure, gave exit to a bloody-looking fluid (very different in appearance from the pale, dirty, red muco-purulent fluid above described).

The transition from the one to the other of the three above-described pathological conditions, was at some places gradual, at others abrupt and well defined. The right lung weighed 2 lb. 4 oz.; its inferior lobe resembling the corresponding part of the left lung, but a much larger portion—more than half—was in a state of granular consolidation.

Of the granular non-circumscribed form of lobular consolidation, the following account of the inferior lobe of the right lung of a man, æt. 23, who died on the 20th day of disease, presents an example. Near the base of the lobe were two or three masses of consolidated tissue, of a dark colour, which sank in water, and readily broke down under pressure. Their cut surface was granular; the tissue between tough and crepitant, as in its normal condition.

The following particulars of the lungs of a female, aged 32, who died on the 34th day of disease, exhibit a condition of the pulmonary tissue which appears intermediate between the non-granular and the granular consolidation.

The right lung weighed 15¼ oz.; was crepitant throughout; felt more solid behind than before; was of a dirty red colour; and floated in water when cut in pieces. The left lung weighed 15½ oz. (i.e. was comparatively heavy); its most depending portion (the subject being on its back) felt solid, contained little air, sank in water, broke down readily under pressure, but had not the appearance of solidified lung in the second stage of either the so-called vesicular or intervesicular pneumonia.

Lobar granular consolidation was, in three instances, conjoined with the foregoing conditions; i.e. in one of the three cases with abruptly defined lobular granular consolidation; in one with granular consolidation, the outline of which was not abruptly defined; and in the third it was conjoined with circumscribed non-granular consolidation.

Typhus Fever.—Thirty-five cases are eligible for analysis. In two of these thirty-five the lungs were healthy in all particulars. In a third case, the posterior congestion was so slight, that it could scarcely be considered a deviation from health. The remaining thirty-two cases may be thus grouped.

1st, Three cases of simple congestion of the posterior part of the lungs. In two of the three, both lungs were equally affected; in one the left lung was more congested than the right.

2nd, Three cases of congestion of the posterior part of the lungs, with diminished consistence of the congested parts. In one of the three, both lungs were equally affected; in another, the right was more deeply diseased than the left; in the third, the left lung only was in this condition, the posterior part of the right being simply congested.

3rd, Eleven cases of congestion of the posterior part of the lung, with non-granular consolidation of the most depending (the subject being on its back) layer of pulmonary tissue. Both lungs were affected in five of the ten cases; but, in two of the five, one lung was more extensively solidified than the opposite. In six cases one lung only was thus diseased. In one case only was there any attempt at circumscription.

4th, In four cases, the most obvious departure from a normal condition was a great excess of almost colourless serosity in some portion of the pulmonary tissue. In one of the four there was marked congestion, with diminished consistence of the most depending part of both lungs, the right being more affected than the left; the most congested portions contained the greatest amount of serosity. In a second, there was simple congestion of the most depending part of the lungs, with great excess of serosity in the superior lobes. In another case, in which there was moderate congestion of the most depending part of the left lung, there was little serosity in the inferior lobe, while the upper half of the superior lobe, anterior as well as posterior part, was saturated with frothy serosity. The right lung, in the same subject, was more congested posteriorly; in the same part of both lobes the excess of serosity was great; but the apex contained more than the other parts. While, in the fourth case, the excess of serosity was limited to the apex of the right lung, from which it flowed, as if from a sponge saturated with moisture. There was no congestion of the vessels of the superior lobe in this case.

5th, In eight cases there was lobular consolidation. In two of the eight, the consolidation was non-granular and abruptly defined. In one of the two it was limited to the left lung; in the other it affected both lungs. In two there was a similar form of solidification; but the line of demarcation between the crepitant and non-crepitant tissues was only marked at places,—in one the right, in the other the left lung, only was affected. In two of the eight, granular and non-granular consolidation of the pulmonary tissue was present in the same subject. There was no distinct line separating the solidified from the crepitant tissue in these two cases, —in one of them, both lungs were nearly equally affected. The solidified masses in this case appeared to be in a state intermediate between the granular and non-granular consolidation; in the other, granular lobar solidification was present in both lungs. In the remaining two of the eight cases of lobular consolidation, the diseased lobules were granular; in one central, occupying the left lung only; in the other confined to the left lung, while the right, in the same subject, was affected with lobar granular consolidation.

6th, Lobar granular consolidation of the upper portion of the inferior lobe of either lung, existed, uncomplicated with the lobular form, in one case.

In one of the last-mentioned cases, there was commencing gangrene of the pulmonary tissue; and, in another case, not included in the thirty-five, there was well-marked circumscribed gangrene. The latter occurred in a boy æt. 8 years, who died on 22nd day of disease. In this same boy a portion of the cornea of both eyes sloughed out before death. The right lung presented the following appearance: It was closely collapsed; in the pleura were about 3 oz. of purulent fluid, possessing a highly-offensive odour. From the centre of the closely collapsed superior lobe projected a mass, which felt about the size of a pigeon's egg, one half of which, however, was buried in the pulmonary substance. The smoothness of the projecting mass contrasted strongly with the corrugated appearance of the general external surface of the superior lobe. On cutting through this mass, its centre was found to be occupied by black semi-fluid matter of very offensive odour; stretching across this black pulpy mass were delicate bands of some consistence. This gangrenous mass was about an inch in diameter, and was distinctly bounded by a border of *white* soft pulpy matter, about half a line in thickness. The pulmonary substance surrounding this white margin, for some lines in every direction was softened, of a purplish red colour, contained no air, had a smooth and uniform non-granular section. Externally, this condition of the pulmonary tissue extended to the pleura. From the inferior lobe of the same lung a prominence, similar to that described above, projected. On cutting into it, some offensive gas escaped, and the anterior wall collapsed. The cavity, laid open by the section, contained some dark semi-fluid black matter and gangrenous shreds,—the whole circumscribed by a white line,

similar to that described, as bounding the gangrenous mass
in the upper lobe. The external wall of the cavity was *very*
thin, and on the pleural surface was a black spot about the
size of a split pea, with well-defined outline. In the vicinity
of the above were two smaller masses, closely resembling the
last described.

It is unnecessary to repeat the descriptions of granular
and non-granular lobular consolidation; but, as congestion of
the posterior portion of the lung, with non-granular consolidation of the most depending part of the organ, did not present itself among the cases of typhoid fever, it is necessary to
describe the appearances exhibited by lungs in that condition.
The posterior portion of the lung, in the cases included under
this head, was congested, and its consistence diminished; the
most depending layer of pulmonary tissue (the subject being
on its back), which extended, in different cases from a quarter
of an inch to two inches into the substance of the lung, was
solidified, very dark bluish chocolate in colour, gorged with
non-aerated dark claret serosity, which flowed freely from the
cut surface; it was scarcely softened; the whole of the solidified layer sank in water. The consolidation did not, unless it
extended far into the pulmonary substance, affect the extreme
base, the apex of the inferior lobe, nor the root of the lung,
i.e. that portion which is immediately in contact with the
vertebral column, but was limited to the part of the organ
which lies in the hollow formed by about the 4th, 5th, and
6th ribs, as they curve backwards, outwards, and forwards,
from the bodies of the dorsal vertebræ. The solidified and
crepitant tissue passed, imperceptibly, the one into the other.
The transition from the pale anterior portion of the lung to
the congested posterior, and from that to the most depending
solidified tissue, was in the greater number of cases gradual,
and not abrupt, as in the circumscribed non-granular lobular
consolidation. As was stated (p. 118), only one lung, in six of
the cases grouped under this head, was affected; therefore,
although position was the determining cause, some other
agent was concerned in the production of this morbid condition—a condition by no means peculiar to fever.

In order to exhibit the difference observed in the lungs
of the subjects dead from typhoid and typhus fever, it will be

necessary to sum up the particulars detailed in the preceding analysis.

In thirty-four cases of typhus fever, there were four examples of granular consolidation, *i.e.* nearly one-ninth of the whole.

In fifteen cases of typhoid fever, there were four cases of granular consolidation, *i.e.* about one-fourth.

Three cases of lobular non-granular congestion in the thirty-four cases of typhus fever, *i.e.* about one-twelfth, while six, or three-fifths, of the cases of typhoid fever, exhibited the same lesion.

Congestion with consolidation, evidently determined by position, was present in nearly one-third of the cases of typhus fever, and in no single instance of typhoid fever.

The comparative frequency of the granular and of lobular non-granular consolidation in the cases of typhoid fever, is too marked to be the result of accident. It is evidently a feature impressed on the pulmonary organs by the disease itself, as will be more evident on examining the conditions of the pleura in the two diseases.

It is also worthy of remark, that in no case of typhoid fever was gangrene of the lung present, while it occurred in two cases of typhus. The occurrence of six cases of congestion of the posterior portion of the lung, with or without diminished consistence, is also a distinctive feature ; for, be it remembered, the one class of patients had been confined to bed as long as the other,—nay, the cases of typhoid fever proved fatal at a later period of disease.

BRONCHIAL TUBES.

Typhoid Fever.—Notes respecting the condition of the bronchial tubes were made only in twelve of the cases included among those here analysed.

In four of the twelve the lining membrane was pale in colour; in the remaining two-thirds it was vividly injected, or *bright* red.

Typhus Fever.—The condition of the bronchial tubes was noted in twenty-two cases.

In two cases they were pale in colour; in two slightly

congested; in eighteen they were noted to be more or less deeply congested, or *dusky* red.

PLEURÆ.

Typhoid Fever.—Of those cases which proved fatal before the 35th day of disease, the chest was examined in fifteen.

There were present unequivocal signs of recent inflammation of the pleura in six cases, *i.e.* in the proportion of 40 per cent. These signs were recent adhesions, or the effusion of lymph.

Typhus Fever.—Thirty-six cases are eligible for analysis. In three of these cases there were signs of recent inflammation of the pleura; but in one of the three the lesion consisted in the presence of pus in the cavity of the pleura, secondary to gangrene of the lung. In two cases only was there any recent lymph, and in one of these it was merely sufficient to render the serosity turbid, and in the other to cause trifling adhesions. Thus, if these three cases be considered as cases of recent inflammation, pleuritis only occurred in the proportion of 8·3 per cent.; while, if the two latter only are considered, but in the proportion of 5·5 per cent. It has been just shown, that 40 per cent. of the subjects dead from typhoid fever exhibited unequivocal signs of recent inflammation of the pleura.

For the purpose of clearly estimating the value of the differences in the symptoms and lesions of structure analysed in the preceding papers, it will be necessary here briefly to recapitulate those differences.

Age.—Typhoid fever was limited, in the cases here considered, to persons under 40 years of age; nearly one-third of the forty-three cases of typhus were more than 50 years of age.

Mode of Attack.—As a general rule, the attack of typhoid fever commenced more insidiously than that of typhus fever. This observation, like all others in this paper, applies, of course, only to fatal cases.

Duration.—The average duration of the fatal cases of typhoid fever was 22 days. Of the fatal cases of typhus fever, 14 days. Half the cases of typhoid fever survived the 20th day of disease. Not a single case of typhus fever survived the 20th day of disease.

Eruption.—The difference in the appearance of the eruption in the two diseases was as great as it well could be, considering that both were of a reddish hue.

Miliary Vesicles, or Sudamina.—These vesicles were present in an equal proportion of the cases of both diseases under 40 years of age. But in no cases of typhus fever, more than 40 years of age, were they detected.

Subsequent experience leads me to believe that miliary vesicles are rarely seen on individuals more than 40 years of age; and very rarely indeed, if ever, on patients more than 50 years old. I have during the last year (1849-50)—*i.e.* since my attention was directed to this point—seen these bodies on no one of the many patients more than 50 years of age, labouring under various diseases, that have come under my observation.

Expression, Manner, Hue of Face, etc.—As the rule, in the cases of typhoid fever here analysed, the expression was much less indicative of prostration, and more anxious, than in the cases of typhus fever. In the former disease, the complexion was tolerably clear, and the flush, when present, was of brightish pink colour, limited to one or both cheeks, and often distinctly circumscribed. In typhus fever, on the contrary, the complexion was thick and muddy, the flush of the face uniform, and of a dusky red colour.

Headache was a constant symptom in all the cases of typhoid and typhus fevers; but it disappeared by about the 10th or 12th day in the latter, and not till the termination of the second, or middle of the third week, in the former.

Delirium commenced in three only of ten cases of typhoid fever before the 14th day; while it began in fourteen out of fifteen cases of typhus fever before the 14th day. As a rule, the delirium was decidedly more active in typhoid than in typhus fever.

Somnolence.—In eight out of nine cases of typhoid fever, somnolence commenced after the 14th day of disease. In seventeen out of eighteen cases of typhus, before the termination of the second week.

Coma-Vigil.—One-fifth of the cases of typhus fever experienced coma-vigil; not a single case of typhoid fever experienced that condition.

Spasmodic Movements were nearly equally frequent in the two diseases.

Retention of Urine, and Involuntary Discharge of Urine and Stools, occurred with equal frequency in the two diseases; but at a much earlier date in typhus than in typhoid.

Loss of Muscular Power.—Little more than a fourth of the patients attacked with typhus fever kept their bed entirely before the 7th day of disease. All the patients affected with typhus, whose cases are here considered, took altogether to their beds before the 7th day of disease.

The prostration was rarely so extreme in the cases of typhoid fever as in those of typhus fever. Extreme prostration, when it did occur in typhoid fever, was not observed till from the 14th to the 30th day, while in a large majority of the cases of typhus fever it was marked between the 9th and 12th day of disease.

Epistaxis was present in five of fifteen cases of typhoid fever—in not one of twenty-three cases of typhus fever.

Hearing was equally and similarly affected in the two diseases.

Eyes.—The conjunctivæ were *very much* more constantly and intensely injected in the cases of typhus than in those of typhoid fever; the pupils were absolutely larger than natural in a majority of the cases of the latter disease, while they were abnormally contracted in a large majority of the cases of the former affection.

Tongue.—Although individual cases of the two diseases may have closely resembled each other in the appearance of the tongue, yet, taking the whole of either group of cases, this organ presented a singularly different aspect in the one from what it did in the other. It was much more frequently moist throughout the disease in typhoid than in typhus fever. When dry, it was often red, glazed, and fissured in the former; rarely so in the latter. Again, in typhoid fever, when the tongue was brown, its hue was much less deep—it was of a yellowish, instead of a blackish, brown. The small dry tongue, with red tip and edges, smooth, pale brownish-yellow fur, fissured—the surface seen between the fissures being deep red—may be considered differentially as a diagnostic sign of typhoid fever. One only of twenty patients affected with typhoid fever, but eight of forty patients labouring under typhus fever, were unable to protrude the tongue when bidden.[1]

Intestinal Hemorrhage occurred in one-third of the patients affected with typhoid fever—in none of those suffering from typhus fever.[2]

The other abdominal symptoms and signs need no recapitulation.

Appetite and Thirst.—No difference in the two diseases.

Pulse.—The frequency of the pulse fluctuated much more, from day to day, in the cases of typhoid than in those of typhus fever.

Cough and Physical Chest Signs.—Sonorous rale was very much more frequently present in the cases of typhoid than in those of typhus fever—*i.e.* it was present in eleven out of twelve cases of the former, and in seven only of twenty-one cases of the latter. Dulness of the most depending part of the chest, from intense congestion of the lung, was observed in nine cases of typhus fever—in no case of typhoid fever.

Sloughing appeared to be nearly equally frequent in the two diseases.

Erysipelas occurred in seven of the twenty-three—*i.e.* in nearly a third of the cases of typhoid fever; in two only of the forty-three cases of typhus fever—*i.e.* in less than one-twentieth of them.

Cadaveric Rigidity ceased much more quickly in the subjects dead from typhus fever than from typhoid fever.

Discoloration of the Walls of the Abdomen, and of the Skin covering the larger Veins, was much more frequently present in those dead from typhus than typhoid fever.

[1] This clearly indicates the difference in the amount of prostration in the two diseases.

[2] I may remark that, in one case only of typhus fever, received into the London Fever Hospital during the last three years (1847-49), has blood passed from the bowels. The case referred to was that of an old man, who had hemorrhoids, which occasionally bled when he was in health. During the time specified, notes of near 2000 cases have been taken.

Emaciation had made greater progress in the typhoid than in the typhus subjects.

Spots.—The spots observed during the progress of the cases of typhus fever continued after death; no trace of the spots visible during life could be detected after death from typhoid fever.

Head.—After typhoid fever, the pia mater and arachnoid separated from the convolutions with abnormal facility in one only of nine cases examined with reference to the point. The vessels of the pia mater were abnormally filled with blood in one-third of the cases, but intensely congested in one only of fifteen cases; the cerebral substance was congested in one-seventh of the cases. After typhus fever, the pia mater and arachnoid separated with abnormal facility in nine of eleven cases of which notes on the point were made. The vessels of the pia mater were congested in nearly half, and intensely congested in one-fifth, of the whole of the cases; while the cerebral substance itself was abnormally congested in half the cases.

Hemorrhage into the Cavity of the Arachnoid, which was not found in a single case of typhoid fever, had occurred before death in one-eighth of the cases of typhus fever.

The amount of serosity found within the cranial cavity was decidedly greater after typhus than typhoid fever.

Pharynx.—After typhoid fever, this organ was found ulcerated in one-third of the cases. After typhus fever, ulceration of the pharynx was not detected in a single case.

Larynx.—Ulceration of the larynx was found in one of fifteen subjects dead from typhoid fever—in one of twenty-six from typhus fever.

Œsophagus.—After typhoid fever, ulcerated in one of fifteen cases in which it was examined. After typhus fever, the œsophagus was free from ulceration in all the twenty-four cases in which it was examined.

The epithelium separated from the œsophagus spontaneously at an earlier period after death from the latter than the former disease.

Stomach.—In none of the fifteen cases examined after death from typhoid fever was the mucous membrane of the stomach softened throughout its whole extent; in no case did softening of the cardiac extremity approach perforation. In four of thirty-seven cases of typhus fever the whole mucous membrane of the stomach was softened; and in four others there was such extreme softening of the whole of the coats of the great *cul-de-sac*, that they were perforated by the slightest violence.

Small Intestines and Mesenteric Glands.—The presence or absence of lesion of these organs was the ground on which the cases of typhoid and typhus fever here analysed were divided from each other,—consequently they were invariably diseased in the one and normal in the other.

Large Intestines.—After death from typhoid fever, the mucous membrane of the large intestines was found ulcerated in rather more than a third of twenty cases. In no instance after death from typhus fever.

Peritoneum.—As peritonitis was in typhoid fever secondary to, and dependent on, the entero-mesenteric disease, it may here be excluded from consideration.

Spleen.—This organ was enlarged in all the cases of typhoid fever—softened in one-third of the cases only. Before the age of 50, it was as large after typhus as typhoid fever; after that age, it was decidedly smaller in the former than in the latter affection. After the age of 50, it was as soft in typhus as in typhoid fever; before that age it was less frequently softened.

Gall-Bladder.—There was ulceration of the lining membrane of the gall-bladder in one of fourteen cases of typhoid fever; in none of thirty-one cases of typhus fever. In the latter disease the bile was much thicker, and of a darker green colour, than in the former.[1]

Liver, Pancreas, Kidneys.—These organs were more flabby in the cases of typhus than in those of typhoid fever.

Urinary Bladder.—This viscus was ulcerated in one of the cases of typhoid fever; in none of the cases of typhus fever.

Pericardium.—This cavity contained a small amount of yellowish transparent serosity in all the cases of typhoid fever examined. The contained serosity was red, from

---

[1] The condition of the bile, as found after death in these two diseases, is worthy of more careful investigation. The difference in appearance is, in a large majority of cases, well marked.

transudation of a solution of hæmatosin, in five of thirty-one cases of typhus fever, in which the pericardium was examined before the termination of the fever.

Heart.—The muscular tissue of this organ was much more frequently and decidedly flabby, and its lining membrane was much more frequently and deeply stained of a dark red colour, in the cases of typhus fever than in those of typhoid fever.

Lungs.—Granular and non-granular lobular consolidation were very frequent in the subjects dead from typhoid fever— rare in those dead from typhus fever. The reverse was the fact with reference to consolidation from congestion of the most depending part of the lung.

Pleura.—Recent lymph or turbid serosity was found in six of fifteen cases of typhoid fever—*i.e.* between half and one-third, or in the proportion of 40 per cent. The same lesions, but much less in amount, were found in two only of thirty-six cases of typhus fever—*i.e.* one-sixteenth, or in the proportion of 5·5 per cent.

The particulars here briefly recapitulated, and still more those fully detailed in the foregoing pages, appear to me to prove indisputably that the symptoms, course, duration, anatomico-pathological lesions, and the tendency to cadaveric changes, are different in typhoid fever from what they are in typhus fever.

To account for the differences in symptoms which exist in continued fever, with and without entero-mesenteric disease, the two following assertions have been put forward :—

1st. That typhoid fever is merely typhus fever complicated with lesion of a particular organ ; and therefore it is to be expected that certain symptoms referable to, and dependent on, that lesion will be present, and so far modify the symptoms of the disease. If the symptoms and signs referable to the intestinal disease as a cause—*i.e.* the condition of the tongue, the diarrhœa, increased resonance, and fulness of the abdomen, gurgling in the iliac fossa, pain and tenderness in the same region, or even the daily fluctuations in frequency of the pulse—were the only symptoms by which typhoid fever was separated from typhus fever, although the idea might cross the mind that they were two diseases, no sufficient ground for their separation would be present, unless the specific cause of the one was proved to be different from that of the other. But, putting aside the symptoms strictly referable to the abdominal lesion, the general symptoms of the two diseases, in the cases here analysed, differed widely; such differences having no apparent connection with the local affection, but being probably, like it, dependent on some common cause acting on the whole system simultaneously.

Thus the remarkable differences in the kind, not simply amount,[1] of the rash in the two diseases; and the tendency to local inflammations, to erysipelas, and to ulceration, observed in the cases of typhoid fever here analysed, cannot, with any show of reason, be considered to have been dependent on the disease of Peyer's patches—i.e. in the same way as the abdominal signs undoubtedly were; and it is to be carefully borne in mind that the external, the hygienic, conditions of either group of cases, were precisely the same in all respects. They occupied the same wards, partook of the same diet, slept on the same beds, under the same amount of clothing, and had the same physicians to attend them, and the same nurses to wait on them.

Moreover, of the symptoms common to the two, the headache continued longer, and the delirium and somnolence came on, as we have seen, much later, in typhoid than in typhus fever; and the delirium, too, possessed a more active character. These differences, also, cannot be explained by the presence of intestinal disease in the former, and its absence in the latter affection.

The short comparative duration of the cases of typhus fever, here considered, is another remarkable point of difference, totally inexplicable by the hypothesis, that typhoid fever is typhus fever with intestinal ulceration. Had the cases eventually recovered, it might have been said, that the intestinal lesion prolonged the disease in the cases of typhoid fever; but that all the fatal cases of fever, with a local lesion of so severe a nature as that recorded to have been present in the cases of typhoid fever, should have had a much longer

---

[1] I have elsewhere shown that the rash and the intestinal disease cannot be considered supplementary of each other. See *Medical Times*, December 1849, and January 1850 (reprinted in the present volume, *vide infra*).

course than all those other fatal cases of fever in which no organic change of structure could be detected after death, appears to me inexplicable, on the supposition that the former is simply the latter disease, with this serious lesion superadded. Let me repeat, by this hypothesis we are asked to imagine that death is retarded in fever by extensive ulceration of the small intestines, and enlargement, softening, and even suppuration of the mesenteric glands. Surely it behoves the supporters of such a statement to bring forward cogent proofs of the identity of the specific cause of the two affections ere they ask us to admit its truth.

The same mode of reasoning appears to me equally conclusive, when we consider the comparatively early period of the disease at which the patients, suffering from fever, lost the ability to make muscular exertion. For to suppose that the presence of abdominal complication in fever invariably prevented the extremely early supervention of debility, is, *a priori*, still more absurd than to suppose such lesions to have retarded death. How, again, are we to explain, if we regard typhoid as typhus with abdominal complication, the differences observed in the ages of the patients, in their general manner; the muddy hue of the skin, and uniform flush of the face, the injected conjunctivæ, and contracted pupils in typhus fever; and the comparatively clear complexion, the pink flush limited to the cheeks, the pale conjunctivæ and the large pupils, in typhoid fever?

In what way, also, are we to account for the differences observed in the physical breath-signs, on the supposition that the one is merely the other, with abdominal complication?

Death itself, moreover, adds new proof to the non-identity of the general affection in the two diseases. The comparatively rapid loss of muscular rigidity, the discoloration of the surface, the more flabby condition of the heart, liver, and kidneys, the extreme softening of the stomach, and the early separation of the epithelium, after typhus fever, are all cadaveric changes, by which death makes us cognisant of a condition of the system at large, which condition must have existed anterior to the cessation of life from that disease; and which condition could not have been present in the cases of typhoid fever, or death would have made it manifest.

I need not here more than advert to the difference observed in the lesions which death simply enabled us to lay bare. The almost constantly congested brain and membranes in typhus fever; the frequent presence of the signs of pre-existing serous inflammation in typhoid fever; the difference in the nature of the pulmonary lesions in the two —are inexplicable on the supposition that the one disease is the same as the other, excepting so far as concerns the abdominal affection.

Thus tried by facts—*i.e.* by recorded symptoms and lesions,—the assertion that typhoid fever is merely typhus fever with abdominal complication, is completely refuted.

2nd. But another mode of explaining the differences which exist between the two diseases has been given—*i.e.* that the differences observed depend on variations in the 'epidemic constitution.' These cases afford a complete answer to this assertion. For the majority of the cases here analysed of both diseases were observed during the same epidemic constitution. If the reader will refer to p. 9, he will find that nineteen of the cases of typhus fever I have used in this analysis were collected between May and November 1848; and that thirteen of the cases of typhoid fever were collected during the same months of the same year. For such as prefer broad general assertions to the details of particular but more limited facts, I may remark, that during three years' attentive watching of nearly all the cases admitted into the London Fever Hospital, in which time there have been epidemics of relapsing fever, typhus fever, and cholera—and, consequently, according to those whose opinions I am here examining, as many changes in epidemic constitution—I have seen no alteration in the general or particular symptoms of either typhus or typhoid fevers, or the lesions observed after death from either—*i.e.* from November 1846 to November 1849. The cases of typhoid fever—which disease is rarely absent for a fortnight from the wards of the hospital, —preserved their symptoms unchanged, and presented the same lesions, whatever the epidemic constitution that prevailed; the same is true of typhus fever. Cases of the latter disease are also rarely absent from the wards of the same institution. It is there common to see patients occupying beds side by side, and presenting respectively the well-marked characters of either disease.

But to return to the particular cases here analysed. Allowing to epidemic constitution all the power of modifying disease claimed for it by certain writers, it must be granted that whatever influence this epidemic constitution exercised over the group of cases without intestinal lesion, it ought to have exercised over the group of cases with intestinal lesion, because the cases of the two groups were scattered indiscriminately over the space of two years only. If, I repeat, the two affections were really the same disease, then the same epidemic constitution ought to have impressed on both the same general features, implanted in both the same local lesions, and given to both the same tendency to cadaveric change, and this allowing for all the modifying influence which the accidental presence of the abdominal lesion in the one and its absence from the other group might have occasioned. The analysis of every sympton and every lesion shows that the two affections were not thus assimilated by the prevalence of any particular epidemic constitution. But if this epidemic constitution, by any stretch of the imagination, could be supposed to change from week to week, to cause the case attacked to-day to have typhus fever, the individual who takes the disease to-morrow to have typhoid fever, still, it could not account for the fact,—as well established as any fact in medicine,—that typhoid fever rarely, if ever, affects persons more than fifty years of age; while age exerts little influence in determining the occurrence of typhus fever.

Thus, then, the assertion that typhoid fever is merely typhus fever modified by the prevailing epidemic constitution, is as irreconcilable with facts, as that the former disease is simply the latter with abdominal complication.

To conclude,—At the commencement of this analysis I proposed to examine whether typhoid fever and typhus fever differed from each other in the same way as small-pox and scarlet fever differed from each other; and, for the purpose of comparison, I laid down certain grounds, as those on which we founded our belief in the non-identity of the two last-named diseases. Those grounds were:—

1st, In the vast majority of cases the general symptoms differ—*i.e.* of small-pox and scarlet fever.

[This holds equally true with respect to the general symptoms of typhoid and typhus fevers.]

2nd, The eruptions, the diagnostic characters, *if present*, are never identical—*i.e.* in small-pox and scarlet fever.

[The particulars detailed in the foregoing papers prove that this is as true of the eruptions of typhoid and typhus fever, as of those of small-pox and scarlet fever.]

3rd, The anatomical character of small-pox is never seen in scarlet fever.

[Just in the same way the anatomical character of typhoid fever—*i.e.* lesion of Peyer's patches and the mesenteric glands —is never seen in typhus fever.]

4th, Both — *i.e.* small-pox and scarlet fever — being contagious diseases, the one by no combination of individual peculiarities, atmospheric variations, epidemic constitutions, or hygienic conditions, can give rise to the other.

[I have here not attempted to determine how far this holds true with respect to typhoid and typhus fevers; but I have considered it in a paper read before the Medico-Chirurgical Society of London, December 1849,[1] the contents of which I may anticipate so far as to state, that to my mind the origin of the two diseases from distinct specific causes, is as clearly proved as that scarlet fever and small-pox arise from distinct specific causes.]

5th, The epidemic constitution, favourable to the origin, spread, or peculiarity in form or severity of either—*i.e.* small-pox and scarlet fever—has no influence over the other, excepting that which it exerts over disease in general.

[The facts detailed in these pages prove that this holds as true of typhoid and typhus fevers as of small-pox and scarlet fever.]

If, then, the above are the grounds—and, after mature deliberation, I am able to assign no others—for the separation of small-pox from scarlet fever, I think it is indisputably proved, that typhoid fever and typhus fever are equally distinct diseases;—not mere varieties of each other, but specifically distinct,—specific distinction being shown in

[1] See page 139 *et seq.*

typhoid and typhus fevers, as in small-pox and scarlet fever, by the difference of their symptoms, course, duration, lesions, and *cause*.

Before concluding, I ought to observe that, with respect to some secondary points—*e.g.* the chronological relation between the laryngeal and pharyngeal affections—it may be considered that I have drawn general conclusions from a too limited number of facts. But a few facts, impartially observed, minutely recorded, and carefully analysed, are, I believe, more likely to give correct results than a multitude of general observations; and, moreover, I believe most men would be astonished if they had in numbers all the cases of any given disease they had ever seen, yet concerning which they have generalised. The method I have adopted, however prolix it may be, however difficult to conform to, however tedious the details into which it leads, has this advantage, that if the observer be honest and capable of noting what is before him, thinking men may judge of the value of his facts, the force of his reasoning, and the correctness of his conclusion; whereas, general observations, while they are totally incapable of proving anything, are exposed to all the fallacies of definite statements, because the one, like the other, rests ultimately on the accuracy of the facts observed. If the observations, on which any reasoning is founded, be erroneous, no cloaking of those observations in general terms can render the conclusions correct. It has been objected to definite numerical statements, that they mislead the reader by an *appearance* of accuracy, in cases where there has been great inaccuracy in observation. This objection appears to me to lie against the condition of the reader's mind and not against the method. For if the reader fails to examine, 1st, the trustworthiness of the author, and 2ndly, the legitimacy of his conclusions, the fault is, obviously, mentally his own, and in noways to be ascribed to the method. Because chemists have, by the imperfection of their analyses, arrived at incorrect conclusions as to the ultimate constitution of various organic bodies, we surely would not have them henceforth confine themselves to the general impressions produced on their minds by a series of experiments or observations. The more complicated the problem to be solved, the more careful ought we to be that *every* step in its solution is made correctly. How complex questions, such as arise in medicine, are to be determined mentally—*i.e.* without the aid of figures—by ordinary men, I am at a loss to conceive. Yet physicians think to solve, by mental reveries, problems in comparison with which the most difficult that the most renowned mental calculators ever answered were mere child's-play; and not only do they think to solve these problems, but to carry in their minds for years the complicated materials by which they are to be solved.

Who can tell what general statements are worth, without knowing on what evidence they rest? One man's many is another's few. Last month (October) I saw thirty cases of fever, —to me these were few; to men with smaller opportunities of observing that disease, they would have been many. One man's frequent is another's seldom.

So much for the method I have adopted.

Finally, as an apology for the length to which this analysis has extended, I may quote the following passage from the learned professor of physic in the Transylvanian University: —"This question of the essential likeness or unlikeness of these two diseases,—typhus and typhoid fever,—is one of the most important and interesting questions of specific diagnosis that has ever occupied the attention of physicians;" and may observe, that if ever the question is to be settled, it must be by a careful analysis of all the symptoms, and all the pathological lesions, observed in all the cases of the two diseases which fall under the observation of the same physician during any given period of time, and then by tracing a number of cases of either disease back to their specific cause.

ON THE IDENTITY OR NON-IDENTITY

OF THE

SPECIFIC CAUSE OF TYPHOID, TYPHUS, AND RELAPSING FEVER

1849

ON THE IDENTITY OR NON-IDENTITY OF THE SPECIFIC CAUSE OF TYPHOID, TYPHUS, AND RELAPSING FEVER[1]

THERE are certain diseases which have peculiarities common to all, so characteristic, that, although we are ignorant of their intimate nature, and even of their exact seat, yet they naturally group themselves together and form a class admitting of one general description. This class exhibits equally natural subdivisions. The species, of which these subdivisions are formed, are distinguished from each other by peculiarities even more marked, if possible, than the class in which they are included is from all other classes. The great class to which I refer is that of—

Acute febrile diseases, having a determinate duration, and dependent for their origin on specific causes.

It includes, as distinct species, smallpox, measles, scarlet fever, typhus fever, typhoid fever, and relapsing fever. For many years the first three were confounded under one name, and it was only after the publication of Dr. Withering's essay that measles and scarlet fever were regarded as distinct affections, *i.e.* distinct as to their course, their symptoms, their lesions, and their causes. The three last-enumerated diseases are yet, by many, looked on as but varieties of one disease, which merely presents differences in its phases according to epidemic constitutions, individual peculiarities, and hygienic conditions. The great work of Louis on the Typhoid Affection, by affording a standard of comparison, materially lightened the labour of separating from that disease those which had previously been grouped with it.

[1] Read before the Royal Medical and Chirurgical Society on Dec. 11, 1849, and published in vol. xxxiii. of the Society's Transactions.

The paper of Dr. Gerhard, in the *American Journal of Medical Sciences* for 1837; the cases collected by Dr. Shattuck,[1] and so ably analysed by M. Valleix;[2] and the excellent paper of Dr. Stewart,[3] in 1840, rendered it highly probable, although they did not prove,[4] that typhoid fever and typhus fever were absolutely distinct from each other, *i.e.* were two species of disease, and not varieties of one affection.

In the *Monthly Journal* of the present year I have attempted to determine absolutely the question of their identity, by an analysis of the course, the symptoms and the lesions of structure found after death in a certain number of fatal cases, collected by myself during one epidemic.[5] It appeared to me that the conclusion which flows from that analysis is, that, so far as concerns their course, symptoms, and lesions, no two diseases can be more distinct. But not only do the diseases, *i.e.* smallpox, measles, and scarlet fever, with which I have classed these fevers, differ from each other in course, symptoms, and lesions, but they differ also with respect to the nature of their exciting cause. That cause is specific. We can generate inflammation of any organ at will by a variety of means; but by the application of *one* cause only can we excite smallpox, measles, or scarlet fever. In like manner, typhoid fever, typhus fever, and relapsing fever must require for their production the application of distinct specific causes, if they be distinct diseases belonging to the same class as smallpox, etc.

The peculiarity which entitles a cause to be termed specific, is that of exciting in those exposed to its action one,

[1] 'Observations of Typhus and Typhoid Fever,' a paper communicated to the Paris Medical Society of Observation in 1838, and published in *American Medical Examiner*, February and March 1840,

[2] 'Du Typhus Fever et de la Fièvre Typhoide d'Angleterre,' *Arch. Gén. de Méd.*, Oct. et Nov. 1839.

[3] 'Some considerations on the Nature and Pathology of Typhus and Typhoid Fever, applied to the solution of the question of their identity or non-identity,'—*Edinburgh Medical and Surgical Journal*, October 1840.

[4] See Christison on Fever, *Library of Medicine*; *Watson's Lectures*, 2d edit.; and especially vol. xii., *British and Foreign Medical Review*, in which the arguments adduced by the above-mentioned and other authors in favour of the non-identity of typhoid and typhus fever are ably criticised, and the following conclusion arrived at: 'That they are the *same species* of disease, but *different* varieties of that species.'

[5] See pp. 1 to 135 of present volume.

and only one, species of disease. Further, all specific causes, the products of individuals labouring under disease, can excite in other individuals only diseases resembling in all essential characters those present in the individual from whom they themselves sprung. Herein lies the test, the *experimentum crucis* by which the absolute non-identity of smallpox, measles, and scarlet fever is proved; for if the same cause, *i.e.* the poison generated by either, could not only produce the disease from which it had its origin, but also the other two, then the three affections would be regarded as varieties of one disease, and not as distinct species; just as *scarlatina simplex* and *anginosa*, and *scarlatina sine eruptione*, are varieties of each other; and just as *rubeola vulgaris, rubeola sine catarrho*, and perhaps it may be said, certain catarrhs without rubeoloid eruption are varieties of each other. We know, however, that smallpox, measles, and scarlet fever, owe their origin to different specific causes, and therefore we assert that they are distinct diseases. If the same difference in the specific cause of any two other affections be observed, then, however trivial the differences in their symptoms, they too must be held to be distinct diseases: *à fortiori*, will this be true of diseases differing from each other so widely as typhoid, typhus, and relapsing fever, in course, symptoms, sequelæ, and pathologico-anatomical lesions?

The object of this paper is to inquire whether the specific cause of the three diseases just enumerated is identical?

The materials used for the solution of the question are the cases admitted into the London Fever Hospital during the years 1847, 1848, and 1849.[1]

The diagnosis of relapsing fever rests on the peculiarity of its course and symptoms; of typhoid and typhus fevers, on the skin eruption when present. The following are the diagnostic symptoms of these affections:

RELAPSING FEVER.—Sudden rigors, headache, skin hot and dry, tongue white, urine high-coloured, bowels regular, occasional or frequent vomiting, loss of appetite, absence of

---

[1] To the medical officers of this institution, and especially to Dr. Tweedie, I am indebted for the liberality with which I have been permitted to make unrestrained use of the cases admitted into its wards.

abnormal physical abdominal signs. In severe cases, jaundice, profuse sweating on about the seventh day, followed by apparent restoration to health; on from the fifth to the eighth day, reckoning from the apparent convalescence, repetition of the original symptoms, with greater or less severity; again terminating in sweating, and then permanent convalescence.

TYPHOID FEVER.—*Rose spots.*—The eruption in typhoid fever appears from the seventh to the twelfth day of the disease, very rarely later, and still more rarely at an earlier period. The characteristic spots are frequently preceded for a day or two by a very delicate scarlet tint of the whole skin.[1] The eruption itself consists of small spots irregularly scattered over the anterior and posterior surface of the trunk. The number of spots on the surface at one time ordinarily varies from six to twenty; sometimes there are very few, at other times, but infinitely more rarely, they are so thickly scated that scarcely an interval of normal cuticle is left between them.

The separate spots are circular, and of a bright rose colour; this hue passes insensibly at their basis into that of the surrounding cuticle. Their usual diameter is about two lines. They are somewhat elevated; but, although perceptible to the finger passed lightly over the surface, they possess none of the seed-like hardness of the first day's eruption of small-pox, nor are they so prominent and perceptible to the touch as the papulæ of lichen. Their surface is rounded, lens-shaped, never acuminated. No trace of vesication can be detected on their apices. If tolerably firm pressure be made on these spots, they entirely disappear; but they resume their distinctive colour and elevation as the finger is being withdrawn. The above characters are preserved by each spot from its first appearance till it disappears. When, however, the duration of a spot is prolonged to five or six days, it usually becomes before that time very small, and less bright in colour; still, however, it disappears

---

[1] This tint closely resembles, as I have elsewhere remarked, that of the skin of a person soon after leaving a hot-bath. It is important to be acquainted with it, because when it is more marked than usual, and sore throat is also present, it may be mistaken for the rash of scarlet fever.

on pressure. The ordinary duration of each spot is about two days, but it varies from two to six days. Fresh spots appear every day or two from the outset of the eruption, till from the twenty-first to the twenty-eighth day of disease. This successive daily eruption of a few small, very slightly elevated, rose-coloured spots, disappearing on pressure, each spot continuing visible for three or four days only, is, so far as I know, peculiar to, and absolutely diagnostic of, typhoid fever.

TYPHUS FEVER—*Mulberry rash.*—The eruption in typhus fever appears on from the fifth to the seventh day, and reaches its maximum amount in a day or two. It occupies the trunk and extremities, and occasionally the face. It consists of distinct spots and a subcuticular rash.

The frequent absence of one of these elements of the mulberry rash, the different proportions they bear to each other, the depth of hue of either, as well as the changes they undergo in their physical characters, cause considerable variations in the appearance of the rash in individual cases.

(1) *Distinct Spots.* The spots vary in number. Sometimes they are very few, and pretty equally diffused over the whole surface; at others, while there are but few spots on the anterior surface of the trunk, the posterior is covered; or again, they may be innumerable anteriorly as well as posteriorly, ordinarily they are very numerous. Their size varies from a mere point to two, three, or four lines in diameter. Sometimes two or three spots coalescing, give rise to very large irregularly-shaped patches. Each spot passes through two, and in many cases, three stages.

First stage.—The spots on their first appearance are slightly elevated, somewhat flattened on their surface; have a dusky pinkish-red colour, somewhat like the stains of mulberry juice; and disappear completely on pressure, resuming their distinctive appearances as the finger is being withdrawn. *Second stage.*—In from one to three days these spots undergo a marked change; they are no longer elevated above the level of the cuticle; their hue grows darker and more dingy; and instead of disappearing on pressure, they only fade, *i.e.* when the finger is firmly pressed on them they grow paler, but do not entirely disappear.

In some cases the spots, after reaching this stage, pass into faintly marked, reddish-brown stains, and then vanish. *Third stage.*—In many cases, and especially those that are severe, the spots reach a third stage; their centres become dark purple, and are unaltered in appearance by the firmest pressure, although their circumferences still fade; frequently entire spots, circumference as well as centre, change into petechiæ.

The duration of each of the above-described spots is from its eruption till the termination of the disease. But a few large, almost scarlet patches, are occasionally seen on the back of the hand on the fifth or sixth day of the disease; these usually disappear altogether in a day or two.

(2) *The Subcuticular Rash.*—When the trunk is covered with mulberry rash, many of the spots are usually pale, very imperfectly marked as spots, and run into each other; these spots are seen indistinctly, as if seated beneath the cuticle; or as the vulgar say, 'are not well out.' They give to the skin a mottled aspect, and on this mottled surface, as on a ground, the darker, more distinct, and decidedly marked spots are situated. Like the distinct spots, the subcuticular rash is deepest coloured on the most depending parts of the body.

The subcuticular rash may precede or be preceded for a day or two by the distinct spots, *i.e.* the eruption is for a day or two very pale, and then some spots grow more distinct, or a few well-marked spots first appear, and then after a day or two the rash becomes more abundant. The diagnostic characters which separate the spots of typhoid from those of typhus fever are then derived from the colour, shape, duration, and the changes in physical characters which each spot severally experiences in the course of these diseases.

Rose spots, diagnostic of Typhoid Fever, from a boy on the 16th day of disease, by W J

FIG 2

1st Stage of the Mulberry Rash diagnostic of Typhus Fever, showing the slightly
elevated spots and the subcuticular rash, from a man on the 5th day of disease by W.J.

Fig. 3

2 3d stages of the Mulberry Rash diagnostic of Typhus Fever, showing the non elevated
and subcuticular rash, on the 10th day of disease. From nature, by W. H. O. Corley, M D

Number of Cases admitted into the London Fever Hospital, during the separate months of 1847, with

All the cases in which two or more persons suffering from typhus fever, typhoid fever, and relapsing fever, were admitted from the same house, into the London Fever Hospital, in 1847. This table exhibits the age, sex, degree of intimacy of the individuals, and the nature of the disease under which they laboured.

Month.	Rose Spots.	Mulberry Rash.*	Months.	Ages of Males.	Ages of Females.	Degree of Intimacy.	Nature of Disease.	Remarks.
			May	30, 32	28	Lodgers	Typhus fever	All mulberry rash.
			July	25	20	Husband and wife	Relapsing fever	No spots.
			July	17	20, 33	Brother, sister, and sister-in-law	Typhus fever	
			September	14, 19		Brothers	Typhoid fever	Both had rose spots.
			September	21	24	Brother and sister	Typhus fever	Both had mulberry rash.
			September		16, 21	Niece and aunt	Typhus fever	Both had mulberry rash.
			October	22	24	Husband and wife	Relapsing fever	No spots.
			October	16	34	Mother and daughter	Relapsing fever	No spots.
			October	55	35	Husband and wife	Relapsing fever	No spots.
			October	40	36	Husband and wife	Relapsing fever	No spots.
			November	13	13	Brothers	Typhus fever	Both had mulberry rash.
			November		21, 23	Sisters	Typhoid fever	Both had rose spots.

* I have no means of determining these particulars for 1847.

K

Number of cases admitted into the London Fever Hospital, during the separate months of 1848, with

All the instances in which two or more cases of typhus, typhoid, and relapsing fever were admitted from the same house, into the London Fever Hospital, in 1848. This table shows the age, sex, degree of intimacy of the individuals, and the nature of the disease under which they laboured.

Month	Rose Spots	Mulberry Rash
January	8	30
February	8	27
March	5	43
April	4	48
May	3	47

Month	Ages of Males	Ages of Females	Degree of Intimacy	Nature of Disease	Remarks
January	22	22	Husband and wife	Typhus fever	The man had mulberry rash, the wife no spots.
February	30	24	Brother and sister	Typhus fever	Both mulberry rash.
	14	11, 33	Mother and daughter	Typhus fever	The child had no spots.
	13, 50	7, 11, 43	Mother and three children	Typhus fever	All mulberry rash.
	5, 15	35	Father, son, and sister-in-law	Typhus fever	All mulberry rash.
		13, 44	Mother and three children	Typhus fever	The infant was convalescent, the mother had mulberry rash, the two older children no eruption.
March	8	30	Mother and son	Typhus fever	Child had no eruption.
	13, 19	16, 20, 45	Mother and four children	Typhus fever	All mulberry rash.
	5	13, 44	Mother and two children	Typhus fever	Mother mulberry rash, children no eruption.
April		8, 18, 20, 24	Sisters and lodger	Typhus fever	All mulberry rash.
	18, 27		Slept in the same room	Typhus fever	Both mulberry rash.
		26, 49	Mother and daughter	Typhus fever	Both mulberry rash.
		9, 17, 35	Mother and daughter	Typhus fever	All mulberry rash.
		12, 42	Mother and daughter	Typhus fever	Both mulberry rash.
	20	16	Brother and sister	Typhus fever	The boy had mulberry rash, the girl no eruption.
May	20, 21	19	Brothers and sister	Typhus fever	The sister had no eruption, brothers mulberry rash.
		11, 8, 33	Occupied the same room	Typhus fever	The child had no spots, the others mulberry rash.
	19, 58	39	Father, mother, and son	Typhus fever	All mulberry rash.

Month					Slept in the same room	Disease	Remarks
June	10	36	17, 25	·	Slept in the same room	Typhus fever	Both mulberry rash.
			11, 38	·	Father and son	Typhus fever	Father mulberry rash, son no spots.
July	11	37	12, 15, 42	29	Father, sons, lodger	Typhus fever	All mulberry rash.
			19	20	Brother and sister	Typhus fever	Both mulberry rash.
			9, 13	30, 40, 45	Inmates of the same ward at workhouse	Typhus fever	All mulberry rash.
August	11	25	15, 44	·	Brothers	Typhus fever	Elder mulberry rash, younger no spots.
			47	11, 36	Father and son	Typhoid fever	Both had rose spots.
			12, 17	47	Mother and daughter	Typhus fever	Both mulberry rash.
			11, 14	50	Husband and wife	Typhus fever	Both mulberry rash.
			4, 10, 13, 42	6½	Brothers	Typhus fever	Both mulberry rash.
September	22	32	47	5, 6	Mother and children	Typhus fever	All mulberry rash.
			10	11, 33	Father and children	Typhus fever	Father and daughter had mulberry rash, the three boys no spots.
			11	12	Sisters	Typhoid fever	Both had rose spots.
				13	Husband, wife, and child	Typhus fever	All had mulberry rash.
					Brother and sister	Typhoid fever	Both had rose spots.
					Brother and sister	Typhoid fever	Both had rose spots.
October	16	18	16, 46	·	Father and son	The father typhus fever. The son typhoid fever.	Mulberry rash. Rose spots.
November	13	38	19, 21, 29	7, 14, 20, 22, 60	Inhabitants of one house	Typhus fever	Rose spots. The youngest child had no spots, the other seven had mulberry rash.
December	7	10	26, 54	23, 49	Whole family	Typhus fever	All mulberry rash.
			7, 23, 52	16, 34	Whole family	Typhus fever	All mulberry rash.

All the cases in which two or more persons suffering from typhus fever, typhoid fever, and relapsing fever, were admitted from the same house into the London Fever Hospital in 1849. This table exhibits the age, sex, degree of intimacy of the individuals, and the nature of the disease under which they laboured.

Number of cases admitted into the London Fever Hospital, during the separate months of 1849, with—

Month	Rose Spots	Mulberry Rash
January	9	24
February	6	18
March	5	22
April	4	15
May	4	16
June	11	12
July	16	6
August	15	8
September	15	11
October	23	6
November	10	5

Month	Ages of Males	Ages of Females	Degree of Intimacy	Nature of Disease	Remarks
January	9, 37		Father and son	Typhus fever	Both had mulberry rash.
	25	22, 30	Husband, wife, and lodger	Typhus fever	All had mulberry rash.
	26, 30	25	Husband, wife, and lodger	Typhus fever	All had mulberry rash.
	14, 50	47	Husband, wife, and child	Typhus fever	All had mulberry rash.
February	10, 48		Father and son	Typhus fever	Both had mulberry rash.
	9, 14	16, 38, 53	Mother, children, and aunt	Typhus fever	The child, æt. 9, had no spots. All the rest had mulberry rash.
March	10, 17		Brothers	Typhoid fever	Both rose spots.
	6, 8, 29		Father and sons	Typhus fever	All mulberry rash.
		53, 61	Occupied the same room	Typhus fever	Both mulberry rash.
	24, 24, 28, 29, 31	26	Same room, lodging-house	Typhus fever	All mulberry rash.
April	6, 21	35, 40	Mother, children, and nurse	Typhus fever	All mulberry rash.
	12	9, 16, 21	Brother and sisters	Relapsing fever	
May	21	21	Husband and wife	Typhus fever	Both had mulberry rash.
June		12, 44	Mother and daughter	Typhus fever	Both had mulberry rash.
		20, 30	Sisters	Typhus fever	Both had rose spots.
July		18, 18, 51	Visitors, lived in the same court	Typhoid fever	All had rose spots.
	21, 15	9	Brothers and sister	Typhus fever	All had mulberry rash.
	42	49	Husband and wife	Typhus fever	Both had mulberry rash.
August			Brothers	Typhoid fever	All had rose spots.
	10, 13, 16	13, 54	Mother and children	Typhus fever	All had mulberry rash.
	16	13, 16, 54	Mother and daughter	Typhus fever	All had mulberry rash.
September	40	47	Husband and wife	Typhus fever	Both had mulberry rash.
October		23	Master had fever, diarrhœa, and passed blood	Typhoid fever	Rose spots.
November	40, 40	12, 34	Husband, lodger, wife and child	Typhus fever	All had mulberry rash.
	9, 12, 22		Brothers	Relapsing fever	

Into these tables are collected *all* the cases in which more than one of a family, or more than one inhabitant of a house, suffering from typhoid, typhus, or relapsing fever, were admitted into the London Fever Hospital, during the periods specified.[1]

It will be observed, that in 1847 there were admitted into the London Fever Hospital two or more cases of typhus fever from each of five separate localities; that two cases of typhoid fever were received from either of two localities; and two cases of relapsing fever from each of five distinct localities. Twelve cases of typhus fever having been brought from five houses, four cases of typhoid fever from two houses, and ten cases of relapsing fever from five houses, in the course of six months. During the same time not a single example was observed of either disease communicating the other, or of cases of the three diseases, or even of two of them, being generated by the same cause. All these diseases, be it remembered, were prevailing in this city at the same time.

During the year 1848 there were admitted into the London

[1] I ought to qualify the expression ' *all* the cases,' because it was not till the year 1848 that the diagnosis between these diseases was made with reference to *all* the cases admitted into the hospital. The consequence is, that not only are there no data for determining the numbers of each of the three affections received into the hospital during 1847, but there are no data for determining, in many instances, to which of the three diseases any given case ought to be referred; *i.e.* the past histories of particular cases were only partially obtained, the exact locality from which the patient came was not recorded, the name of the street, or even parish, being often all that was ascertained. I have, therefore, been obliged to omit very many cases received into the hospital in 1847 ; but I have included *all* those of which the records available for my purpose permitted the diagnosis to be made, and the locality from which the patient came, to be learned. In 1848, comparatively very few cases were admitted of which the diagnosis was not recorded, and the exact residence ascertained ; and during 1849, the greatest care was taken to ascertain the locality from which each case was received. Since the middle of 1848, the diagnosis of the cases here used has been made or verified in nearly every instance by myself. In 1849 in every case. Before the middle of 1848, the characters of the spots were in many cases recorded by my friend Mr. Sankey, or his assistant, Mr. Humphrey – *i.e.* if two of one family entered the hospital, the notes of one of the cases were frequently taken by either of those gentlemen, while I kept record of the other ; this fact I regard as valuable, because it was only on collating these notes, eighteen months after they were made, that I became aware of many of the facts embodied in this paper.

Fever Hospital two or more cases, one of which presented the symptoms of typhus fever, from each of thirty-four localities. These thirty-four foci of disease yielded on the whole 101 cases. During the same year, more than one-fourth of the cases of fever received into the hospital were examples of typhoid fever, therefore one-fourth, *i.e.* twenty-five of the 101 cases ought, if typhoid and typhus fevers are but varieties of each other, to have presented the symptoms of typhoid fever;[1] but, as the above tables show, in one instance only were two patients, one of whom laboured under typhoid, and the other typhus fever, brought from the same house. The cases referred to are those of a man, æt. 46, who was admitted October 10th, 1848, with well-marked typhus fever, and his son, æt. 16, who had been received into the hospital on September 19th, with equally well-marked typhoid fever. The diagnosis of the latter case was made by my friend Mr. Humphrey. I verified the diagnosis in the case of the father. But in this apparent exception to the rule, the mother of the boy had visited him in the hospital, and therefore might have carried the contagion of typhus fever to her husband. The father, moreover, had been little exposed to the contagion emanating from the son, because the latter, a vagabond, at variance with his father, was from home when he was taken sick.

From January 1st to November 26th, 1849, there were received into the hospital two or more cases, of which one presented the symptoms of typhus fever, from each of eighteen separate localities. These eighteen localities afforded fifty-one cases. During the same eleven months nearly half the cases

[1] Although one could not have expected the cases of typhoid and typhus fevers, that is to say, supposing their cause was identical, admitted from any locality, to have borne to each other the exact proportion that the total numbers of the cases of either disease, admitted into the hospital during the same period of time, did to each other, yet an approach to that proportion ought absolutely to have been present in a majority of instances; while if occasionally the cases of either disease were proportionally too few, they would on other occasions have been, if derived from the same cause, proportionally too many. I have, therefore, used the relative proportion of the cases of the two diseases admitted into the hospital as a standard. It appears to me that correct conclusions are, in a question of the nature considered in the text, more likely to be arrived at by cumulative evidence, such as is above adduced, than by the application of the calculus of probabilities to any one number of cases, however large that number might be.

received into the hospital were suffering from typhoid fever. The whole number of cases admitted was 262; of typhoid fever, 116—of typhus fever, 143—therefore nearly half, or exactly 22·5 of the 51 cases admitted from the eighteen localities, ought to have had typhoid fever, *i.e.* if the cause of the two fevers is identical, while, as the above tables show, not one of the 51 presented the symptoms of that disease.

We see from these tables, moreover, that in 1848 two cases of fever, one of which presented the symptoms of typhoid fever, were admitted from each of five distinct localities; now, as rather more than three-fourths of the cases admitted into the hospital during the same year laboured under typhus fever, the remaining five of the ten ought to have had typhus fever, but one only did so. To this apparently exceptional case I have before referred.

From January 1st to November 26th, 1849, two or more cases, one of which was suffering from typhoid fever, were received into the hospital from four localities, in the whole ten cases. Seeing that rather more than half the cases admitted into the hospital during the same period had typhus fever, the remaining six cases ought to have presented the symptoms of typhus fever, if, as I have before observed, the cause of the two diseases is identical. But in not a single instance was a case of typhoid fever and a case of typhus fever admitted into the hospital, from the same house, during the eleven months of 1849.

The foregoing tables demonstrate, that in every month of 1848 and 1849 several cases of typhoid fever and typhus fever were admitted; that the epidemic constitution favourable to the spread of typhus fever had little influence in diminishing or increasing the absolute number of cases of typhoid fever;—thus, during the first eight months of 1848, 60 cases of typhoid fever, and 292 cases of typhus fever, were admitted into the hospital; and during the corresponding months of 1849, 70 cases of typhoid fever, and 121 only of typhus fever; so that, while the cases of the latter disease had diminished nearly three-fifths, the cases of the former had increased only one-sixth.

As some writers have asserted that there are certain transition cases to be observed, marking the passage of one epidemic constitution into another, I ought here to remark, that with reference to the characteristic peculiarities of typhoid fever, and the rose spots in particular, they were as well marked in the autumn of 1846 as during the epidemic of relapsing fever in 1847, or of typhus in the autumns of 1847 and 1848, or as they are at the present moment. The spots have undergone no change, have experienced no modification; although the epidemic constitution on which the difference in the rash is said to depend, must have varied more than once. The same is true of the mulberrry rash of typhus fever. It presented, in a few cases observed in 1846, the same characters as during the epidemic of 1847-48; the same characters during that epidemic as at the present moment, when the number of the cases of typhoid fever bear to that of typhus fever the proportion of three to one.

So with regard to the intestinal lesion. In all the fatal cases examined in the three years referred to, in which the mulberry rush existed during life, Peyer's patches, and the mesenteric glands were absolutely free from disease, and in every fatal case in which rose spots were noted during life, serious lesion of the agminated and mesenteric glands was discovered after death. The lesion, like the eruption, was quite unmodified by that epidemic constitution which favoured the spread of typhus fever in 1847 and 1848;—for example, although the constitution of the autumn of this year (1849) favoured the spread of typhoid fever, yet, when a man and his wife were admitted in August with typhus fever, the mulberry rash preserved its characteristics unmodified, and when they died, as both did, Peyer's patches and the mesenteric glands were found to possess their normal anatomical characters.

There are a few cases included in the preceding tables, which may here be more fully adverted to with advantage. In November and December 1848 forty-eight cases of typhus fever, and twenty of typhoid fever, were admitted into the Hospital, i.e. nearly one-third of the patients were affected with typhoid fever. At the latter end of October, 1848, a boy, 14 years of age, went to reside with a family named Mitchell, in Adden Place, St. Pancras. The Mitchells were at that time in health. The boy left his own home because his brothers were 'down with the fever.' This lad was, early in November, admitted into the Hospital, suffering from typhus fever. Early, also in the same month, the man Mitchell, aged 29 years, with whom the boy lodged, the man's daughter, aged 7 years, and a female lodger, aged 22, were also admitted with typhus fever. The other members of Mitchell's family, expelled from Adden Place, then removed to 21 Hertford Street, at least a mile from their former residence. At this time, so far as I could learn by personal inquiry, there was no fever in Hertford Street, and *certainly* none in the house in which they had taken up their residence. On November 22nd, the two sisters of Mitchell's wife, aged respectively 14 and 22, who had removed from Adden Place with Mrs. Mitchell and her infant, aged 4 years, were received into the Hospital, both suffering from typhus fever. On December 8th the landlady of 21 Hertford Street, aged 60 years, was admitted with very severe typhus fever; and on December 20th the son-in-law of the landlady was also admitted with the same disease. I subsequently saw Mitchell's infant, aged 4 years, at its own home; it was similarly but very slightly affected. The only member of the family that escaped was the woman Mitchell, and she had had 'spotted typhus fever,' according to her own voluntary statement, some few years before.[1] Here was a group of persons, whose ages varied from four to sixty years, and whose constitutional predispositions also must have varied infinitely, for there were several of them unconnected by blood, exposed to the poison of typhus fever (introduced among them by the lad aged 14) at a time when typhus fever was only twice as prevalent as typhoid fever. What was the result? Did one-third of the eight have typhoid fever? No, not one.

---

[1] I may here observe that I have never known the same individual to be affected twice with typhus fever. The same person has been admitted twice, or, indeed, oftener, into the London Fever Hospital. But on reference to the Hospital records, or to my own notes, I have invariably found that such persons had at the one time a different disease from that present at the other. Thus two boys were admitted, Sept. 1849, with typhus fever; they had been inmates of the Hospital in 1846. Reference to the Hospital records of that year proved that they then had relapsing fever. I know no evidence, I repeat, to prove that typhus fever attacks the same individual *twice* more frequently than typhoid fever.

In December 1848 ten cases of typhus fever and seven of typhoid fever were admitted into the Hospital. Five cases came from one house; these five individuals varied in age from 7 to 52 years,—their degree of relationship was, grandfather, daughter, and three grand-children. All five had well-marked mulberry rash, were unequivocally affected with typhus fever. It is evident that, as at this time, the number of those admitted with the two diseases was pretty nearly equal; two of these five ought, if the cause of the two diseases is identical, to have had typhoid fever, with rose spots.

In March and April 1849 eight cases of typhoid fever, and thirty-one cases of typhus fever, were admitted into the Hospital. Between the 19th of March and the 10th of April eight persons were brought to the Hospital from one room, suffering from fever. Did one-fourth present the rose spots of typhoid fever? No, not one—all had well-marked typhus fever.

In September, October, and November 1849 eighteen cases of typhus fever, and forty-eight cases of typhoid fever, were received into the Hospital, i.e. nearly three times as many cases of typhoid fever as of typhus fever. During the same three months a mother and her two daughters, aged respectively 54, 16, and 13; a husband and wife, aged 40 and 47; a husband, wife, child, and lodger, aged severally 40, 39, 12, and 40—i.e. in all nine persons, were brought from three localities. At least five ought to have had typhoid fever, if that affection and typhus fever are due to the same specific cause. Was it so? No, in every case the persons secondarily affected, whatever their age or sex, had the same disease as the individual from whom they caught it.

In April 1849 a girl suffering from relapsing fever was brought from a house in Fulham—in a few days her brother and two sisters were admitted into the Hospital. Did either of the three latter have typhus fever, which was the prevailing disease, or typhoid fever, which was then also very much more widely spread than relapsing fever? No; all had the same fever.

Although not absolutely necessary for the purpose of my argument, I may observe that I have visited, in a few instances, the houses [1] from which more than one individual affected with typhoid fever or typhus fever were brought to the Hospital, without being able to detect any hygienic differences in the condition of the people, or in the localities themselves to modify the exciting cause.

Before concluding, it will be well summarily to repeat that in 1848 one-fourth of the cases admitted into the Hospital had typhoid fever; while, from thirty-four foci of typhus fever, yielding 101 cases, there was brought to the Hospital once only a case of typhus fever and a case of typhoid fever from the same house; and during the same time, among five localities, affording nine cases of typhoid fever, one locality only, viz. the house from which the father and son before referred to were brought, yielded a case of typhoid and one of typhus fever. That in 1849, although eighteen foci of typhus fever yielded fifty-one cases, and four foci of typhoid fever afforded ten cases, not a single example of the two diseases being received into the Hospital from one house occurred. With reference to the exceptional case, I must observe, that for exceptional cases to be of any value in proving the identity of typhus fever and typhoid fever, they must be met with more frequently than similar exceptional cases are met with in diseases having a specific cause, universally acknowledged to be different.

Now, the following facts prove that, with respect to measles, scarlet fever, and typhus fever, such exceptional cases are as frequent as with respect to typhoid and typhus fevers. During the last three years I have seen a case of typhus fever brought into the Hospital from a house in which all the children were suffering from measles; another case of typhus fever brought from a house in which the children had scarlet fever; a girl admitted with scarlet fever, who had been on terms of intimacy with another girl, admitted shortly before with typhoid fever. And in these cases no direct contagion for the diseases under which the patients laboured could be traced. It is also important to observe that the cases of scarlet fever admitted

---

[1] These houses were situated in courts or streets in the City, Bethnal Green, St. Pancras, and Holborn. I visited too few and made too imperfect inquiries to draw any *strict* inferences, but my *general* impression is stated in the text.

during the time specified were nothing like so numerous as the cases of typhus fever or of typhoid fever.

The facts contained in this paper appear to me to prove incontestably, so far as induction can prove the point, that the specific causes of typhus and typhoid fevers are absolutely different from each other, and to render in the highest degree probable, that the specific cause of relapsing fever is different from that of either of the two former. I have elsewhere, as I stated at the opening of this paper, attempted to prove that the course, the symptoms, the lesion, and the sequelæ of typhoid and typhus are different, and as relapsing fever differs from both too widely, so far as symptoms and course are concerned, to be confounded with them, it follows that if small-pox be separated from measles, and both from scarlet fever, because their course, symptoms, lesions, and specific causes are different, so must, for like reasons, typhoid fever, typhus fever, and relapsing fever be separated from each other, and regarded as absolutely distinct diseases, not merely varieties of each other, as are scarlatina anginosa and scarlatina *sine eruptione*, but distinct species of disease, as are scarlatina, rubeola, and variola.

I have, throughout this paper, expressed myself as if the specific cause respectively of typhoid fever, typhus fever, and relapsing fever was an influence emanating from the bodies of those affected with either disease. With respect to the contagious nature of typhus fever, I know no one who entertains a doubt. If typhoid fever be contagious, it is infinitely less so than typhus fever. My experience leads me to regard it as contagious. Those who believe typhoid fever to be non-contagious while they admit the contagious nature of typhus fever, cannot for a moment doubt the difference in the specific causes of the diseases. It would not, it ought to be observed, have weakened the force of the facts adduced if I had regarded these diseases as non-contagious, because the question here considered is not how the individuals respectively got the disease, but if the same cause, whether contagion or any other, can produce typhoid fever, typhus fever, and relapsing fever.

APPENDIX.

Dr. Barclay inquired of Dr. Jenner, whether he regarded all cases
of fever, in which there was not any eruption, as instances of relapsing
fever; and further, whether cases of continued fever, without an
eruption, were or were not liable to relapse?

Dr. Jenner replied in the affirmative, relative to the occurrence of
continued fever without eruption. About one-fourth of the cases
under fifteen years of age were unattended with spots; and also three
out of 21 from that age to the twenty-second year; after that age the
eruption showed itself in all cases. There was not any eruption in
one-fourth of Louis's cases.

Dr. Stewart could not but feel gratified, that the views he had
ventured to lay before the medical world nine years ago on the subject which this evening occupied the attention of the Society, had
been so fully borne out by the interesting researches of Dr. Jenner.
He felt assured, when he published those views, that time and observation would thoroughly establish the fact;—for it was a *fact*, and
not a theory,—that the eruptions of typhus and typhoid fevers were
essentially and invariably distinct, and never passed the one into the
other. One point to which he had directed attention in the paper
alluded to, and which he thought had not yet been sufficiently in-
vestigated, was the frequent occurrence of true relapses in typhoid
fever. By this he meant, that not unfrequently, after the disease
seemed to have run its course, and convalescence was almost established, a new attack was ushered in with fresh rigors, followed by
febrile excitement, fresh rose-coloured exanthem on the skin, a repetition of all the previous symptoms, and, as might be proved by dissection in the event of death, which sometimes takes place after a
second and even a third attack, with fresh intestinal lesion, and the
development, amid the cicatrices of former ulcers, of new, highly
swollen and elevated glands, both aggregated and solitary. Such a

phenomenon as this was never met with in typhus. There might be sequelæ in typhus, but never true relapse. There was another point of great importance, of which he was lately reminded by his friend Dr. Gueneau de Mussy. The common answer of those who held the identity of the two diseases to those who showed them the intestines, in typhus uniformly free from ulceration, and even from anything that could be called disease, was, that the malady had run too rapid a course for the characteristic appearances to be developed. The fact being, that the peculiar lesion of typhoid fever attained its maximum of development about the third or fourth day, from which time the process of disintegration seems to commence. The more rapid, therefore, the course of the disease, the more fully developed ought the glands to be. The inquiries instituted by Dr. Jenner, and detailed in his paper regarding the localities from which the cases came were certainly of deep interest; and he (Dr. Stewart) apprehended, that the most important question now demanding investigation, and the decision of which would go far to settle the controversy, was, whether an attack of the one disease generally protected those who had had it from the other, or whether, on the contrary, there were well-authenticated cases of both fevers having attacked the same individuals. It was not strictly correct to affirm, that one attack of exanthematic typhus uniformly protected against another, for there was a considerable number of instances to the contrary. A very noted one, he believed, was Dr. Christison, who had had three or four attacks of true typhus, and was now obliged to refuse attendance on cases of that disease, as each succeeding attack was more severe than the preceding.

Dr. Barclay was not satisfied with the answer he had received respecting the occurrence of fever without spots. His own experience showed that that state of the skin was very common in fever, and the appearance of an eruption in fever was rare. Out of 111 cases that had occurred during one year, at St. George's Hospital, there were only 59 of all kinds of eruption. He himself found considerable difficulty in distinguishing between the different kinds of eruption attendant on, and said to characterise, typhoid and typhus fevers, as in some cases he had noticed the rose-coloured eruption become of a dark hue, while in others no such change took place. He could diagnose between typhus and typhoid fevers, by the condition of the glands in the intestinal canal, and by the state of the tongue and of the abdomen, the excretions, etc., but not by the appearance of the patient's skin. The conclusion he drew respecting the eruptions was, that when the spots were dark-coloured, it was much less common to meet with intestinal ulceration. He had ascertained, by the examination of bodies after death, that when the rose-coloured eruption existed, there is always ulceration of the intestinal canal; in the dark-coloured eruptions that condition is always absent.

Mr. Sankey remarked, that when he first became connected with the London Fever Hospital, he held the same opinions as Dr. Barclay. His ideas were confused, and he did not know when he should and when he should not find abdominal lesions. He had found the same degree of confusion respecting these eruptions in the latest works on medicine. Watson, in speaking of the rashes, evidently confounded the two forms which appear in typhoid and typhus fevers. His description is that of the typhus eruption; but he mentions one symptom which belongs solely to the typhoid. This state of mental confusion was removed by the perusal of the last edition of Louis's work on 'Fever,' to which his attention had been directed by Dr. Jenner. He did not hesitate to say, that when the distinguishing characters of the two rashes are clearly understood (and they may require some well-marked cases placed side by side to elucidate them), there will never again be the least chance of their being confounded together; indeed, he added, the nurses of the hospital had learned to diagnose between the two forms of fever from the characters of the eruptions. So accurately can the diagnosis be made when either of these kinds of spots is present, that out of from 200 to 300 autopsies, there has not been a single error in the diagnosis, as to the existence or absence of disease in Peyer's glands. As stated in the paper, for two or three years past, the majority of cases at the Fever Hospital were instances of typhus; there were not, in fact, any cases of typhoid fever, and, consequently, ulceration of the intestines was not met with. While typhus was thus raging in London, the parish authorities of St. Margaret's, Westminster, their own infirmary being crowded, sent many cases to the Hospital, chiefly of the newly-arrived Irish; these cases were all typhus. Before the epidemic was on the decline, fever broke out in the Westminster-school, and in the precincts of the Abbey. Two domestic servants of one of the prebendaries were admitted into the hospital, and their cases were clearly typhoid fever. It was supposed, at first, that the epidemic had spread to the precincts, but he (Mr. Sankey) stated to Dr. S. Smith, who had been directed to investigate its characters, that it must have arisen from some other cause than contagion, as it was essentially different from the cases previously under treatment from that neighbourhood, and, in all probability, was connected with some local cause. This proved to be the case, as a foul and obstructed drain was discovered passing at the rear of all the houses in which fever had broken out. He (Mr. Sankey) could corroborate Dr. Stewart's remarks as to the early occurrence of intestinal ulceration in typhoid fever, for he had seen, a few years ago, a case of extensive intestinal disease in a woman who was working on the Friday, and died of typhoid fever the succeeding Monday. The solitary and agminate glands were perfectly hypertrophied on that, the fourth day of the fever. He could readily conceive that confusion with respect to the eruption might arise, unless several cases, from 20 to 25, were seen and examined at the same time. A number of cases were sent into the hospital as instances of fever, which in reality were not such, but cases of bronchitis, pneumonia, etc., with febrile disturbance. In fact, a disease has often been named fever, because it cannot be clearly made out to be anything else—by a process of reasoning by exclusion. If the disease be not (or, what is the same thing, be not discovered to be) inflammation of this or that organ, then it has ever been taught that such disease should be called fever ; so that the word fever has been, as it were, a shelf on which to deposit those cases which do not readily fit any place in the nosological system.

Dr. Baly remarked that if the assumed fact Dr. Jenner had related, of the connection of certain eruptions with certain forms of fever, be admitted as proved, then the additional fact, that cases of typhoid and typhus fever were rarely sent to the hospital from the same house, became very important, and would seem to show that they depend on different causes. They had had 117 cases of fever in the Milbank prison, while typhus and typhoid fever were prevalent without. Of these 117, about 20 cases ended fatally. In all these, there was great mischief in Peyer's patches and in the mesenteric glands. The cases in the prison were well-marked instances of typhoid fever. He (Dr. Baly) was not very intimately acquainted with the characters of the eruption in typhoid fever, so as to be able to distinguish it from that of typhus, but from his general knowledge he was quite sure that a large number of cases may occur without any eruption at all.

Dr. West observed, that one form of fever which had not as yet been alluded to, the infantile remittent of children, had been considered by Barthez as identical with the typhoid of Louis, and in that opinion, he (Dr. West) agreed. It presented the same characters during life, and the same changes after death, as the typhoid described by Louis. The characteristic rash was, however, often absent. Among the poorer classes of society this form of fever is often very severe and even fatal. In no instance could he recollect seeing a case of typhus fever in the house, nor, on the other hand, could he recollect a case of typhus occurring when infantile remittent already existed in a house. These facts were, as far as they went, confirmatory of Dr. Jenner's view.

Dr. Webster inquired of Mr. Sankey if he meant to imply that medical men sent cases of pneumonia and bronchitis into the Fever Hospital, under the mistaken idea that they were cases of pure fever?

Mr. Sankey wished it to be understood, that in making these remarks, he meant other diseases than those the author of the paper and himself would call true fever. For, indeed, if every member of the profession were agreed as to what cases were fever, and what were not: if the point were not an open question, there would be no discussion. The rules of the hospital expressly provide for the admission of all cases of febrile disturbance of a contagious nature, or likely to become such. In fact, cases of small-pox, acute rheumatism, pneumonia, bronchitis, etc., had been admitted even lately.

Dr. Heale was old enough to recollect the time when fever was said not to exist unless some acute lesion of an internal organ were present. He did not think it, therefore, very disparaging to mistake instances of bronchitis, pneumonia, etc., for cases of fever, especially when there was much febrile excitement. It was more likely to occur among the sick poor, the parochial surgeon being anxious to get rid of the charge of a case of complicated illness.

Dr. Webster inquired whether the author of the paper considered typhoid and typhus fevers at all contagious? It might be produced by other causes; and he instanced a case of eight people living in one room, all of whom were taken to the hospital with fever.

Dr. Barclay had tabularised the respective ages of patients in St. George's Hospital, labouring under fever, in whom the two different forms of eruption had appeared. From the age of ten to twenty, there were 5 rose-coloured and 3 dark-coloured; from twenty to thirty, 7 rose and 3 dark; thirty to forty, 5 rose and 3 dark; and from forty to fifty, 4 rose and 5 dark. The age of the patient influenced the duskiness of the eruption, the occurrence of which he considered to be casual, and depending on other causes than the peculiar character of the fever.

Dr. Mervyn Crawford thought the difference of opinion between the physician to the Fever Hospital and that of St. George's, was owing to the fact that in the former hospital the patients were congregated together, and exposed to the influence of a virulent fever poison, and in the other the patients were disseminated throughout the wards, and the poison was much milder in consequence. He himself, like Dr. Barclay, was unable to recognise the exanthem. He believed the eruption was an accidental circumstance, dependent on an unhealthy locality and want of ventilation.

Dr. Jenner replied, that in common with all writers on typhoid fever, he had seen cases of that disease in which there was no eruption, and referred, in confirmation, to the analysis of cases he had published during the present year in the *Monthly Journal of Medical Science* (Edinburgh), and that in last week's *Medical Times* he had also shown, that the eruption was frequently absent in cases of typhus in children; that the paper he that evening had the honour of laying before the Society only spoke of the eruptions as diagnostic *when they were present*. Dr. Jenner then adverted to the fact, that the skin eruption was sometimes absent in scarlet fever and in measles, and to the bearing of this fact, as showing the invalidity of any arguments by which it was attempted to associate typhus and typhoid fevers, because the eruption was occasionally absent in these two diseases, and then stated, that in many cases the mulberry rash of typhus, on its first appearance, so closely resembled the rose-spots of typhoid fever, that, to one unused to observe them closely, they might appear, in rare cases, identical; but that his experience, grounded on notes of about 2000 cases of fever, made on the patients' admission into the hospital, and repeated on the subsequent days of their stay, warranted him in asserting, that if any spots, the characters of which were doubtful when seen on or about the eighth day of disease, presented at a later period the characters assigned in his paper, and figured in the wax model as those diagnostic of typhus, then if the patient died, no lesion of Peyer's patches would be found. With reference to the cases alluded to by Dr. Baly, Dr. Jenner remarked, that to be of value in determining the question on which the discussion had turned, *i.e.* the diagnostic value of the eruption, it was absolutely necessary to confine the remarks to fatal cases examined after death. Dr. Baly had not stated whether such examination had been made with respect to the cases he had seen. With reference to Dr. Crawford's opinion, that the impure nature of the atmosphere of a hospital in which so many cases of fever were accumulated, might account for the dusky nature of the rash in the cases of typhus, and that, probably, difference in the locality in which St. George's and Middlesex Hospitals and the London Fever Hospital were situated, might also aid in accounting for the discrepancy in the opinions of Dr. Jenner and others, he (Dr. Jenner) observed that the latter institution received patients from all localities indiscriminately; from almost every parish in and around London, from

Bethnal-green, Holborn, St. Pancras, Marylebone, Kensington, and Fulham; from Greenwich, Clapham, Wandsworth, and Harrow; and that, consequently, locality could not account for the peculiarities observed in the disease; and, moreover, that he (Dr. J.) had visited the houses of the people in very different localities, and could not observe any difference in the hygienic conditions of their inhabitants. As to impurity of atmosphere, those who had visited the Fever Hospital could not attribute anything to that cause, but those who had not must detect how little force the supposed impurity could have exerted, when they remembered that it was in that hospital, the air of which was *fancied* by Dr. Crawford to be so impure as to convert the rose rash into the mulberry, that such conversion was averred by Dr. Jenner *never* to take place. Dr. Jenner stated, that his observations fully confirmed those of Dr. West, that the ordinary remittent fever of children was really typhoid fever; and that, although several children in the same house occasionally suffered from that disease at the same time, or soon after each other, he (Dr. Jenner) had never seen it give rise in such houses to typhus fever. Dr. Jenner reminded Dr. Stewart, that, in the papers before referred to, he had himself mentioned a fatal case of typhoid fever, in which there was a distinct relapse, accompanied by a second crop of eruption. Dr. Jenner did not consider Dr. Christison having suffered from fever three or four times was any proof that typhus fever recurred in the same individual more frequently than typhoid fever, because that gentleman might have had typhus fever, typhoid fever, and relapsing fever, and as he drew no distinction between them, he would call them all continued fever, and thus might be said to have had fever several times. Dr. Jenner dwelt on the importance of the agreement in the observations of Dr. Gerhard, in America, in 1837; Dr. Shattuck, in London, in 1839; Dr. Stewart, in Glasgow, 1840; and his own in 1849, and referred to Dr. Bartlett's recently published work, in which that author states, that he had seen cases of typhus and typhoid fever lying in Dr. Gerhard's wards in 1847, side by side, each disease marked by its own peculiarities, and added, that the preservation of its own peculiarities by each disease, when side by side in the same ward, was of frequent occurrence, on a large scale, in the London Fever Hospital.

Dr. Stewart begged to be allowed two remarks, notwithstanding the lateness of the hour, in reference to what had fallen from Dr. Crawford. That the peculiar symptoms referred to were not attributable, as Dr. Crawford suggested, to the concentration of the malignant virus was plain, from the experience obtained at the Edinburgh

Infirmary. Along with his much lamented friend, Dr. John Reid, who had kindly furnished him with some interesting data for his paper in 1840, he had frequently visited the wards of that hospital, where the fever patients were distributed, as in the Middlesex Hospital, among those labouring under other complaints, and yet precisely the same symptoms presented themselves there as in the Fever Hospital, where, if Dr. Crawford would look in, the next time he was at Islington, he would find as pure air, and as well-aired wards, as in any hospital in London. But there was one observation of Dr. Crawford's that was of the utmost moment—that we should consider fevers not only with regard to time, but with regard to place. Dr. Crawford stated, that he had found no typhus at Munich, but he (Dr. Stewart) when he visited the Hospital at Stuttgart along with Dr. Kless, found both it and typhoid fever in the wards. At Paris, as Dr. Crawford mentioned, there was never a case to be met with, and when Dr. Shattuck's cases were published in 1840 (only half a dozen), they made quite a sensation in the medical world. And now, there could be no doubt that there was a growing conviction in Paris, that the diseases were essentially distinct. In London, again, there were peculiar facilities for the careful study of this important subject; for in no two great cities in the world were the numbers of the patients affected with each complaint so nearly equal.

TYPHUS FEVER, TYPHOID FEVER,

RELAPSING FEVER, AND FEBRICULA,

THE DISEASES COMMONLY CONFOUNDED

UNDER THE TERM

CONTINUED FEVER.

ILLUSTRATED BY CASES COLLECTED AT THE BEDSIDE.

1849–1851

TYPHUS FEVER, TYPHOID FEVER, RELAPS-ING FEVER, AND FEBRICULA, THE DISEASES COMMONLY CONFOUNDED UNDER THE TERM CONTINUED FEVER,

Illustrated by cases collected at the bedside.[1]

INTRODUCTION.

Some years since I was, in conjunction with one of the most able physicians of the day, a man of great experience, in attendance on a young lady supposed to be labouring under acute idiopathic peritonitis. Death ensued. Fortunately permission was obtained to examine the body. We discovered tolerably extensive ulceration of Peyer's patches, and enlargement of the mesenteric glands; in fact, the anatomical characters of typhoid fever. It was evident that an error in diagnosis had been made. The question then arose, which under such circumstances the practitioner always ought to ask, was the art of medicine defective in not affording means for the diagnosis, or were we behind the age in the information we possessed?[2] I was so struck with the importance of the question, that I determined to investigate the subject of fever on a large scale, if ever opportunity served.

[1] This essay was comprised in a series of twenty-one papers contributed to the *Medical Times*. The first paper appeared in the issue of that journal for November 17, 1849, the last on February 8, 1851.

[2] In justice to the accomplished physician referred to, as well as to myself, I ought here to anticipate, and state that this case presented peculiarities which defied diagnosis so long as the idea of continued fever, severe enough to prove fatal, was confined to cases presenting a brown tongue, delirium, and extreme prostration.

Through the kindness of the medical officers of the London Fever Hospital, I have during the last four years been enabled to undertake such researches in an extensive field, and with the greatest facilities for prosecuting the inquiry.

The object of these papers is to illustrate what appears to me to be the state of our knowledge at the present moment on the subject of the diseases commonly called continued fever. I lay little claim to originality. I had no theory to substantiate when I undertook the investigation; I have now no theory to propound. I lost a case which had baffled my knowledge in discovering its nature, and I was only anxious that I might never again commit the same mistake. If, during these researches, I have been led to adopt views not generally acknowledged as correct in this country, it is only because I am unable to withstand the evidence which nature offers of the truth of those views, *where alone* the truth can be elicited, at the bedside and in the dead-house.

There are two opinions entertained on the subject of continued fever. The first, which is that generally held in this country, may be stated thus—continued fever is one disease, capable of assuming different forms or types, as inflammatory, ataxic, etc.; the stress of the fever may fall on any one organ, and so give rise to the varieties termed bilious fever, brain fever, etc.; the symptoms of this disease vary infinitely according to atmospheric, individual, and hygienic peculiarities; consequently there can be no definition of fever applicable to more than the epidemic prevailing at the time the definition is given; by these atmospheric and hygienic peculiarities are to be explained the differences in the disease, as observed in Paris and Edinburgh, and its variations at different times in the latter city. Some even go so far as to maintain, that hygienic conditions may develop the poison of plague out of that emanating from a person labouring under typhus fever.

The second and much less commonly received opinion, I say less commonly, but in reality it is not taught in a single systematic work on fever in this country, may be thus stated:—

Under the term continued fever are confounded three, if not four fevers, each having its origin in a specific cause; and granting all to be contagious, the poison of one fever is altogether incapable, whatever may be the individual or hygenic conditions existing, of exciting the other. Each is a general disease, capable of being complicated with local lesions; one of the four, however, is constantly attended by a lesion peculiar to it. This morbid structural change so invariably accompanies the general symptoms of that particular fever, that even if the local symptoms which ordinarily indicate the existence of that change be absent, yet, if the *general* symptoms of that fever are present, we may predicate, with absolute certainty, that the lesion alluded to is present also.[1] Perhaps the truth is, however, scarcely expressed by the assertion, that the general state is attended by the local lesion; for the latter is as much a part of the disease, as sore throat is a part of scarlet fever; nay, even more so, for angina is not so constant a concomitant of scarlet fever as lesion of Peyer's patches is of typhoid fever.

The two opinions, which I have above endeavoured briefly to state, may be illustrated thus,—Suppose a common lodging-house, each room of which is in a different hygienic condition, if a person labouring under any form of continued fever,—say those who maintain the identity of the fevers I believe to be different—be admitted into room No. 1, he may produce or excite in the inhabitants of that room typhus fever, with the mulberry or measly rash, or spotted typhus, as it is sometimes called; if he then be removed into No. 2 in the same house, the occupier of that room, inhaling the same poison as did the inhabitant of No. 1, may have short or relapsing fever; the dweller in No. 3, febricula; while the resident in No. 4 may catch from the same person continued fever, complicated with ulceration of Peyer's patches and enlargement of the mesenteric glands; and if—some go so far as to maintain—highly unfavourable hygienic conditions exist in another room in the same house, then may the unfortunate who inhabits it have true Oriental plague, as a consequence of inhaling the breath of the man labouring under typhus fever. They further maintain that an eruption on the skin may be present or absent in either, in all, or in none, of these cases; that if present, it may consist of a few rose-spots, an abundant exanthematous or mulberry rash,

---

[1] The bearing of this fact on prognosis is of incalculable importance.

petechiæ or true plague buboes; and that it would be impossible, judging from the *eruption alone*, to predicate the presence or absence of lesion of Peyer's patches and enlargement of the mesenteric glands.

Those who maintain the non-identity of certain continued fevers, say, on the contrary, if a man labouring under typhus fever, *i.e.* a continued fever, having a determinate duration, and attended by a peculiar rash, but unaccompanied by lesion of Peyer's patches, be admitted into room No. 1 of a common lodging-house, he can excite in the inhabitant of that room no other disease than typhus fever; that this disease, like all others, may vary in severity; that the dweller in the infected atmosphere may, according to various external, and also individual peculiarities, have a mild or a severe attack, but that the disease will present the symptoms—however different they may be in degree or in number—and, if it prove fatal, the pathological appearances observed in typhus fever, and that the disease will preserve its characters, varying only in severity and number, whether it be communicated to the dwellers in one or all of the rooms of the house; that if a person labouring under what they term another disease, viz. typhoid fever,—*i.e.* a fever having a determinate duration, accompanied during life by a peculiar eruption, and presenting after death lesion of Peyer's patches and enlargement of the mesenteric glands,—be admitted into the house, he, too, may communicate fever,[1] but then it will be typhoid fever, that as in the first case rose spots and lesion of Peyer's patches were present, so the same eruption, if any, and the same lesion, will occur in all the cases which have fever from contact with, or proximity to the first case, and this whatever be the individual peculiarities, or external hygienic conditions in which they are placed; exactly as a person labouring under scarlet fever, if admitted into the different rooms of a lodging-house, would excite in the inhabitant of those rooms, scarlet fever, and that disease only, however much the hygienic conditions of its rooms might vary, and however different the individual peculiarities of their inhabitants.

---

[1] I assume here, for the sake of elucidating my position, that typhoid fever is contagious. I am, of course, aware, that the contagious nature of typhoid fever, unlike that of typhus, admits of reasonable doubt.

Individual and hygienic peculiarities might modify the severity of the disease; but, *if any* eruption occurred, it would be that characteristic of scarlet fever; if any serious lesion, it would be sore throat. The duration of the scarlet fever thus produced would be the same in a large proportion of the cases, though some might have their illness prolonged by local complications, and others might have the disease in so mild a form that they might consider themselves well ere the symptoms characteristic of the diseases, to the eye of the experienced physician, had entirely disappeared. But, however much the hygienic conditions of the rooms might vary, no modification in the poison exhaled could be produced by which it could be converted into a different poison capable of exciting another contagious disease, *i.e.* one able, like the first, to reproduce itself. Thus a person suffering from scarlet fever cannot produce a poison capable of exciting small-pox, nor *vice versâ*.

The question is not one barren of practical results, as they are termed (as if *all truths* were not practical), for, of what avail can be any observations respecting treatment, general or particular, so long as two, three, or four diseases are called by one name? Let me, in illustration, refer to the fact, that measles and scarlet fever were long confounded under the same name. What value could be attached to any observations respecting the efficacy of the treatment of a class of cases in which were confounded two diseases so different in their essential nature as scarlet fever and measles? —diseases, of which not only does the medicinal treatment differ, but the hygienic conditions suited for the one are diametrically opposed to those fitted for the other. For one moment suppose the two, as not many years since they were, thus confounded; a medical man treats a hundred cases, of which ninety are examples of scarlet fever, ten of measles; he will arrive at the conclusion, that cold sponging is highly beneficial in the treatment of the disease, and he adduces his experience in confirmation of the statement. Now, let us reverse the case, and suppose that another practitioner has one hundred cases of these two diseases, confounded under one name, to treat, and that, of these one hundred cases, ninety are examples of measles, ten of scarlet fever. He uses cold sponges, opens the windows, allows his patient to lie exposed while the eruption is out, etc. He loses a large proportion of his one hundred cases, and finds, on examination after death, pneumonia in every case. He instantly avers, that the treatment declared by the first to be so advantageous, is most deadly, and forthwith advocates a line of treatment diametrically opposed to that which had proved so efficacious in the first practitioner's hands. The same holds true with respect to continued fever: if three or four diseases are united by one name, and then a line of treatment is stated to be successful in continued fever, with what confidence can we receive the statement?

In the epidemic (of relapsing fever) which visited Edinburgh in 1817-20, bloodletting was practised in every case, and was supposed to cut short the fever because, soon after the bleeding, the symptoms disappeared; now observation has proved that a disease, presenting all the symptoms noted in that epidemic, will get well in a short time if left to the unaided effort of nature, and that the inference drawn, that it was possible to cut short true typhus fever by bloodletting, was most erroneous, the disease which was then treated by bloodletting being a totally distinct disease from typhus, but confounded with it. One consequence of the supposed success obtained in bloodletting in that epidemic, was the extensive employment of the same remedy in the true typhus, and incalculable loss of life as a result. Bloodletting is practised with advantage in the common continued fever of Paris; in Scotland wine is the mainstay, and bleeding is stated to be most injurious. ' Mere difference in epidemic constitution,' say the advocates of the identity of the disease in those cities. 'Two distinct diseases, requiring different modes of treatment,' say those who regard them in the light in which I am in these papers about to describe them. There cannot remain a doubt on the minds of those who have treated both diseases on a large scale, during the *same epidemic constitution* and under the *same hygienic peculiarities*, that typhus fever, *i.e.* the ordinary fever of Edinburgh, requires wine to be administered, and often largely; while typhoid fever, *i.e.* the continued fever of Paris, and a very common disease in London, demands wine much less frequently, and bears abstinence from stimulants much more easily, nay, often derives marked benefit from it.

Having attempted thus briefly to show that it is of no trifling importance to distinguish two or more diseases confounded under one name, before anything like practical directions for treatment can be offered, I may state, that my intention is merely to give such descriptions and illustrations of the diseases commonly termed continued fever, as shall enable the practitioner to discriminate them from each other with facility. In proof of the ease with which the diagnosis between the two most important,—viz., typhus and typhoid fevers,—can be made, I may state, that the nurses of the London Fever Hospital rarely fail to distinguish between the two; and I am constantly answered, when asking them if any new cases have been admitted, by 'Yes, Sir, a case of typhoid or a case of typhus fever,' as it may happen, and it is not common for me to have to correct their diagnosis.

I have no intention of attempting to *prove* in *these* papers what *I affirm*,—viz., that each of the diseases here described are really distinct from each other, in the same sense as are scarlet fever and small-pox. That I have already done elsewhere, so far as concerns the symptoms and lesions of typhoid and typhus fevers;[1] and I have now in my possession the materials for giving the final proof of their non-identity, by showing that their exciting cause is different. These materials consist of an analytical examination of all the cases in which more than one patient has been admitted from the same house into the London Fever Hospital during the last three years.

The plan I propose to adopt in these papers is, in the first place, to detail a few cases illustrating the ordinary uncomplicated form of each disease; then to sketch briefly the

---

[1] See a series of papers by the author in the *Monthly Journal of Medicine*, for April, June, and subsequent months of 1849, 'On the Identity of Typhoid and Typhus Fevers,' etc. (reprinted in present volume, pp. 3 to 135). I may add, that during more than three years' almost daily attendance at the London Fever Hospital, I have not seen nor heard of one exception having occurred among fatal cases to the rule, that fever, accompanied by the rose spots, is also attended by disease of Peyer's patches and the mesenteric glands, and that fever, with mulberry rash, offers, after death, no lesion of the same organs.

principal features of that disease in a severe form, with the pathological appearances usually observed in the uncomplicated disease; and, finally, to illustrate the various anomalies and complications of that disease, incidentally referring to the treatment.

For the accuracy of the facts and observations, and for the soundness of the opinions expressed, I am alone responsible. The treatment of the cases has been conducted by the Physicians of the Hospital, Dr. A. Tweedie and Dr. Southward Smith.

§ 1. TYPICAL CASES OF TYPHUS FEVER.

CASE I.—Shortly after exposure to the contagion from a person suffering from fever, accompanied with mulberry rash, and without lesion of Peyer's patches, as proved by examination after death:

Ensued:—Sudden debility—headache — rigors — constipated bowels—mulberry rash—mental confusion—delirium —dry, brown tongue—extreme prostration—rapid pulse— death on the thirteenth day.

Thirty-six hours after death.—Persistence of spots noted during life—Partial loss of cadaveric rigidity—Congestion of the brain and pia mater—Blood beneath the lining membrane of pharynx—Intestinal mucous membrane normal— Mesenteric glands healthy—Liver flabby—Spleen softened— Lungs intensely congested posteriorly—Heart flabby.

J. M., a locksmith, aged from 65 to 70, an aged-looking, thin man, with grey hair, was admitted into the London Fever Hospital, February 1, 1849, under the care of Dr. Tweedie. His residence was an empty house, of which he had charge, 14 London Street, Islington. He had been in the habit of visiting a family named Penny, who lived about one mile from his home. Two of these people were admitted into this hospital a little while since, with well-marked symptoms of typhus fever. The father, aged 46, died, and Peyer's patches and the mesenteric glands were healthy. The son, aged 15, is still in this hospital; he, too, had well-marked mulberry rash. This man, J. M., cleaned out the house of the Pennys, which was in a most filthy state, the week before his present illness commenced. He is of sober habits, but has lately suffered from great want.

January 25, 1849, he was suddenly seized about 3 P.M., with a sense of weariness, pain in his limbs, headache, rigors, and chillness. His bowels were confined, so that he took two doses of calomel, 5 grains each, an aperient draught, and some jalap. He took to his bed on the first day of his illness and has not left it since. His wife, from whom this history was obtained, noticed his mind to wander three days before his admission. He had had no epistaxis. The following was his state when the first notes of his case were made, on the eleventh day of disease :—

He had passed a very restless night, and had but little sleep. He was dozing at the time of the visit, talking in his sleep. There was twitching during sleep of the muscles of the face, arms, and neck. His mind, when he awoke, was found to be very confused. He had no idea where he was, nor how long he had been in the hospital; but he knew those around him. His complexion was particularly muddy. His face was pale ; there was no increased vascularity of the conjunctivæ, and the pupils were natural. He was quite unable to leave his bed unassisted, and even turned with some difficulty. His lips were dry ; the tongue dry and covered with dark brown rough fur. His bowels confined for the two days preceding his admission, had acted twice since from castor oil; there was no appetite, some thirst, no fulness, resonance, tenderness, nor gurgling of the abdomen. The pulse was 120; very weak. There was much cough ; the respiration was 30, and quiet. He expectorated a little frothy, tenacious mucus.

Physical chest signs.—Some slight want of resonance posteriorly over the most depending part of lungs. At the same place was heard unequal, coarse, sub-mucous rale, and breath sound appeared as if muffled.

The skin was warm, dry, and spotted.

The spots were very numerous, and there was an abundant subcuticular rash; some of the spots faded on pressure, others were unaffected, none disappeared, none were elevated. They were darker in hue on the back than elsewhere. The dorsum generally was much congested ; there were no miliary vesicles.

Gin, 4 oz.; mist. am. carb. 4tis horis; jus bov. On the 12th day the pulse had risen to 160, and was very weak ; the respiration was 36. He had passed a very restless night ; lay night and day with his eyes open muttering unintelligibly. The expression of prostration was much more marked, and he turned in bed with great difficulty. He opened his mouth when told to show his tongue, but made no effort to protrude it. The twitching of the muscles continued,—the conjunctivæ were considerably more injected than natural.

The gin was increased to 6 oz. He died at 3 A.M. on the 4th of February, *i.e.* the 13th day of disease.

The body was examined 36 hours after death, and the following appearances noted :—

Cadaveric rigidity disappearing from upper extremities still tolerably marked in the knees and toes. Abdomen concave. Some greenish discolouration of the flanks and abdominal parietes. Scattered over the whole surface of the trunk and extremities were numerous purplish spots (*i.e.* those noted during life). The posterior surface of the body was much discoloured. The spots above referred to were on the discoloured parts darker than elsewhere.

Head.—There was considerable subarachnoid effusion. Opacity and thickening of the arachnoid, especially over the anterior lobe. The pia mater was congested. The arachnoid and pia mater separated in one mass from the convolutions, and without removing any of the grey matter. There was a little serosity in the lateral ventricles, and about 1 ounce at the base of the brain. The red points throughout the grey and white matter were more numerous than usual. The substance of the brain, including the central parts, was firm.

The *tongue* was covered with dry brown mucus. The *pharynx* was pale, and there was a little effused blood beneath the mucous membrane of the uvula. The *œsophagus* was dusky purple. The cartilages of the *larynx* were ossified ; its lining membrane was pale. The mucous membrane of the trachea was pale and healthy.

There was no fluid in either pleura.

The *left lung* was bound by old adhesions at the apex to the costal pleura ; it contained several cretaceous masses. The posterior part of the inferior lobe contained *much* frothy, dirty, reddish serosity ; most abundant in the *most depending part.* The texture of this part was softened, its colour *dark* brownish red.

The *right lung* was united to the costal pleura by universal old adhesions ; it generally resembled the left.

The bronchial tubes contained much frothy mucus ; their mucous membrane was dusky red ; its thickness and consistence appeared natural.

The *pericardium* contained about 1 drachm of transparent yellow serosity. The heart was slightly enlarged ; its lining membrane was stained on the right side. The valves were healthy, the substance flabby.

Much dark fluid blood, and some loose black coagula escaped from the venæ cavæ and pulmonary veins. Tha right auricle and ventricle, and the left auricle, were distended with black loosely coagulated blood ; the left ventricle contained a little fluid blood.

In the pulmonary artery and aorta respectively was a smooth clot moulded to the sigmoid valves.

The pyloric half of the lining membrane of the *stomach* was covered with thick mucus. There was no mammillation of that membrane, the consistence and thickness of which was natural. Its colour was *pale* dusky red. The colour, consistence, and thickness of the mucous membrane of the *small and large* intestines was natural throughout. Peyer's patches were very indistinct. There was no enlargement of the mesenteric glands.

The *liver* was flabby, otherwise normal. The *gall bladder* was distended with thick dark greenish bile; its lining membrane appeared healthy.

The *pancreas* was pale and healthy.

The *spleen* weighed 8 oz., and was very much softened; rapidly becoming pulpy on exposure.

The kidneys were healthy in appearance.

The urinary bladder was not examined.

CASE II.—After exposure to the contagion of fever, accompanied with mulberry-rash, and without lesion of Peyer's patches, as proved by examination after death:

Ensued:—Sudden frontal headache—loss of appetite—extreme chilliness—bowels regular—very scanty epistaxis—mulberry rash—little loss of strength till ninth day, then sudden and extreme prostration—mental confusion—somnolence—delirium—dry brown tongue—absence of abdominal symptoms—quick pulse—profuse sweats—death on the fourteenth day.

Twenty-nine hours after death:—Persistence of spots noted during life—marked cadaveric rigidity—clots in the cavity of the arachnoid—congestion of the pia mater and cerebral substance—intense congestion of the most depending part of the lungs—heart flabby—absence of intestinal and mesenteric lesion — liver flabby—spleen softened—separation from basement membrane of the epithelium of œsophagus, kidneys and bladder.

George W., aged 49, a native of London, a labourer in the docks, was admitted into the London Fever Hospital, August 15th, 1849, under the care of Dr. Tweedie. A thin man, with light hair and eyes, and fair skin. His wife was received into the hospital at the same time with himself.[1] He stated that his previous health had been very good, that he had never been confined to his bed before. He affirmed that he was of temperate habits, but this was doubtful.

Present Illness.—About 3 P.M. on Friday, August 10th, 1849, he was seized with frontal headache. On the following day his appetite failed him, and the pain in the head increased in severity. On the 3rd day he complained of chilliness, and felt so cold that he 'could have crept into the fire.' He lost a few drops of blood from the nose as he came to the hospital on the 15th. His bowels were regular from the outset, and there had been no vomiting.

Present Symptoms.—August 16th, 7th day of disease. He slept well last night (*i.e.* first night in the hospital). His mental powers appear unaffected. The expression of his countenance is nearly natural. He complains of much frontal headache; there is a little vertigo. His special senses are unaffected. The conjunctivæ are somewhat more injected than natural; the pupils are normal.

He walked up stairs on admission last evening unassisted, and now leaves his bed with facility. His position in bed is unconstrained.

His tongue is white, and rather dry in the centre. He has passed, since his admission, four formed stools. He has trifling pain about the umbilicus. There is no fulness, resonance, tenderness, nor gurgling of abdomen.

The pulse, 96, is full and soft. There is no cough. The physical chest signs are normal.

The skin is warm, dry, and spotted. The spots are not very numerous on the trunk, but are found in greater number on the extremities. They are not elevated; some disappear; some *fade only* on pressure. Those on the fore-arm and backs of the hands are larger and of a brighter hue than elsewhere; the large majority of these disappear on pressure.

Mist. am. acet.; jus bov.

On the 8th day somnolence commenced; at the same time his mind became dull and his memory defective; his estimate of time being prolonged. The somnolence and mental confusion increased. On the 10th day he complained that he felt his mind was wandering, that he had '*appeared* to travel hundreds of thousands of miles during the night.' There was no actual delirium at this time. He knew the name of the day on which

---

[1] This woman's case is detailed subsequently (Case XXI. p. 234). She laboured under well-marked typhus fever, and died on about the twenty-eighth day from the outset of her illness.

he entered the hospital, but thought he had been in eight instead of five days. The conjunctivæ were at this time considerably injected, and the somnolence was almost constant. On the 11th day he was delirious night and day when aroused from somnolence; the stools and urine were passed into bed.

The somnolence was less constant on the 12th day. The pulse, 96 on the 8th day, was 108 on the 9th, and 120 on the 10th day, which rate of frequency it maintained till the last note was taken on the 13th day.

His tongue on the 9th day was dry brown, and continued unchanged in appearance till his death. He left his bed with difficulty unassisted on the 9th day, but on the 11th day he could scarcely turn without aid. On the 12th day he appeared somewhat improved, less somnolent, and more sensible, for he asked to be assisted on to the close pan. He turned in bed also, unassisted, at will. His bowels continued regular, acting twice daily. The stools were solid. The following notes were made on the afternoon of 13th day of disease, i.e. that preceding his death:—

'Pulse 120, extremely weak. He is sweating profusely. The nurse states that he has perspired so much that his clothes have been soaked through. The skin is cool; the spots are well out, and little affected by pressure on the back. The backs of the hands have a somewhat livid hue. He slept little during the night, but has dozed the greater part of to-day. He is delirious when awake. The conjunctivæ are injected, the left very much less so than the right. He opens his mouth when told to show his tongue, but makes no effort to protrude it. He is unable to move unassisted in bed. There is some catching of the hands, and *subsultus tendinum*.'

He has passed two watery stools into bed.

The treatment adopted was stimulant. On the 8th day of disease 8 oz. of porter was administered; on the 9th it was increased to a pint. 4 oz. of gin were added on the 10th day, and carbonate of ammonia, in doses of 5 gr., was administered every four hours in addition to the other stimulants on the 11th day.

He sank gradually, and died at 10 A.M. on the 23rd August, i.e. the 14th day of disease.

The body of George Warren was examined at 3 P.M., August 24th, i.e. twenty-nine hours after death.

Height, 5 ft. 5 in.; length of trunk, 21½ in.; breadth of shoulders, 15 in.

The cadaveric rigidity was well marked. Numerous purplish spots, the remains of those observed during life, were visible on the anterior surface. The posterior surface of the trunk and extremities were of a port-wine hue, dotted over with spots of a much deeper colour, the latter the remains of spots seen before death. The discoloration gradually faded as it approached the anterior surface. The parietes of the iliac fossæ were of a very pale greenish hue; the abdomen concave. The muscles were dark; there was about half an inch of fat on the walls of the abdomen.

Head.—The dura mater appeared normal. On the convex surface of the right hemisphere of the brain, within the cavity of the arachnoid, near the junction of the anterior and middle lobes, and about 1½ inch from the longitudinal fissure, was a crimson and black clot (*i.e.* its colour varied with its thickness), thin, flat, about an inch in diameter. A similar clot was found between the anterior lobe and the *falx cerebri.* Over the convex surface of the left hemisphere, also within the cavity of the arachnoid, were scattered six clots, each about the size of split peas. A little bloody serosity escaped on dividing the dura mater. The arachnoid covering the convex surface, especially of the middle lobes of the brain, was considerably thickened, and had a milky, semiopaque appearance. There was a little colourless serosity beneath the arachnoid, slightly elevating that membrane at places, and also infiltrating the pia mater. There was considerable injection of that membrane between the cerebral convolutions. The arachnoid and pia mater separated from the cerebral surface *in one mass*: no portion of the grey matter, however, came away with them. The grey matter of the convolutions had a pinkish hue, more marked next the white substance than on the free surface. The red points in the white substance were rather more numerous than is normal. The lateral ventricles contained about one drachm of transparent, colourless serosity. The vessels of the plexus choroides and the venæ corp. atriat. were distended with blood. The cerebral substance, including the commissura mollis [1] and other central parts, was of good consistence. About half an ounce of serosity was found at the base of the skull, but no clots.

The *tongue* was pale brown, and covered, as was the *velum pend. palati*, with thick mucus.

The *pharynx, œsophagus, larynx,* and *trachea*, were healthy in appearance, but there was no trace of epithelium on the œsophagus, and the larynx contained some thick mucus.

There was no fluid in either *pleura*.

The apex of the left lung was firmly adherent to the costal pleura, and in the substance of the apex were several collections of mortar-like matter.

---

[1] When examining the brain I have always noted the consistence of the commissura mollis, because that is one of the first parts of the organ to suffer from cadaveric softening.

The posterior portion of the inferior lobe was of a deep brownish-purple colour, and gave exit, on section, to a considerable quantity of red, slightly aerated serosity; on pressure this fluid gushed out. The pulmonary tissue was, however, crepitant, and floated in water. The most depending parts were the deepest in hue and contained the least air. The anterior portion of the lung was pale and somewhat emphysematous.

The right lung resembled the left in all particulars, except that the congestion of the posterior part of the inferior lobe was more marked; and here and there, from its most depending part, very small pieces could be cut which sank in water; there was no line of demarcation between the consolidated and non-consolidated tissue; the latter sank in water when slightly pressed before immersion.

The bronchial tubes contained very little mucus; their lining membrane was of a dull red colour.

There was no enlargement of the bronchial glands.

The pericardium appeared healthy; it contained about three drachms of transparent yellow serosity.

The *heart*, slightly enlarged, was very flabby, both sides being equally affected. The endocardium was stained of a dull reddish colour. The right auricle and ventricle contained a moderate-sized, black, and soft fibrinous clot. The left side of the heart was empty. The valves were healthy. Some fluid dark blood, and two or three very small loose black clots, escaped from the venæ cavæ and pulmonary veins when the heart was removed.

The mucous membrane of the *stomach* was mammillated throughout, from cardiac orifice to pylorus, excepting only a narrow band along the smaller curvature. There were numerous rugæ along the greater curvature. The consistence of the mucous membrane was firm; its thickness somewhat increased. Strips of half an inch were readily obtained from the anterior surface of the stomach, and seven-eighths from the great cul-de-sac. Its colour throughout was a delicate, pale, yellowish red grey.

The *small* and *large intestines* were pale and healthy in consistence. Strips of mucous membrane, of ordinary length, were readily obtained.

Peyer's patches were normal in appearance. The mucous membrane covering them was of good consistence. The mesenteric glands were scarcely visible.

The *liver* was very flabby, and tore with facility. It was of a pale yellowish liver colour.

The gall bladder contained about half an ounce of exceedingly thick bile, green in mass. Its lining membrane appeared normal.

The *spleen* weighed seven and a half ounces. It was decidedly softened.

The *pancreas* was pale and healthy.

The *kidneys* were healthy. A milky fluid was expressed from the mammilla. The mucous membrane of the urinary bladder was somewhat congested posteriorly. It contained about half an ounce of milky fluid.

The turbidity of the fluid expressed from the kidneys, and of that contained in the bladder, was due to the large number of epithelium scales they contained. Those in the fluid from the bladder were evidently detached from the lining membrane of that organ.

CASE III.—After exposure to the contagion of fever, accompanied by mulberry rash :

Ensued :—Sudden attack of pain in limbs—Severe rigors —Heat of Skin—Slight headache—Some loss of mental power—Sudden debility—Bowels regular—Frequent vomiting—Muddy hue of face—Mulberry rash—Tongue somewhat dry and brown—Pulse quick—Absence of abdominal signs —Deafness, twelfth day—Marked improvement on thirteenth day—Recovery—Death on about fortieth day from small-pox.

J. H., aged 26, an agricultural labourer, not in want of food, but residing in a crowded small room, at Islington, was admitted into the London Fever Hospital, November 3rd, 1848, under the care of Dr. Tweedie. His brother was received into the hospital at the same time, labouring under typhus fever, and covered with well-marked mulberry rash. He was a strong-made, moderately stout, dark man, who had never suffered a day's illness till the present attack.

On Saturday, October the 28th, 1848, he was seized with pains in the limbs, severe rigors, several times repeated, and each time followed by heat of skin, but there was no sweating ; there was, at the same time, slight frontal headache. He vomited several times before his admission. His bowels were regular from the outset. He took to his bed on the Sunday morning, because he ' felt too ill and weak to keep about.'

The following note was made on the 8th day of disease :— ' He slept well last night. The mind is dull, the expression heavy ; the face is dusky red, and has a somewhat muddy aspect. There is no headache nor delirium. He suffers from vertigo when in the erect position. The conjunctivæ are very much injected, the pupils natural. With the exception of a bitter taste, and a sense of unpleasant odour, there is no affection of the special senses.'

His position in bed is unconstrained, but he leaves it unassisted, with great difficulty.

His lips are dry; there are sordes on the teeth; the tongue is covered with a thick white fur,—its border and tip are red. There is complete loss of appetite; the thirst is considerable. He passed three stools this morning, after a dose of castor-oil. There is neither fulness, resonance, tenderness, nor gurgling of the abdomen. The pulse was 120 of moderate power. There was a little cough, and he had expectorated since his admission about two drachms of mucus, streaked with bright blood. There were no abnormal physical chest-signs.

The skin was hot, dry, and spotted. The spots were numerous; some obscure, others well marked. They were of irregular shape; the majority faded; a few disappeared on pressure.

Abrad. Capill.: Mist. am. acet.; jus bov.

The notes made on the 9th and 10th days show but little change in his condition. On the 11th day, the spots were observed to be decidedly darker in hue, and less affected by pressure. He moaned much in his sleep, and his tongue was dry in the centre. On the 12th day there was slight deafness, and the pulse fell from 120 to 108; but the tongue was rather tremulous, and the skin continued, as from the first, hot and dry, and the conjunctivæ much injected.

On the 13th day, a decided improvement took place, the pulse had fallen at the time of the visit to 96; the skin was warm and soft, the complexion clearer, the tongue steady, the conjunctivæ less vascular, and the spots paler. On the following day the pulse again fell to 76, the tongue began to clear, the appetite had partially returned, the conjunctivæ were pale, and of the spots merely a trace remained, in the form of a brownish stain; but, at the same time, the deafness increased. This, however, disappeared in about three days, and his appetite was so good that he was placed on convalescent diet. He continued to gain strength for ten days, when he was suddenly seized with rigors, vomiting, etc.; and in three days an eruption of small-pox pustules appeared. He was removed into the Small-pox Hospital. He had the disease in the confluent form, and died in about eight days.

Through the kindness of the medical officers of the institution, I was permitted to examine the body. It is sufficient to observe that the intestinal canal and mesenteric glands were quite free from any trace of lesion. The agminated glands were carefully examined, and I am certain no remains of cicatrisation could have escaped observation.

CASE IV.—After exposure to the contagion of fever, accompanied with mulberry rash, and without lesion of Peyer's patches, as proved by examination after death:

Ensued :—Headache—pain in the limbs—delirium — somewhat relaxed bowels—absence of abdominal signs— quick pulse—mulberry rash—deafness on the 15th day —Convalescence on the 16th day.

Thomas B., aged 6, a moderately stout fair child, was admitted into the London Fever Hospital, April 30th, 1849, under the care of Dr. Tweedie.

His mother, brother, and the nurse of his mother, were all received into the hospital the same week, and all had the mulberry rash.

His present illness commenced on the 20th April, with headache and pains in the limbs. Delirium was observed on the 8th day of the disease. His bowels were relaxed (from medicine?) for the four days preceding his entrance into the hospital.

The following notes were made when I first saw him on the eleventh day of disease :—He is very delirious, screaming and crying. He says that he has no pain in his head. The complexion is thick, and there is a mottled appearance of the face, as if from eruption seen through the cuticle. There is no running from the eyes nor nose. He can just stand alone, but staggers a little. His tongue is slightly furred, and dry in the centre. He has passed no stool since his admission this morning. There is no appetite, and but little thirst. The abdomen is free from pain, tenderness, or gurgling. The pulse is 120; rather weak; there is no cough, and no abnormal physical chest-signs.

The skin is warm and dry. The trunk and extremities are covered with roundish dusky red spots, not elevated above the surrounding skin, which fade on pressure, and an abundant sub-cuticular rash. There are no miliary vesicles.

Mist. am. acet. : jus bov.

The delirium continued the two following days, and he passed restless nights. The mulberry rash was much paler on the 15th day; there was a little appetite, and, on the same day, slight deafness was observed for the first time. The tongue, dry and brown in the centre on the fourteenth day, was moist and clean on the fifteenth. The bowels acted twice daily; the stools were not watery. The pulse continued at 120 till the 16th day of disease, when the following note marked his convalescence.

Pulse 96. He slept well; tongue is moist and clean; appetite returning; one stool; no abnormal abdominal signs; skin cool, soft. Spots *scarcely* visible.

I would here direct particular attention to a few points connected with the four cases above detailed.

1st. The ages of the patients were respectively, seventy, forty-nine, twenty-six, and six years; *i.e.* there was about twenty years difference in the ages of each of the four cases.

2nd. Each case was clearly and indisputably traceable to contagion as a highly probable exciting cause.

3rd. These cases agree with each other, and with those from which they caught the disease in the presence of the diagnostic symptom, *i.e.* the mulberry rash, and in the absence of the anatomical character of typhoid fever, *i.e.* of lesion of Peyer's patches, and enlargement of the mesenteric glands.

4th. These four cases further agree with each other in the duration of the disease under which they laboured.

5th. The two patients who died during the course of .the fever, offered no lesion after death to account for the fatal termination ; the patient who fell a victim to small-pox presented no trace of lesion referable to the fever; and the child who recovered exhibited no symptoms that could lead us to suppose that any one organ suffered in such a manner, as that if the child had died, serious structural change would have been seen on examination of the body after death.

Having detailed four cases of uncomplicated typhus fever, which might be regarded as models of that disease, I shall now give a general description of typhus fever in its severe form, before considering the special symptoms on the varying severity of which the modifications the disease exhibits chiefly depend.

§ 2. GENERAL DESCRIPTION OF THE SYMPTOMS AND PATHOLOGICAL APPEARANCES OBSERVED IN TYPHUS FEVER.

Typhus fever attacks persons of both sexes and of all ages, from early infancy to extreme old age.

After a few days' trifling sense of languor, or slight malaise of mind and body, the patient is seized, more or less suddenly, with rigors and chilliness, usually followed by heat of skin, and occasionally by sweating; pains in the back and limbs, and frontal headache. The rigors and sense of chilliness are in many cases repeated, at irregular intervals, for two or three days. The patient hovers over the fire one hour, although his skin may at the time feel hot to his attendant, and the next hour complains of the heat of the room; or when near the fire feels hot and oppressed, when away chilly and uncomfortable. The appetite is lost, and there is frequently more or less thirst from the outset; the tongue is white, large, and pale, and often slightly tremulous;[1] the bowels confined or regular; the urine rather scanty and high-coloured; nausea and vomiting are often among the earliest symptoms. There is total want of sleep, or, on the contrary, heaviness and drowsiness. Sleep, if it occurs, is disturbed by dreams, or interrupted every few minutes by sudden starts, is unrefreshing. The sick man frequently declares that he has 'not had a wink of sleep,' when those watching testify that he has slept for hours.[2] Unable to think or to fix his attention, he feels 'downright ill,' and so extremely weak, that, however pressing the calls for his exertion, the patient usually takes to his bed by the second or third day, and not unfrequently on the first. There is both absolute loss of muscular power, and an almost intolerable sense of exhaustion; the latter being at first, perhaps, out of proportion to the former. Vertigo and noise in the ears are frequently among the earliest and most loudly complained of symptoms, especially the former. The debility increases rapidly, so that by the seventh day the patient can rarely leave his bed without some assistance. By this time, if not before, the muscular movements are unsteady, the raised arm shakes, and the protruded tongue trembles. The inability to fix the thoughts soon passes into defect of memory;[3] this into delirium, at first between waking and sleeping, then by night; and finally

[1] The early loss of muscular power, of which the tremulous tongue is one example, is a symptom of grave import so far as concerns the prognosis. In no disease is the effect of previous habits of intemperance more clearly seen, in causing muscular tremors, than in typhus fever.

[2] This fancied wakefulness has been erroneously termed *coma vigil.*

[3] It is a singular fact, that the patient invariably supposes time to be prolonged; thus, if taken ill on a Monday, he will say, on the Monday succeeding, that he has been ill ten or twelve days, or perhaps weeks, and never assert that his illness has lasted only four or five days. At the same time

by night and day. When delirium first sets in, the patient is able to correct himself, *i.e.* on thinking he becomes conscious of his mental error, but this power is soon lost, and he believes in the existence of all the phantasma his imagination conjures up, or his erring senses paint.

The headache ceases on from the 7th to the 10th day of disease; if not before, almost invariably as soon as delirium commences.[1]

About the 5th or 6th day an eruption appears on the skin; at first consisting of numerous roundish, slightly elevated, dusky pink spots effaceable on pressure by the finger, quickly resuming their colour, however, when the finger is removed; on the 2nd or 3rd day after their appearance, these spots, instead of being effaced, merely fade, *i.e.* grow paler, on pressure. At the same time, with the spots referred to, there is present a much paler rash, which appears to be seen through the cuticle, as if the spots composing it were, as the vulgar say, 'not well out.' The latter is the subcuticular rash, the whole eruption the mulberry rash.

[NOTE.—As a clear perception of the characters of the eruption in typhus fever is of the highest moment in forming a diagnosis, attention is especially directed to the following particulars :—Seen on about 9th day, the patient in a well-marked case of typhus fever appears covered with a dusky red rash, having somewhat the hue of mulberry stains. On more minute inspection, and careful watching from its commencement to its disappearance, the rash is found to be divisible into two parts :—

---

he may, and generally does remember the name of the day on which he was taken ill, or on which any given event happened. If the medical attendant tells the patient that any given day is Wednesday, if he asks, at his visit on the following day, 'How long is it since you saw me?' the sick man will probably answer, 'three or four days;' but, if he asks, 'On what day did you see me last?' he will probably be answered correctly, 'on Wednesday,' especially if any event occurred at the first visit to make an impression on the patient.

[1] This is a point of great practical importance, for if headache is voluntarily complained of by the patient, or even if declared to be severe in answer to the question of the physician, after delirium has commenced, strong suspicions, to say the least, of inflammatory action within the cranium should be entertained, and remedies adopted in accordance with that view of the case. While headache, before delirium has commenced, is in itself not the slightest proof of increased vascular action within the cranial cavity.

I. DISTINCT SPOTS.

Each spot passes through three stages. *First stage.*—On their first appearance the spots have a dusky pinkish hue, and are very slightly elevated. They vary in size from a point to three or four lines in diameter. They are somewhat flattened on the surface, and have an irregular outline. They have no well-defined margin, but pass insensibly into the hue of the surrounding skin. They disappear on pressure, but resume their characteristic appearance as soon as the pressure is removed. The largest spots appear to be formed by the coalescence of two or more smaller, and the shape of the former is, as a consequence, more irregular than that of the latter. *Second stage.*—In from one to three days the spots undergo a marked change; they are no longer elevated above the level of the surrounding cuticle; their hue grows darker and more dingy; and instead of disappearing, they only fade on pressure, *i.e.* when the finger is firmly pressed on them they grow paler, but do not entirely disappear. In some cases the spots, after reaching this stage, pass into very faintly marked, reddish-brown stains, and then disappear. *Third stage.*—In other cases the spots reach a third stage; their centres become dark purple, and are unaltered in appearance by the firmest pressure, although their circumferences still fade; or the entire spots, circumference as well as centre, change into petechiæ.[1] A few may be found in the third stage, while the majority are in the second.[2] The spots are generally very numerous on the trunk and extremities, but occasionally there are very few. They are rarely seen on the face. Their number reaches its maximum on the 2nd or 3rd day at latest. Each spot remains from its first eruption till the disease terminates, excepting a few large almost scarlet patches, occasionally seen on the back of the hand, on the 5th or 6th day of the disease, which usually disappear altogether in a day or two.

II. THE SUBCUTICULAR RASH.

When the rash is very abundant, usually many of the spots are pale, imperfectly marked, and run into each other; these spots are seen indistinctly, as if situated beneath the cuticle. They often give to the skin a mottled aspect, and on this mottled surface, which I have termed the subcuticular rash, as on a ground, the darker, more distinct spots are situated.

The appearance of the rash in typhus fever varies, then,

[1] By petechiæ I mean spots not elevated above the cuticle; of a dusky crimson or purple colour, quite unaffected by pressure, with well-defined margins.

[2] I have sometimes observed the spots to possess the characters of the second or third stage on their first appearance.

according to the number of the spots, their stage, the abundance of the subcuticular rash, and the depth of colour of either. Sometimes there is present only a faint subcuticular rash, sometimes only a few well-marked spots; or again, the subcuticular rash may be abundant, the well-marked spots few in number, or the latter may be very numerous, and the former all but absent. For the whole eruption I have elsewhere (see *Monthly Journal*, April 1849) proposed the term *mulberry rash*, and by that term I shall designate the eruption characteristic of typhus fever in these pages.]

The skin throughout the course of the disease is often particularly sensitive, the lightest touch occasioning pain. At the termination of the first, or at the commencement of the second week, the tongue grows dry in the centre, and at the same time its white fur is replaced by pale dirty brown mucus. Usually about the 9th or 10th day, but sometimes much earlier, the delirium becomes decided, although the attention may still be fixed by a sharp question. At this time the patient is in some cases violent, and, unless restrained, leaves his bed to wander about the room. The expression, which at first was simply indicative of languor, weariness, or of a semi-drowsy condition, resembling that of a man unwilling to be aroused from half-drunken slumbers is now that of complete stupidity and decided prostration. The complexion, which from the first was thick and dirty, in the course of the second week becomes absolutely muddy; the conjunctivæ injected, and the pupils contracted. The face is now often flushed, the flush being dingy and pretty uniform over the whole face; occasionally, however, somewhat more marked on the cheeks than elsewhere. The eruption grows darker in hue, the centres of many of the spots towards the termination of the second week, are unaffected by pressure, and here and there are to be seen some spots with well-defined outline, quite unalterable in appearance by the firmest pressure of the finger, i.e. true petechiæ. The posterior surface of the trunk is considerably congested, and the spots are there much darker and less affected by pressure than on the anterior surface.

About the 10th or 11th day, somnolence sets in and gradually passes into stupor and even coma, when the expression indicates profound prostration. The patient lies on his back unable to turn or assist himself in the slightest degree, and the urine is often passed involuntarily, or is retained, requiring the use of the catheter for its removal. The tongue is thickly coated, dry and dark brown, or even black, appearing as if baked; perhaps unable to be protruded; the teeth are covered with sordes; the patient is unable to be roused for more than a minute or two, and then mutters incoherently; the conjunctivæ are intensely injected, and the pupils contracted; the skin is cool, and occasionally moist; miliary vesicles, or sudamina, are sometimes observed about the end of the second week; usually in the groins, at the epigastrium, and under the clavicles.[1] The abdomen continues flaccid and indolent throughout. The bowels usually act once or twice a day, the stools being somewhat relaxed.

The pulse, from the outset of the disease, is quickened, and it increases in rapidity until the disease terminates fatally; or, after reaching a certain point, its frequency as gradually subsides till health is restored. A little cough and some sonorous râle are now and then present.

The disease generally terminates, if it proves fatal, from the twelfth to the twentieth day.[2] Before death the prostration increases to the last degree; *subsultus tendinum*, or perhaps involuntary twitching of the muscles of the face and arms make their appearance; the face becomes dusky or even livid; the breathing very quick; the pulse so rapid and feeble that it can scarcely be felt, or, it may be, quite imperceptible; some want of resonance of the most dependent part of the chest may often be observed at this stage of the disease; the respiratory murmur at the same part appears muffled, as if heard through a thick veil, and there is sometimes a little coarse unequal crepitation. The urine, which is secreted in large quantities—from three to four pints daily,—is retained,

[1] My impression is that sudamina are rarely if ever seen on patients more than fifty years of age.

[2] The question of critical days is not here considered. It requires for its solution a most careful analysis of numerous fatal and non-fatal, complicated and uncomplicated cases. The uncomplicated cases must evidently be analysed separately from the complicated, because the latter are often protracted long after the fever has run its course, or are cut short by the severity of the local disease almost irrespective of the fever. Ordinary hospital records, from the little trouble taken to fix the day on which the disease commences, are obviously of no avail in settling a question of so much delicacy as the one to which I here refer.

or passed into bed with the stools involuntarily. The skin
at this time is often bathed in a profuse sweat, the temperature being below the natural standard; the spots are scarcely,
or not at all, affected by pressure, especially on the dorsum;
the whole skin of the posterior surface of the trunk is deeply
congested. The patient lies on his back unable to move, or
he sinks, if his head be at all elevated, towards the bottom of
the bed. A slough frequently forms about the middle or the
end of the second week on the lower end of the spine or on
the posterior spine of the ilium.

Occasionally for a day or two before the fatal termination
of the disease, the condition termed *coma vigil* is observed.

A person labouring under *coma vigil* presents a very
peculiar appearance. He never sleeps. He lies on his back
with his eyelids widely separated; his eyes, staring and fixed
on vacuity; his mouth partially open; his face pale and
expressionless. He is totally incapable of being roused to
give a sign of consciousness; the breathing is often scarcely
perceptible; the pulse rapid and feeble, or unable to be felt;
the skin cool, perhaps bathed in perspiration. Life is only
known to have ceased by the eye losing its little lustre, and
the chest ceasing its slow and feeble movements. I have
never seen recovery from absolute *coma vigil.*

If, instead of death, the disease terminates in recovery,
the improvement in the condition of the patient is frequently
sudden. On from the thirteenth to the seventeenth day he
falls into a profound quiet sleep, and after from twelve to
twenty-four, or even more, hours, awakes decidedly improved
in all respects. The complexion is clearer; the delirium has
disappeared; the pulse fallen in frequency; the conjunctivæ
are no longer injected; the tongue is moist at the edges;
there is perhaps a little appetite; the skin is softer; the spots
paler; the general powers improved. In a few days the
tongue cleans, the appetite becomes ravenous, and the patient
rapidly regains strength.

APPEARANCES FOUND AFTER DEATH FROM UNCOMPLI-
CATED TYPHUS FEVER.

The cadaveric rigidity disappears shortly after death. The posterior surfaces of the trunk and extremities are of a deep port-wine colour; the abdominal parietes rapidly assume a greenish hue, and the course of the large superficial veins in the neck, arms, and lower extremities is often marked by lines of a dusky, dirty violet colour. If miliary vesicles formed during the last days of life, they are still seen.

On the surface of the trunk and extremities are found the remains of the spots noted during life. If the spots were before death rendered paler on pressure, they are less distinctly marked, and have a less deep hue than during life; if they were unaffected by pressure, they retain the exact appearance they presented before death. Those on the most depending part of the subject are by far the deepest in hue.

If a portion of the skin is removed and examined with a lens, the persistence of the spots, which faded or grew paler on pressure is found to be due to staining of the surface of the cutis; while the whole of that texture, and even the sub-cutaneous tissue, is dyed deep purple, in those spots which were unaffected by pressure during life.

There is usually a moderate amount of serosity beneath the arachnoid, and in the meshes of the pia mater; and considerable congestion of the latter membrane, especially between the convolutions. The sinuses and larger vessels are filled with dark fluid blood. The arachnoid and pia mater separate with abnormal facility, and in much larger portions than natural, from the convex surface of the brain. Both membranes may generally be removed in an unbroken mass. The red points in the grey and white substance are rather more numerous, and larger than is usual after death from other diseases. The amount of fluid in the lateral ventricles and at the base of the brain is slightly increased. The consistence of the brain is nearly natural.

The pharynx and larynx are normal. The œsophagus is healthy, but its epithelium is found in a great measure detached. The mesenteric glands retain their normal appearance. The mucous membrane of the cardiac extremity of the stomach, nay, the whole of its coats in that part, are frequently softened, and the entire lining membrane is smooth, presenting but few rugæ: in other particulars, the organ appears to possess the characters of health. The intestines, large and small, are normal in colour, thickness, and consistence; the liver moderately congested and flabby; the pancreas in a similar condition; the spleen varies somewhat in its state, according to the age of the subject; before forty-five or fifty it is usually much enlarged; after that date it is still often enlarged, but not so markedly as in the earlier period of life. Softening of this organ appears to follow the reverse order, as it is softer in aged than in young subjects.

The kidneys are congested and flabby, and the epithelium lining the tubes of their cortical substance separates from the basement spontaneously very shortly after death. The bladder is healthy, but a little turbid fluid is frequently formed in it; the turbidity is owing, in many cases, to a separation of the epithelium covering the mucous membrane of the organ.

The heart is particularly flabby; its contents are either fluid, or loosely coagulated black blood, and a small soft fibrinous clot stained reddish violet. The lungs are intensely congested posteriorly, and occasionally solidified at the same part. The solidified portion being that which, in the recumbent position, is the most dependent; the distance it extends into the lung varies from $\frac{1}{4}$ to $1\frac{1}{2}$ inch. It is tough, non-crepitant, non-granular and contains much dark reddish serosity. The crepitant portions adjacent are generally gorged with reddish frothy serosity. The bronchial tubes usually contain much frothy mucus, and their lining membrane is considerably congested. The bronchial glands appear healthy.

The peritoneum, pleuræ, and pericardium are normal in all particulars; but, if the examination after death has been delayed, the pericardium contains some red serosity; this red colour of the serosity is the consequence of transudation of a solution of the colouring matter of the blood. Large patches of epithelium may be detected by the microscope floating in it, but *no* blood corpuscles.

N

§ 3. EXAMINATION OF THE CONDITION, SYMPTOMS,
AND COMPLICATIONS ON THE VARIATIONS IN WHICH
THE DIFFERENCES OBSERVED IN INDIVIDUAL CASES
OF TYPHUS FEVER DEPEND.

AGE—ITS INFLUENCE ON THE COURSE AND SYMPTOMS.—
The model Cases I., II., III., IV. of typhus fever above
narrated were aged respectively 70, 49, 26, and 6 years,[1]
and I shall have repeatedly to detail or to refer to the
cases of individuals, whose ages respectively varied between 4 and 80 years. So far as personal observation
enables me to speak, without actual numbers, I cannot say
that either youth or age, as such, are predisposing causes of
typhus fever. But there are certain modifications in the
disease dependent apparently on age, which it will be well to
point out.

The mortality from typhus fever is much greater among
individuals at an advanced period of life than before forty. It
is rarely fatal till after puberty. The only cases under puberty
that I have examined after death, are detailed below (Cases v.,
VIII.). Both it will be observed proved fatal after the termination of the fever, from severe local complication set up during
the progress of the original disease, i.e. the typhus fever.

CASE V.—Well-marked mulberry rash—severe febrile
symptoms—sloughing of cornea—death either on or about
the twenty-second day of disease—*Twenty-six hours after
death* pus in right pleura—consolidation and circumscribed
gangrene of right lung—no trace of intestinal or mesenteric
lesion.

William L., aged 8 years, an extremely dark-complexioned
child, almost a mulatto—judging from his appearance, he had
some negro blood in his veins—was admitted into the London
Fever Hospital under the care of Dr. Tweedie, June 19th, 1847,
the fourth day of disease. On his admission the skin was free
from rash. I saw him twice only, and made no note of the case
during life, excepting so far as related to the eruption.

The mulberry rash, which by the termination of the first week
of the disease was well marked, and at the end of the second week

[1] Children under six years of age are not received into the London Fever
Hospital.

scarcely rendered paler by pressure, was by the nineteenth day very pale. From the notes of a friend I am able to state that the febrile symptoms were very severe, even before it is probable that the chest affection supervened. A few days before death, an aperture was formed in the inferior half of either cornea, about two lines in length and a line in breadth ; each aperture resulted from the separation of a slough. The irides protruded through the openings.

The following appearances were observed on examination of the body of W. L., twenty-six hours after death.—Great emaciation. The left pleura contained a little serosity. The left lung was free from adhesions. The lung itself, pale and crepitant anteriorly, was of a deep purple colour posteriorly. Here and there, from the posterior part of the inferior lobe, small portions of pulmonary tissue could be cut, which sank in water, contained no air, and broke down more readily than natural under pressure. This lobe contained about its centre two or three small masses of tubercle just commencing to soften.

The right pleura contained about 3 oz. of fluid resembling pus, of highly offensive odour.

The right lung was closely collapsed and corrugated externally, with the exceptions to be mentioned. The pulmonary pleura was opaque and dull white. From the centre of the closely collapsed superior lobe projected a mass about the size of half a pigeon's egg, firm and smooth; an equal quantity of the mass was buried in the substance of the lung. Its smoothness contrasted remarkably with the corrugated appearance of the lobe generally. On dividing this mass, its centre was found occupied by black semifluid matter of highly offensive odour. Stretching through the semifluid matter were delicate bands of some consistence. This absolutely gangrenous portion was about one inch in diameter; and was distinctly bounded by a border of soft white pulpy matter, rather less than a line in thickness. The pulmonary substance external to this white line was for some extent in every direction— soft dark purplish red, contained no air, and had a smooth and uniform section. The consolidated tissue extended outwards to the pleura.

Projecting from the inferior lobe was a prominence resembling externally that observed in the superior lobe; but on cutting into it some highly offensive gas escaped, and its anterior wall collapsed. In addition to the gas, this cavity contained some semifluid black matter and gangrenous shreds; the whole bounded by a white line similar to that described as bounding the gangrenous mass in the upper lobe. The external wall of the cavity was formed by little more than the pleura. On the free surface of the latter, corresponding with the centre of the cavity, was a black spot about the size of a split pea, with well-defined outline. There was no appearance of any attempt at the separation of this black spot from the surrounding pleura. In the vicinity of the last-described gangrenous mass were two smaller masses resembling it in appearance.

The heart, liver, spleen, pancreas, and kidneys presented no deviation from their normal state.

The *stomach, small and large intestines*, were healthy throughout; the colour, consistence, and thickness of the mucous membrane were normal; there was no disease of Peyer's patches; the solitary glands of the large intestines were distinct, but not diseased.

The mesenteric glands were rather large, but pale and firm.

The other organs were not examined.

This case offers a well-marked instance of circumscribed gangrene of the lung. There were, it will be seen, several distinct gangrenous centres. Was this the result of the pneumonia, to which the gangrene was probably secondary, having been disseminated or lobular at its outset, and only becoming generalised or lobar by the junction of the circumferences of the several centres of inflammation? The condition of the opposite lung appears to lend a colouring of probability to this view of the case. At any rate, in conjunction with Case VIII., it illustrates the tendency of inflammatory action set up in the course of typhus fever, to assume a low type. The sloughing of the cornea of both eyes is of interest. If any inflammatory action of the conjunctivæ preceded it, I am unable positively to say. So far as memory serves me there was little or none. Pressure, the ordinary determining cause of sloughing in typhus fever, was here out of the question, from the situation of the sloughs.

With reference to the symptoms of typhus fever, this case illustrates the fact, that the eruption appears on about the same day of the disease, and continues about as long in children as in adults; that it may be very abundant in children, and well marked in those of dark skin.

But the points on which I wish to rivet the reader's attention are, 1st, that continued fever occurred in a child not more than eight years of age: 2nd, that the fever was accompanied by abundant mulberry rash; 3rd, that the child died on the twenty-second day of disease, within a few days after the termination of the fever, *i.e.* if the nearly total disappearance of the rash, not from sudden retrocession, but from gradual fading, be considered (as I am inclined to consider it, from an examination of very numerous uncomplicated fatal and non-fatal cases) as a mark of the termination of the fever; and yet, that in this youthful subject, affected with severe fever, which ran its full course, no trace of intestinal lesion was discovered. The gangrene of the lung terminated the life of the boy too soon after the fever for any such lesion to have disappeared, had it ever existed.

In children the rash of typhus fever is often absent. When several cases of typhus fever occur in one house, if the mulberry rash is absent from any members of that family, in a large majority of cases, it is the children who are free from eruption. The following observations appear to me to prove the above assertion, so far as induction from a limited number of carefully observed facts can prove it.

I have notes of 152 cases, in which more than one member of the same family were seen by myself. There was no eruption in 16 of the 152 cases. Thirteen of these 16 were individuals whose ages varied between 4 and 15 years inclusive; the other 3 of the 16 cases were between 16 and 22 years of age. Fifty-five of the 152 cases were less than 15 years of age; 76, *i.e.* just half, were more than 22 years of age, 21 of the 152 cases being between the ages of 16 and 22 inclusive. Thus the rash was *present* in every individual more than 22 years of age. It was *absent* in 3, or one-seventh of the individuals whose ages varied between 16 and 22 years, while it was also *absent* in 13, or one-fourth of those 15 years of age and under. I ought to remark, that of the 13 individuals last referred to, there was in reality only one whose age exceeded 13 years. Let me express more clearly this very important fact, one, it seems to me, unequivocally proved.

Suppose 100 individuals of all ages to have typhus fever, we may expect the rash to be absent

From one-fourth, or 25 of those under puberty.

From one-seventh, or 14 of those under manhood.

From none above 22 years of age.

I would here just recall to the reader's remembrance, how frequent is sore throat without scarlet eruption in adults, after exposure to the poison of scarlet fever—an analogous fact in an analogous disease.

The cases of typhus fever without rash are, so far as my observations extend, invariably mild, never fatal, but now and then local complications arise in the progress of the fever so mild and harmless *in itself*, by which the patient is cut off. Cases v. and viii. are examples of such fatal complications. Case v. also illustrated the fact, as I before remarked, that even in young children the rash may be intense in hue, and very abundant. Cases vi. and vii. will illustrate the phenomena of the disease when the rash is absent.

CASE VI.—After exposure to the contagion of typhus' fever, there ensued, in a child aged 10: frontal headache—delirium—diminished strength—pale brown dry tongue—absence of abnormal, abdominal, and chest signs—quick pulse. Convalescence on the 12th day.

Henry B., aged 10 years, was admitted into the London Fever Hospital, under the care of Dr. Tweedie, Sept. 19, 1849. A thin, rather delicate-looking child, whose previous health, however, had been very good.

The following notes were made, when he first came under observation on the 6th day of disease:—Slept well; mind unaffected; headache little, if any; expression natural; no flush of face. His strength is slightly impaired, but he can leave his bed unassisted with facility; tongue moist, slightly furred; bowels confined till after a dose of castor oil, which acted three times; a little appetite; no gurgling; no tenderness, and no abnormal fulness nor resonance of the abdomen; pulse 100; no cough; no abnormal chest signs; skin warm and dry; no eruption; that night he got little sleep, was very restless. On the 7th day the restlessness continued, and he complained of frontal headache; the tongue was dry, smooth, and covered with a yellowish brown fur; he passed two stools; he had little sleep at night, was restless and slightly delirious; the mind continued to wander at intervals during the following day. His pulse never exceeded 108, and his bowels continued regular throughout; he was convalescent on about the 12th day.

Several members of this child's family were admitted with well-marked typhus fever. His sister, aged 6½ years, was received into the Hospital at the same time: her illness had commenced on the same day, and she was also convalescent on from the 10th to the 12th day of disease. This little child had marked, but scanty, mulberry rash. The spots were present on the 6th day, at which time the notes of her case were first taken; they had nearly disappeared on the 10th day, when the last notes respecting them were made.

The treatment in these cases was simply expectant. Castor oil was administered when the bowels were confined; the hair removed, and cold applied to the scalp when the pain in the head became severe, or delirium supervened. A large well-ventilated apartment, fresh air, a cool, but not too cold, atmosphere, quiet, abstinence from solids, and a free supply of cold water, milk and water, and weak broth. These are the remedies on which, on a large majority of cases of typhus fever, the judicious practitioner relies for the safety of his patient.

In no disease is the advantage of refraining from meddling more clearly displayed than in typhus fever. In no disease is the prompt use of powerful remedies more clearly indicated than in typhus fever. It is in determining when to act, and when to do nothing, that the skill of the physician as a curer of disease, or rather, with reference to fever, as an averter of death, is shown. Interfere, bleed, or stimulate when nothing should be done, and the patient, but for you safe, is lost. Refrain from depletion or withhold wine, when one or other is required, and the patient sinks into that grave from which judicious treatment might have saved him.

CASE VII.—After exposure to contagion from person labouring under typhus fever, with mulberry rash, there ensued in a child, aged 7: frontal headache, disturbed sleep, heaviness of expression, debility, confined bowels, loss of appetite, quick pulse, hot skin, no rash. Convalescence on the 13th or 14th day.

Sarah M., aged 7, was admitted into the London Fever Hospital, November 2nd, 1848, under the care of Dr. A. Tweedie. A delicate-looking, fair child, who had been ill three days only before she came under observation.

The following were the symptoms at that time:—She had slept several hours the preceding night, but moaned much in her sleep; she complained of much headache, which she described as confined to the forehead, was quite sensible, and remembered the date of her entrance into the Hospital; there was some heaviness of expression; the conjunctivæ were pale, the pupils natural, but she shunned the light; there was no flush of the face. She appeared very weak, but turned in bed with facility; the tongue was moist, slightly furred white; there was much thirst, no appetite, and no stool the preceding 24 hours; she swallowed without any difficulty; the abdomen was somewhat full and resonant, but not tender; she complained of a little pain in the belly: the pulse was 108, weak; there was trifling cough, but no abuormal chest signs; the skin was hot and dry; there were no spots.

There was little change in the symptoms during the progress of the disease—excepting that the skin became moist—till the 13th or 14th day, when her appetite returned, and she was noted to be convalescent.

In this case, too, as in all such cases it ought to be, the treatment is medicinally expectant. The hygienic conditions necessary for the safety of the, in itself, mild case of typhus fever, were rigorously observed, i.e. the child was placed in a large uncrowded apartment, plenty of fresh air was admitted, the temperature kept at about temperate, her linen frequently changed, and solid food withheld, while her thirst was slaked with as much water as she chose to drink.

The whole family, of which No. 6 was one, were, with the exception of the mother, who had "spotted" typhus five or six years before, and a child aged 4, admitted into the London Fever Hospital between November 1st and December 20th. The ages of these patients were respectively 14, 19, 20, 21, 22, 29, 60; in all seven the mulberry rash was well marked. The youngest child I visited at home, and found suffering from symptoms similar to those under which her sister laboured when the foregoing notes of her case were taken. She, too, had no spots; or, if she had, they were too faintly marked to be seen in the dark room in which these people slept. Like her sister she had a very mild attack.

CASE VIII.—After exposure to the contagion of typhus fever there ensued, in a child, aged 10: Faintly-marked, scanty mulberry rash—delirium—debility—moist and white tongue—confined bowels—quick pulse—rapid respiration, dulness of left lung, commencing inferiorly—cavernous breathing—gurgling—pectoriloquy, first at inferior angle of left scapula—fetid sputa—hæmoptysis—death on about the twenty-fourth day of illness. *Twenty-nine hours after death.* —Tubercles in both lungs—consolidation of intervening tissue of left lung—enormous cavity in left lung—tubercles beneath intestinal mucous membrane and in mesenteric glands—tubercles in the spleen—opacity and increased vascularity of pericardium.

Martha A., aged 10, was admitted into the London Fever Hospital, October 3, 1848. A dark-complexioned, delicate girl, rather thin. Her mother, aged 59, brother, aged 16, and sister-in-law, aged 29, were admitted between October 3 and November 4, with typhus fever. All had well-marked mulberry rash.

As nearly as could be ascertained, she had been ill nearly a fortnight when first seen by me, October 4. She had kept her bed since the 25th of September; i.e. I saw her on the 10th day after she took to bed; at that time, i.e. about the 14th day of disease, the following particulars were noted:—

She had passed a very restless night, and had but little sleep. She had left her bed several times while delirious. At the time of the visit she seemed quite sensible, said she had no headache, but complained of vertigo in the erect position. There was slight heaviness of expression; the complexion was muddy: the cheeks covered with a dusky flush; the conjunctivæ were pale. With the exception of a disagreeable taste the special senses were in their normal state. Although, while delirious, she left her bed unassisted, she was, when I saw her, quite unable to leave it.

The tongue was moist and white; there was considerable thirst, but no appetite; the bowels were confined; there was no tenderness, pain, abnormal fulness, resonance, nor gurgling of the abdomen. The pulse was 100, the respirations 36; the nostrils dilated largely during inspiration: there was trifling hacking cough. She complains of a sharp pain, increased by deep inspiration, under the left mamma, which 'took her breath away.' There was a little sonorous, and much mucous rale over the anterior surface of the left side of the chest; posteriorly below the angle of the scapula there was abundant fine crepitation and some friction; at this latter part also, there was slight want of resonance on percussion. The skin was hot and dry, and stated, in my notes, to be free from spots; but on the following day I wrote thus:—'On the abdomen and back were seen, on careful inspection, a few irregular dusky pink spots, which fade on pressure. As these spots are very pale, her skin very dark, and there are numerous flea-bites over the same parts; they might have been overlooked yesterday.' On the same day, i.e. the second of observation, the 15th of illness, the cough had increased in severity; it retained its short hacking character. There was now positive dulness from the angle of the left scapula downwards, and the breathing was tubular in the same situation; from the angle to the spine of the scapula there was abundant fine crepitation. On the 16th day the pulse was 96; the respiration 30; the cough continued, and was accompanied, for the first time, by the expectoration of some purulent fluid, coloured green, from the admixture of vomited matter; the quantity, in consequence of this admixture, could not be ascertained; the mixed fluid was highly offensive; the dulness had reached the spine of the scapula. About the angle of that bone there was abundant moist crepitation, so large as to amount almost to gurgling. At the same spot there was cavernous breathing and pectoriloquy; above there was fine crepitation. Anteriorly, on the same side, there was dulness and fine crepitation as high as the inferior border of the third rib; there was respiratory fremitus and friction sound over the same extent. She expectorated about 3 oz. of nearly homogeneous, offensive, purulent fluid (examined microscopically) on the 18th day. On the 22nd day the following note was made :—' The sputa, which have continued purulent and highly offensive, were this morning streaked with blood; about an ounce of rather dark blood has just (1 P.M.) run from the mouth; no cough preceded or accompanied this discharge. On the 28th day there was dulness from the extreme base of the left lung to the spine of the scapula posteriorly, and to the lower border of the second rib anteriorly. There was no enlargement of that side of the chest, and the intercostal spaces were well marked. The vocal fremitus was greater on the left than on the right side. From near the base posteriorly to near the middle of the scapula, there was gurgling, cavernous breathing, and whispering pectoriloquy; there was large mucous rale as high as the spine of the scapula; anteriorly and laterally there was friction and submucous rale as high as the lower border of the second rib. By the 23rd day the dulness was complete over the whole posterior surface of the left side, and the gurgling and cavernous breathing had reached the spine of the scapula. There was some friction over the lower part of the *right* scapula. She had expectorated from 10 to 12 ozs. of extremely fetid pus, mixed with a considerable quantity of dark, frothy blood, during the preceding twenty-four hours; the nurse stated that till 4 A.M. the expectorated matter was yellow; that while coughing at that hour, much dark, frothy blood was suddenly ejected from the mouth. At the time of the visit the expectorated matter was muco-purulent, streaked with blood. On the following day she expectorated from 8 to 12 ozs. of purulent fluid, containing but little blood. After this the sputa continued very abundant, but became thin, watery, and of a pale dirty yellowish colour, with a little thick purulent sediment.

The pulse, 96 till the 19th day, then rose to 108, and on the 27th was 120; at this latter date the respirations were 52 in the minute. Delirium continued at intervals from her entrance

till her death. She was the whole time extremely restless, and
often fretful, so that often it was impossible to examine her chest.
Towards the last she suffered much from night sweats and hectic
flushes. The tongue became covered with a brown fur posteriorly
about the 19th day. The expression of, as well as the actual
prostration, at the same time increased considerably. The bowels,
which acted regularly till the 36th day, then became much
relaxed ; at the same time she began to complain severely of griping pain in the abdomen. These symptoms continued till her
death, on about the 44th day of disease. On the 38th day
the belly was full and resonant, and continued so till the afternoon
preceding her death, when the last note was made.

She died at half-past seven A.M., Nov. 2nd, i.e. 44th day of disease.

The body of M. A. was examined twenty-nine hours after death.
Cadaveric rigidity was tolerably well marked. The ends of the
fingers were slightly enlarged ; the nails curved. There was
slight discoloration of the posterior surface of the trunk. The
abdomen was slightly convex ; the emaciation extreme.

Head.—A considerable depression of the internal table of the
frontal bone was found, and on inquiry from the mother, was
traced to an accident some six or seven months before the death
of the child (see *Transactions of the Pathological Society of London*,
vol. ii. p. 118). The membrane, excepting at the spots corresponding to the injury, and the substance of encephalon were healthy
in colour, consistence, etc.

The *pericardium* contained about 1 oz. of turbid yellow serosity,
in which floated a few shreds of lymph. The serous membrane
itself was dull, white, and opaque, and there was abnormal vascularity of the parietal pericardium corresponding to the left pleura.
There was no lymph adherent to the pericardium-proper or parietal.

The *heart*, both substance and valves, was healthy.

The *larynx* and *trachea* were normal in appearance.

The *right pleura* contained about 2 oz. of yellowish serosity.

The *right lung* collapsed but slightly. There was a little
recent lymph over the posterior part of the inferior lobe.
The posterior surface of the lung was mottled with deep
purple patches, here and there separated from each other by well-
marked, opaque, white, inter-lobular septa. In the substance of
the apex and anterior part of the superior and middle lobe were
felt numerous irregularly nodulated solid masses. On section
these latter were found to be caused by collections of semi-
transparent grey granulation and opaque yellow tubercles.
Scattered between these masses were numerous solitary, minute,
grey, semi-transparent granulations ; the tissue around the tubercles
was crepitant and apparently healthy. When the posterior part
of the lung was divided, the pulmonary tissue corresponding to the

purple patches described as seen externally, was non-crepitant and saturated with bloody serosity; this condition did not extend for more than from a third to half an inch into the pulmonary tissue.

The *left lung* was very firmly adherent to the pleura posteriorly, and as low as the upper border of the third rib; anteriorly from that point downwards, the anterior part of the lung was separated from the costal pleura by a collection of highly offensive dirty brown fluid, circumscribed by lymph. Opening into this cavity were several small apertures communicating through the under surface of the upper lobe, with an immense cavity reaching from near the base to near the apex of this lung, extending through the division between the two lobes. The posterior wall of this cavity was extremely thin, a mere film, about two-thirds downwards from the apex. The cavity contained a fluid resembling that in the pleura but somewhat more purulent. The walls of the cavity were extremely ragged; large masses of sloughy matter hanging loosely from them. The pulmonary tissue yet un-destroyed was stuffed full of tubercles, and numerous opaque yellow tubercles of cheesy consistence studded the walls of the cavity.

The *bronchial glands* were somewhat enlarged, and contained much dull yellow tubercular matter.

The *liver, pancreas,* and *kidneys* were healthy in appearance.

The *spleen* was studded with tubercles.

The *mesenteric glands* were enlarged, especially in that part corresponding to the middle of the small intestines; they varied in size from a pea to a small bean, and, on section, were found to be studded with small, opaque, yellow tubercles.

The *pharynx, œsophagus, stomach,* and *duodenum* were normal in all respects.

Beneath the mucous membrane, covering one of Peyer's patches, about eighteen inches from the commencement of the *jejunum*, were numerous distinct, firm, slightly elevated, opaque, yellowish spots; the next two or three patches descending the gut were similarly affected; then came six or seven perfectly healthy patches, and then one slightly diseased. The remainder, to the ileo-cæcal valve, were normal in appearance. The whole mucous membrane of the *jejunum* and *ileum* was pale and natural in colour and consistence.

The *large intestines* appeared healthy.

The urinary bladder, uterus, and ovaries were not examined.

A few of the mesenteric glands were studded with small, opaque, yellow tubercles.

The facts in this case especially worthy of attention are—

A. Those respecting the fever. The patient was of that

age when the intestinal affection is common, yet an examination after death showed that she had no such lesion.[1] This illness was prolonged by local complications till the 44th day, although the fever, properly so called, terminated on about the 14th day.   It is of importance, in all cases, to fix the date of the termination of the fever; for no greater error can be committed than to confound the length of the fever with the duration of the illness—to use the two expressions as synonymous terms.   The intestinal lesion, diagnostic of typhoid fever, was absent, although the eruption was very scanty and imperfectly marked; thus in conjunction with other cases detailed by myself in these papers, rendering untenable the opinion first advanced in a most able article on ' Continued Fever' in the twelfth volume of the *British and Foreign Review*, and subsequently adopted by Dr. Watson, that the skin eruption and the intestinal lesions are ' supplementary of each other.'

B. Those respecting the chest affection.—I can only just allude to a few of the many points of interest this case offers for consideration.

What was the order of sequence of incidents in the case?

1st. The child was delicate-looking and thin, and had been for some time before her present illness suffering from cough.   It is true, the ordinary signs of the presence of tubercles in the adult were not detected in the lungs on her admission; but then the elasticity of the thoracic parietes of a child, the pretty equal amount of the tubercles probably existing in the two lungs, precluding comparison, as well as their diffusion at considerable intervals from base to apex, in minute masses, might have rendered their detection impossible,[2] and certainly would have rendered it highly improbable, in a case of fever, when the attention was only secondarily directed to the chest.

2nd. Typhus fever.

[1] When treating of typhoid fever I shall refer to this case, as illustrating the difference in the appearance of tubercular and typhoid deposit in the agminated glands—a difference which, in the majority of cases, forbids their being confounded by a tolerably experienced observer.

[2] ' Miliary tubercles and grey granulations are made manifest by roughness of the respiratory murmur, or by prolonged expiration with clearness on percussion.'—Rilliet et Barthes. *Maladies des Enfants*, vol. iii. p. 247.

3rd. Pleuro-pneumonia. This was probably induced by the exposure which the child experienced in coming to the hospital; the inflammation commenced in the situation usually occupied by lobar pneumonia of the left lung in children, i.e. at the base.

4th. The rapid deposition of fresh tubercular matter. This was proved by the large amount found in the portions of pulmonary texture, undestroyed at the time of death, an amount which must, independent of any inflammatory pneumonic consolidation, have caused absolute dulness of the left side of the thorax; and certainly no marked, even comparative, dulness existed on the child's admission.

5th. The formation of a cavity in the inferior lobe of the left lung, due probably to the softening down of tubercular matter, as well as to the formation of pus and gangrene of the pulmonary tissue; in fact a tubercular gangrenous abscess, and then the sudden opening of this abscess into a bronchial tube.

6th. The rapid extension of the cavity by a kind of phagedenic solution of its parietes.

7th. The formation of a communication between the cavity in the lung and the pleural cavity.

8th. The extension of the inflammatory action from the left pleura to the pericardium, next to rheumatism and kidney disease, the most frequent cause of pericarditis.

The rapid formation and extension of the cavity is matter of extreme interest. The physical signs were so well marked, that the exact date of the first formation of the cavity can be unequivocally fixed. The pneumonia, which was lobar, had produced but imperfect consolidation on the 14th day of disease; perfect consolidation on the 15th day, as shown by complete dulness and bronchial breathing; and on the 16th day there was indubitable evidence of the existence of a cavity communicating with a bronchial tube in the lower lobe of the left lung. In twenty days from the commencement of the pneumonia this cavity occupied the greater part of the lung reaching from base to apex of the organ. The hemorrhage was doubtless owing to the rapid extension of the cavity. The destruction of tissue was too rapid to allow of closure of the vessels. Hemorrhage is much more common from gangrenous than from tubercular cavities.

Having considered the influence which age exerts on the symptoms and termination of typhus fever, I shall now detail a few cases to illustrate the modifications induced in the disease, when particular organs become the seat of special lesions, and also to exhibit the effects of pregnancy on the mortality.

CONVULSIONS, ETC.

CASE IX.—No history—mulberry rash—mental confusion —deafness—delirium—brown tongue—absence of abdominal signs—quick pulse—somnolence—convulsions—coma—death on the fifth day of the stay in hospital. *Eight hours after death.*—Continuance of spots noted during life—clots in the cavity of the arachnoid—slight congestion of the posterior part of the lungs—hemorrhage into the pulmonary substance —congestion of the posterior wall of the urinary bladder— slight enlargement and softening of the spleen—old disease of the kidneys and of the mitral valve of the heart—other organs healthy.

Mary H., aged 60. A rather small-made, thin woman, of whose past condition no particulars could be obtained, was admitted into the London Fever Hospital, under the care of Dr. Tweedie, September 9th, 1847.

On September 10th, the following was her condition:—Her memory was very much impaired; her mind so confused, that, although she thought she was in the hospital, she felt by no means certain; she was slightly deaf; her conjunctivæ were abnormally injected; her pupils were natural; the cheeks were covered with a dingy red flush, not circumscribed; she was unable to leave her bed without assistance; the lips and teeth were covered with sordes; the tongue was dry and brown; there was neither fulness, tenderness, nor gurgling of the abdomen; the bowels acted regularly; the pulse was 100 and full; the heart's impulse strong; the cardiac dulness rather too extensive; a rough murmur was audible with the first sound at the apex; she suffered from a little cough; and some sonorous and sibilous rales were heard over the whole chest; the skin was hot, dry, and spotted; the spots were numerous, of a purplish red colour, varied from one-eighth to one-sixth of an inch in diameter; some of the spots were rendered paler by pressure, some were unchanged by the firmest pressure; these spots were more numerous and darker on the posterior than on the anterior surface of the trunk; here and there, several spots appeared to have coalesced, and so to have formed large irregular purple patches, unaffected by pressure; there were no sudamina on the surface.

She passed a very restless night, *i.e.* between the 10th and 11th; slept but little, and was occasionally delirious; about 2 A.M., she was suddenly seized with general convulsions; she appeared to the nurse insensible during the time the attack lasted, —*i.e.* about ten minutes; there was no frothing at the mouth; her bowels acted once; the pulse rose to 120; the stools and urine were passed into the close stool.

On the following day there was some somnolence, interrupted by delirium, and increased deafness; the skin was cool; the prostration was more decided; all the muscular movements were very tremulous; the stools and urine were passed into bed. There was little change till the night of the 13th, when her speech became unintelligible, and she was again seized with general convulsions, followed by coma. She was lying comatose at the time of the visit, on the fourteenth day of disease, and died that night. On the 10th, 6 oz. of wine were ordered to be administered daily, and, on the following day, the quantity was increased to 8 oz.

The body was examined *eight hours after death*. The weather cool. The cadaveric rigidity was well marked; the trunk was yet warm; the extremities were cold. Of the spots marked before death as fading, a mere trace of a palish red colour remained; the colour of *these* spots was limited to the surface of the cutis. The spots marked during life as unaffected by pressure, retained the dark purple hue they possessed before death. On section, the colour of *the latter* was found to extend through the whole substance of the cutis, and even slightly, under the darkest spots, into the substance of the subcutaneous cellular tissue. The tint was even deeper beneath the cuticle than on the surface. *Examined with a strong lens, the discoloration appeared to be due to dyeing of the tissues; a few minute vessels were seen loaded with blood, converging towards the spots, but none in the discoloured part itself.*

In the cavity of the arachnoid, on the convex surface of the anterior lobe of the left hemisphere of the cerebrum, was a dark crimson clot, about 1 inch in superficial diameter, thin but firm. Continuous with it was a delicate pale, red, fibrinous film, spreading over a large portion of the superior part of the same hemisphere; a second smaller dark clot, situated on a line with the upper edge of the left meatus auditorius externus was united to the first-described coagulum, by the delicate fibrinous film; a similar crimson clot was found on the convex surface of the middle lobe of the right hemisphere.

All these coagula could be detached with the greatest facility, without the least injury to the subjacent arachnoid. The vessels of the pia mater were moderately full of fluid blood; not a drop, however, could be pressed into the cavity of the arachnoid; there was no discoverable lesion of the sinuses; there was no blood at the base of the brain; a little reddish serosity escaped on opening the cavity of the arachnoid.

About 1 oz. of colourless serosity was found in the ventricles, and a little at the base of the brain. There was not the slightest abnormal vascularity of the substance of the organ, of the lining membrane of the ventricles, nor of the plexus choroides. The substance itself of the encephalon was firm and healthy in all respects.

The *heart* was somewhat larger than natural; its substance was firm. There was some old disease of the mitral valve. The blood was fluid, with the exception of a few small, soft, black coagula in the venæ cavæ and right auricle and ventricle.

The *larynx* was healthy; the *bronchial tubes* slightly congested.

The *lungs* were slightly congested posteriorly; in the *anterior* inferior angle of the lower lobe of the right lung was a nodule of pulmonary apoplexy of some size.

The *liver* was healthy, but congested; the gall-bladder contained about 1 oz. of thick dark green bile.

The *spleen* weighed 7 oz.; it was soft and dark.

The *kidneys* were healthy but congested; a few hemorrhagic points were found under the lining membrane of either kidney. The lining membrane of the posterior wall of the urinary bladder was minutely injected, and beneath the mucous membrane were also several hemorrhagic spots.

The *pancreas*, the *œsophagus*, and the *mesenteric glands* were healthy.

Stomach.—The lining membrane of the stomach was smooth; there were no rugæ, and a mere trace of mammillation; the consistence and thickness of the membrane was normal.

Large and small intestines.—The colour and thickness of the mucous membrane lining the intestinal canal were normal; but it was somewhat softened, especially in the small intestines, where shreds of any length were obtained with difficulty.

The large intestines contained some solid fæces; there was very little air in any part of the canal.

The points especially worthy of attention in this case are the passage of the spots into petechiæ, the persistence of the spots after death, especially the condition of the cutis (as observed after death), on which the discoloration causing

O

the spots depended. In addition to the well-marked mulberry rash, itself diagnostic of the disease, whatever other
symptoms are present or absent—the mental confusion,
the muddy hue of skin, the dingy flush of the face, the
injected conjunctivæ, the absence of headache *after* the
commencement of delirium, the prostration combined,
were sufficient to render the existence of typhus fever highly
probable, though certainly in themselves not absolutely
diagnostic.

Convulsions are by no means common in typhus fever.
When they do occur, the case almost invariably proves fatal.
After death, in the case we are here considering, an effusion
of blood was found to have taken place into the cavity of
the arachnoid. Although it cannot be questioned that this
hemorrhage occurred before death, yet it may be doubted
whether it was the cause of the attack of convulsions. The
ordinary result of an effusion of blood into the cavity of the
arachnoid on the convex surface of the brain is coma. It is
not improbable that the convulsions were induced by the
action of the generally diseased blood on the nervous centres,
and that the intra-cranial hemorrhage resulted from the
impeded return of blood from the brain during the convulsions.
The condition of the anterior inferior angle of the right lung
rendered this view of the case highly probable.

My experience leads me to regard effusion of blood into
the cavity of the arachnoid as by no means of infrequent
occurrence in typhus fever. Capillary hemorrhage is
probably favoured as well by the condition of the solids as of
the blood itself. In the case before us there were numerous
minute spots of ecchymosis beneath the lining membrane of
the pelvis, of the kidneys, and urinary bladder. The bile in
this case was, as it generally is after death from typhus fever,
thick and dark green; the spleen was soft and not very much
enlarged;—the age of the patient favoured softening of that
organ, while it was unfavourable to enlargement. (See p. 96.)
The fluid state of the blood, and the smoothness of the mucous
membrane of the stomach are both commonly present after
death from typhus fever. But softening of the mucous membrane of the intestinal canal is very rarely seen to the same
extent as in this particular case. There had been no signs to

indicate its existence during life; and it is probable that it was in a great measure cadaveric. Peyer's patches, and the mesenteric glands, it is to be observed, were in all respects in their normal state.

Hemorrhage sometimes takes place into the substance of muscles where no external violence can have occurred. The rectus abdominalis is a frequent seat of the effusion of blood. The following case illustrates this complication.

CASE X.—No history of early symptoms.

Mary B., aged 70, a thin woman with grey hair, came under observation on the sixth day of disease. No particulars of the symptoms present before her admission into the London Fever Hospital, under the care of Dr. Tweedie, July 21st, 1848, could be obtained. She had resided from some years preceding her admission in Kensington workhouse. Several cases of fever, with mulberry rash, had been admitted shortly before from the same locality.

When first seen, on the sixth day of disease, her mind was wandering. She fancied she had been in the hospital three days. There was no headache; she had slept a little. She was deaf. The tongue was dry and brown; the bowels slightly relaxed. There were, however, no abdominal signs; the pulse was only 80. There was slight want of resonance, and very feeble respiratory murmurs over the most depending part of the lungs, the patient lying on her back; the skin was warm and dry. Mulberry rash was well marked. The prostration was so great that the patient was unable even to turn in bed unassisted. 4 oz. of gin were ordered to be given during the twenty-four hours in divided doses. On the next day the pulse had risen to 120; it was very weak; there was some somnolence; in other respects there was little change; she died at 7 A.M. on the ninth day of disease, apparently from asthenia.

The body was examined *thirty-one hours after death*, the weather being cool; the cadaveric rigidity had almost entirely disappeared; the spots observed during life continued. Beneath and extending among the fibres of the left rectus abdominalis muscle was a loosely coagulated dark bloody clot, 2 inches in length and 1 inch in breadth. It was situated, as above described, midway between the umbilicus and pubes.

The *heart* was flabby; the clots contained in it soft and dark; the lining membrane was stained dusky red; the lungs were deeply congested posteriorly; the mucous membrane of the stomach was smooth and free from rugæ; the consistence, thickness, and colour of the whole gastro-intestinal mucous membrane was normal; Peyer's patches in all particulars healthy; larynx, pharynx, and œsophagus healthy; there was no enlargement of the mesenteric glands. A few small cysts studded the cortical substance of the kidneys; the urinary bladder and uterus were normal in all particulars; the pancreas healthy; the liver very flabby and soft; the spleen somewhat enlarged.

Head.—The pia mater was congested; there was a little sub-arachnoid effusion of serosity; and the pia mater and arachnoid separated from the cerebral convolutions with abnormal facility. The substance of the encephalon itself appeared healthy in all respects.

This patient, like all affected with typhus fever when they make any mistake as to the duration of time, supposed it lengthened; thus she thought three days had elapsed between her entrance into the hospital and my first seeing her, whereas really it was only one day. In addition to the presence of a clot in the substance of the rectus abdominalis muscle, this case illustrates the early period at which death from typhus fever, uncomplicated with local lesion, may ensue. There was nothing found after death to account for the fatal termination. Some congestion of the most depending part of the lung—slight congestion of the pia mater—trifling enlargement of the spleen—and a small quantity of loosely coagulated blood in the substance of a muscle were all the physical changes established during life which the scalpel enabled us to lay bare. The effect on the solids of the general disease, which latter itself our scalpel could not detect, was manifested by the flabby state of the heart and liver, the early disappearance of the cadaveric rigidity, etc.

In Case IX. an example was afforded of convulsions co-incident with an effusion of blood into the cavity of the arachnoid. I shall now detail a case in which that lesion was detected after death, when there had been no symptoms to indicate its presence during life, Case XI.: and then I shall narrate a case, XIII., in which convulsions occurred, but which presented no lesion, excepting some congestion of the brain and its membranes, to account for so serious a symptom; and then Case XIV., in which the cerebral symptoms were very prominent during life, but in which, after death, not the slightest deviation from the normal condition of the encephalon or its membranes could be discovered.

CASE XL—After exposure to the contagion of fever accompanied with mulberry rash.

Ensued:—Rigors frequently repeated—pain in head and limbs—confined bowels—rapid prostration—hoarseness—deafness—disturbed vision—mental confusion—dry brown tongue—difficult deglutition—quick pulse—cool skin—mulberry rash—extreme difficulty of breathing—death on the 16th day.

Eleven hours after death: Persistence of spots—clot in the substance of left rectus abdominalis muscle—clot in the cavity of arachnoid—slight congestion of the posterior part of lungs—softening of the mucous membrane of pharynx—thickening of rima glottidis—pus in larynx—other organs normal.

Mary G., aged 49, a moderately stout woman, subject to constant cough, was admitted into the London Fever Hospital, May 9th, 1848, under the care of Dr. Tweedie. Her daughter left the hospital three weeks before, and Mary G. washed her clothes. She was a native of London.

Present illness began thirteen days before her admission with rigors frequently repeated—pains in the head and limbs, and confined bowels. She took to her bed entirely on the second day of disease, because she felt generally ill and extreme weakness. There had been no epistaxis. She had taken before admission several doses of aperient medicine. Hoarseness first made its appearance, her relations stated, on the 9th day of disease.

The following notes of her case were taken on the 13th day of disease:—No headache, slight deafness (not deaf till present illness), no delirium, memory defective; complains of seeing strange objects about the wards; she is quite conscious that these objects have no real existence; says she has a most disagreeable taste, and a constant sense of unpleasant odours; there is no flush of the face; she is unable to leave her bed without considerable assistance.

The tongue is brown and dry; she swallows either solids or liquids with considerable difficulty; there is swelling and dusky redness of the tonsils, uvula, and velum pendulum palati; she has passed two stools during the last twenty-four hours; there is neither pain, tenderness, fulness, resonance, nor gurgling of the abdomen; no appetite, no thirst.

She can speak only in a faint, hoarse whisper; no tenderness
of the larynx; cough troublesome; some sonorous and mucous
rales over both sides of the chest; percussion normal; pulse 120,
weak; heart sounds normal; skin cool, covered with mulberry
rash; vin. alb. ʒiv., jus bov.   On the 14th and 15th days
there was little change in the local or general symptoms, excepting that the spots were paler somewhat on the 14th day,
and she was quite unable to protrude her tongue; she passed
her stools in bed on the 15th day.   The muscular movements
at the same time were extremely tremulous; the pulse had risen
at the latter date to 128, was very weak, and the skin cool.   She
became very restless during the afternoon of the 15th day.
Death occurred at 4 A.M. on the 16th day.   For some hours
before the fatal termination the breathing was exceedingly laboured.
There were no convulsions, and no coma.

A blister was applied to the throat on the 14th day of
disease, and at the same time the wine was increased to six ounces
in the twenty-four hours.   On the 15th day four ounces of gin
were given, in addition to the wine.

Eleven hours after death the following appearances were observed :—The spots noted during life were still to be detected;
there was no emaciation; at least 1½ inches of fat covered the
abdominal parietes.   Between the left rectus abdominalis muscle
and its sheath, anteriorly and posteriorly, and also among the
fibres of the muscle, which were at that place softer than elsewhere, was a considerable quantity of loosely coagulated blood.
The extent occupied by the clot was about 6 inches by 2 inches.
It commenced an inch above the pubes.

Head.—The bloody points on the external surface of the dura
mater were very numerous.   A little bloody serosity escaped on
opening the cavity of the arachnoid.   On either side, extending
from the greater wing of the sphenoid bone to the tentorium cere-
belli, closely applied to the arachnoid covering the pia mater, and
within the cavity of the arachnoid, was a film of coagulated blood
of a bright red colour, with spots of a dark venous hue scattered
over it at intervals.   The difference in colour depended on the
difference in the thickness of the clot.   There was no trace of any
clot in the longitudinal fissure, and no coagulum at the base of
the brain.   In the meshes of the pia mater was much colourless
serosity, and a moderate amount of the same in the lateral ventricles.   The bloody points on the cut surface of the cerebrum
appeared more numerous than natural.   There was increased
vascularity of the plexus choroides.   The consistence of the cerebral substance was natural.

There was no abnormal congestion of the *pulmonary tissue.*
The lining membrane of the bronchial tubes were finely injected;

the tubes themselves contained much muco-purulent fluid. The *pericardium* and *heart* were healthy. The clots in the heart firm.

The mucous membrane of the *pharynx* was of a dirty yellow colour, and so soft that it could be readily removed by the slightest scraping from the subjacent tissue.

Larynx.—The rima glottidis was narrow, the mucous membrane of the whole larynx finely injected, and covered with a layer of purulent fluid. On and above the chordæ vocales was some solid opaque white matter, resembling lymph in physical character.

The *liver* was flabby; the *spleen*, small, weighing only 4¾ oz., was soft and flabby.

The *pancreas, urinary bladder*, and *uterus* were healthy. The *kidneys* contained numerous small cysts in their cortical substance.

The *œsophagus* was normal in appearance.

Stomach.—The whole of the coats of the great cul-de-sac were so soft that the finger passed through them with the greatest facility. Bluish white bands, from which the mucous membrane had disappeared, extended from the softened portion towards the pylorus. The whole mucous membrane of the stomach was exceedingly soft, but very pale.

Large and small intestines.—The thickness, colour, and consistence of the mucous membrane lining the intestinal canal, as well as the condition of Peyer's patches, were carefully noted. They were healthy in all particulars. The mesenteric glands were in their normal condition.

In this case there was much more blood within the cavity of the arachnoid than in Case x., and yet there were no convulsions. The softened condition of the substance of the rectus abdominalis, and the presence of a clot of blood in it, are points worthy of attention, as showing the relation between the diseased condition of the solids and fluids generally, and the presence of hemorrhage into the cavity of the arachnoid. Clots were found on both cerebral hemispheres The absence of any trace of clot in the longitudinal fissure rendered it probable that the hemorrhage occurred primarily on the two sides, *i.e.* that the blood did not pass before coagulation from the one hemisphere to the other. As is common in cases of hemorrhage into the arachnoid, no trace of the vessels from which the blood escaped could be detected.

A small quantity of coagulated blood is, as I have before remarked, by no means infrequently found within the cavity of the arachnoid after death from typhus fever. Thus this lesion was discovered to exist in one-seventh of the cases of typhus fever which proved fatal during the progress of that disease analysed by myself in the *Edinburgh Monthly Journal* for October 1849,[1] and my impression is, that such proportion does not very far exceed what the whole of the cases I have examined after death would afford. The quantity of blood, however, I ought to remark, is often very small. I have never seen the slightest trace of hemorrhage into the *substance of the brain* after typhus fever. Now, intense congestion of the membranes of the brain is frequently, almost constantly, found after death from typhus fever. Congestion of the cerebral substance much more rarely; and when it does occur is infinitely less intense.

This case also illustrates one form of laryngitis, as found in typhus fever, *i.e.* that form which advances insidiously, and is unattended with those violent symptoms which are consequent on sudden swelling of the submucous tissue of the larynx. The physical obstruction to the entrance of the air was comparatively trifling. It will be observed that from the history of the symptoms, as well as from the more advanced stage of the disease of the pharyngeal than of the laryngeal mucous membrane, that the affection commenced, as it usually does, in the pharynx, and then spread down to the larynx. Deafness was noted in this case, as it was in Cases III., X., and XII. It is a common symptom in typhus fever. The softening of the stomach was cadaveric, a part of that tendency to softening of the tissues so eminently characteristic of the disease I am here considering. The sonorous rale, and the condition of the bronchial mucous membrane, were probably dependent on the chronic bronchitis, of which it appeared this woman had long been the subject.

CASE XII.—Slight rigors, pains in back and abdomen— diarrhœa without medicine—sudden prostration—mental confusion—trifling headache, vertigo—brown and dry tongue —tenderness of abdomen—mulberry rash—convulsions— coma—*death*—persistence of spots—meningeal and cerebral congestion—blood very loosely coagulated—hypertrophy of the heart—other organs healthy.

[1] See *ante*, p. 62.

Thomas B., aged 61, a printer, a thin man, whose previous health had been very good, was received into the London Fever Hospital, May 27th, 1848, on the 8th day of disease, under the care of Dr. Tweedie. He never had a fit of any kind before his admission into the hospital. His illness commenced with slight rigors and pain in the back and abdomen. His bowels were relaxed from the outset and before he took medicine of any kind. He kept his bed on the 2nd day of illness.

On the 9th day of disease the following notes of his case were made:—

He states, when asked, that he has slight headache and some vertigo—he slept but little last night—his mind is somewhat confused. The tongue is dry and brown—the abdomen tender—the bowels much relaxed. He has passed five stools since his admission yesterday—there is no appetite and but little thirst.

The pulse is only 90. With the exception of rather extensive cardiac dulness, there are no abnormal physical chest signs.

The muscular powers are greatly impaired—he is quite unable to leave his bed unassisted, even to reach the close stool. The skin is warm and dry. There is abundant mulberry rash.

During the night he was seized with convulsions, throwing his arms about violently; he appeared at the time unconscious of all going on around him. This fit lasted for about ten minutes. He slept for some time before and after the fit.

When I saw him again on the following morning, i.e. the 10th day of disease, he said he was free from headache—his mind was rather more confused than on the 9th day—the conjunctivæ were injected, the pupils small—the urine was passed into the bed. On the following day he had a second attack of convulsions, which lasted, however, but a very few minutes. During this attack his limbs became very rigid and he foamed at the mouth, and after it he slept for half-an-hour. He was otherwise very wakeful and occasionally delirious. On the 11th day he continued watchful and delirious—there were frequent twitchings of the muscles of the face—the urine and the stools were passed into bed—the pulse was scarcely perceptible. He died at 11 A.M. on the 12th day of disease. He was comatose for some hours before death.

The body was examined twenty-seven hours after death.—The spots marked during life continued visible.

Head.—The dura mater was considerably congested. There was a little fluid in the cavity of the arachnoid, and a small quantity infiltrated the meshes of the pia mater. The arachnoid was rather opaque. The pia mater minutely injected over the whole surface of the brain. Numerous but minute bloody points studded the cut surface of the grey and white matter of the cerebrum. The consistence of the brain was natural. The lateral ventricles were moderately distended with colourless fluid. The vessels of the plexus choroides were loaded with blood.

Chest.—With the exception of a very small soft black clot in the right auricle and ventricle, and a still smaller clot in the left auricle and ventricle, the blood was fluid throughout the body.

Pericardium healthy.

Heart somewhat enlarged and hypertrophied.

Larynx—bronchial tubes—bronchial glands and *lungs* healthy in appearance.

Pharynx and œsophagus normal. .

Stomach.—With the exception of a few rugæ, along the greater curvature, and trifling mammillation near the pylorus, the mucous membrane of the stomach was smooth; the mucous membrane was posteriorly of reddish colour, anteriorly a darker red, and along the greater curvature of a vermilion hue; the redness was punctiform and capillary; the deeper red parts were slightly thickened and firmer than the surrounding; there was no softening of any part of the lining membrane; the larger vessels of the posterior wall of the organ were moderately full of blood; none were visible on the anterior surface of the organ.

The *mesenteric glands* and *intestines* were healthy in colour, thickness, and consistence.

The *pancreas, liver, kidneys, and urinary bladder,* were normal; the *gall bladder* contained some dark green bile; the *spleen* was dark and firm; and weighed 7½ ozs.

Thus with the exception of the congestion of the brain, by no means greater than in many cases when no convulsions occurred, there was no lesion to account for that symptom. The patient died at an early period of the disease, *i.e.* on the 12th day, and no local complication of importance was revealed by the scalpel. The convulsions and death were probably the result of the same cause, the diseased condition of the blood. I would wish particularly to direct the reader's attention to the fact, that diarrhœa, pain in the abdomen, and tenderness of the belly, were among the earliest and most prominent symptoms, and yet there was no lesion of Peyer's patches. The tenderness, probably, depended on the condition of the gastric mucous membrane. I shall have, hereafter, to detail cases, in which constipation was a prominent symptom, and yet extensive ulceration of the agminated glands was detected after death. So that, *by themselves,* pain in the abdomen and diarrhœa, even when present in fever, are by no means *diagnostic* of lesion of Peyer's patches.

CASE XIII.—George C., aged 58, a stout fair-complexioned man, was admitted into the London Fever Hospital, under the care of Dr. Tweedie, July 4th, 1848, labouring under typhus fever, accompanied with the diagnostic mulberry rash. This man's wife and children were patients in the hospital some weeks before; they, too, laboured under typhus fever with mulberry rash. From his admission till about the 14th day of disease, when the following notes of his condition were taken, he was *violently* delirious:— ' He sleeps very much—when roused is very delirious; he cannot be made to take his medicine; will not protrude his tongue; is unable to leave his bed unassisted: he has passed two stools during the last twenty-four hours; his pulse, which, up to this date, has not exceeded 96, is 108, and for the first time irregular; on the following day it reached 120 in the minute; it continued irregular, and, during the last twenty-four hours of life, was inter-mitting. On the 15th day, strabismus was observed for the first time; his eyes were both drawn upwards and inwards; his wife was struck by his appearance, and remarked spontaneously, that she had never seen him squint before his present illness; the spots grew darker as the disease advanced; coma preceded death for many hours; he died on about the 18th day of disease.'

The following was the condition of the organs discovered on an examination of the body twenty-four hours after death:—

There was no opacity of the arachnoid; a little fluid only in the cavity of that membrane; a little colourless serosity in the meshes of the pia mater; slight congestion of the latter; the arachnoid and pia mater separate in one mass from the surface of the convolutions, without carrying away any of the cerebral substance; a little transparent serosity in the ventricles; there were a few more red points than common in the white substance of the brain; the consistence of that organ was perfectly normal.

With the exception of some red serosity in the pericardium, which microscopic examination proved to contain no blood cor-puscles,—a very flabby condition of the heart, the lining membrane of which was stained dusky red,—a nearly fluid condition of the blood throughout the body,—a limited amount of consolidation of the pulmonary tissue of the left lung from central pneumonia,—flabby liver,—dark thick bile,—and smoothness of the lining membrane of the stomach,—common after death from typhus fever, as I have before pointed out, the whole of the organs were in a normal state.

I have narrated the above scanty particulars of this case, in order that the reader may have another illustration of the frequent presence of what are called head-symptoms,—violent delirium, squinting, and coma,—and yet after death-examination be unable to afford the slightest explanation of the morbid vital phenomena, by the demonstration of any change of structure within the cranium. An irregular or intermitting pulse is by no means rare in typhus fever, when no old disease of that organ is detected after death.

I do not give a case illustrative of the pathological appearances observed within the cranium after death from typhus fever, complicated with inflammation of the brain or its membrane, for this reason, because *I have never made an examination, after death, of a case of typhus fever, in which such appearances were present.* The assertion that the symptoms of typhus fever are due to inflammation of the brain, rests on as untenable grounds as that of the same disease in gastro-enteritis.

COMA VIGIL.

CASE XIV.—Maria W., aged 52, was first seen on the 9th day of disease; at that time the symptoms of typhus fever were present. She slept much, and on the 10th day almost constantly, night and day. Somnolence continued till about the middle of the 13th day, gradually, however, becoming less constant. From the time of the visit, on the 13th day, till her death, at 1 A.M. on the 15th day, she never closed her eyes. On the 14th day, the following note was made :—She lies constantly on her back ; eyes open ; has not closed them since the visit yesterday ; cannot be made to open her mouth, or to attempt to protrude her tongue ; gives no sign of consciousness when spoken to. The skin is cool and sweating profusely ; the spots are darker than on admission ; there are no sudamina.

The body was examined twenty-two hours after death. There was some colourless serosity in the cavity of the arachnoid ; a little similar fluid in the meshes of the pia mater ; a moderate quantity in the ventricles. The pia mater, arachnoid, and cerebral substance, appeared healthy in colour and consistence.

Thus, no condition of the encephalon was detected, to account for the peculiar symptom above described.

I have seen one person only recover from this state, and in that case the coma vigil was not complete.

CASE XV.—George P., aged 30, a surgeon, was received into the London Fever Hospital, June 2nd, 1849, on the 8th day of disease, under the care of Dr. Tweedie. He had well-marked and very severe typhus fever. At the time of his admission the mulberry rash was very abundant. On the 16th day the following note was made:—

'He has been since last evening in his present condition. Is now lying on his back, his eyes open, but he is apparently unconscious of all going on around him. He cannot be made to protrude his tongue, or even to make any effort to do so; yet he swallows a little fluid when poured into his mouth. His pupil acts very little by the aid of a candle. Pulse 132, very weak. Urinary bladder distended; urine passing into the bed. The mulberry rash is well marked. A blister was applied to his forehead, and on the following day the pulse had fallen to 108. He had some sleep; assisted himself to drink; protruded his tongue fully when bidden; and the spots were much paler. From this time he rapidly recovered.'

It will be observed, that the condition described as having existed in the two last described cases was very different from somnolence or ordinary coma. It was the opposite of that described as coma vigil by Chomel and some other writers, *i.e.* a condition in which the patient sleeps as much, or even more than in health, and yet declares that he has never closed his eyes.

PREGNANCY.

Pregnancy is by no means a necessarily fatal complication of typhus fever; nor do pregnant women necessarily miscarry, as the two following cases, XVI. and XVII., prove.

CASE XVI.—Mary Ann G., aged 23, a stout, well-made, married woman, was received into the London Fever Hospital, August 18, 1847, on the 9th day of disease, under the care of Dr. Tweedie. Her brother, also suffering from typhus fever, was admitted with her. This woman was between seven and eight months gone with child. She had well-marked severe typhus fever. The mulberry rash was copious and characteristic. Her pulse on the 10th day of disease was 140, and on the 12th day 150; the tongue dry and brown, and the spots dark. On the 15th day of disease the pulse had fallen to 100; the tongue was moist, and the spots were fading. Vomiting became very troublesome during convalescence. She left the hospital in the early part of September.

CASE XVII.—Margaret G., aged 36, night nurse in the

London Fever Hospital, came under observation on the 6th day of disease, March 2nd, 1849, She was then about seven months gone with child; she had severe typhus fever; thus, on the 12th day of disease, her pulse was 140; her mind was confused; the mulberry rash was dark and characteristic; from this time she slowly recovered. Like Case XVI. she suffered much from vomiting during convalescence.

This woman left the hospital at the beginning of April; went her full time, and was then delivered of a living child. I saw her about two months after her confinement; she said that she had a very good time. The child I saw; it was small, and did not look very healthy; but the mother informed me it was strong, and it appeared to her to be thriving. This woman had been confined to her bed for a fortnight in the preceding November, *i.e.* when two months advanced in the same pregnancy, with modified small-pox. I saw her daily during that attack, and for a few days she was exceedingly ill; she was, moreover, the subject of rather extensive valvular disease of the heart.

DURATION.

As some difference exists in the statements of writers respecting the duration of typhus fever, and as the bearing of the question on the non-identity of typhus and typhoid fever is of importance, I shall offer a few remarks, and detail some cases, which may serve to illustrate, in a measure, the cause of this discrepancy.

The analogy between typhus fever and other diseases, such as scarlet fever and measles, which have their origin in specific causes, and are accompanied by a rash, would lead us to suppose that the former, like the latter, might possibly have a determinate duration. Experience proves that it has such limited duration. It is invariably an acute disease; and by no peculiarity of individual or external conditions can it become chronic.

What do we mean by the duration of typhus fever? How is that duration to be ascertained?

In determining the duration of those specific diseases with which typhus fever must be grouped, *i.e.* scarlet fever and measles, observers have been led to take the day of the disappearance of the rash as that of the cessation of the disease, and to class together the morbid phenomena which arise subsequently under the name of sequelæ. But the primary affections may have local diseases of serious import, not constituting an integral part of themselves, set up in their progress. These local diseases are called complications. Now, a complication may be very severe when the primary affection is of little moment, and may continue, or even increase in severity, after the primary affection has run its course. The patient may die of pneumonia or of tuberculosis a month or six weeks after the commencement of measles, there having been no cessation in the severity of the general febrile symptoms from the outset of the illness.

But we should never think of maintaining that the measles continued in this particular case for six weeks. All we could affirm would be that the local complication set up during the progress of the measles continued after the termination of the latter, and so prolonged the illness. Take another case, —one of rubeola *sine catarrho*, or a very mild case of scarlatina simplex; the patient suffers more or less general distress; an eruption appears, and he forthwith declares that he has nothing the matter with him. I have recently seen a man, suffering from scarlatina, with difficulty restrained from following his ordinary employment, and a physician of the very highest authority on the subject of scarlet fever informed me of a case in which a gentleman applied to him to be examined for the purpose of assuring his life, and who, when his life was refused on the ground that he was at that moment suffering from scarlet fever, expressed his astonishment at the information, stating that he felt perfectly well. A physician would consider such a man to be labouring under scarlet fever till the rash disappeared. We may briefly express the matter thus :—So long as the eruption continues, the disease of which it is the diagnostic character exists. The disappearance of the rash, in uncomplicated cases, indicates the termination of the specific disease.

There are two very opposite circumstances under the influence of which the date of the first appearance of the eruption is changed, and its duration shortened.

1st. A very mild attack of the specific disease.

2nd. The development of severe local complications in the course of the specific disease.

The normal duration of the eruption, and consequently of the disease, of the existence of which the latter is the index, is only to be determined from well-developed uncomplicated cases.

Corroborative evidence may be obtained from the examination after death of fatal cases; thus, if a person dies while suffering from scarlet fever, an examination after death may demonstrate no lesion to account for the fatal termination. We consider the individual to have died, in such a case, from the direct action of the poison on the blood or nervous system; this absence of local lesion experience proves only to be observed in cases fatal within a limited period from the outset of the illness; if the patient dies after that period has elapsed, experience proves that local lesions are invariably found sufficient to account for death.

All this is equally true of typhus fever.

CASE XVIII.—Sudden headache—pain in the limbs —rigors—loss of strength—epistaxis—mulberry rash—quick pulse—bowels regular—dry brown tongue—slight somnolence —disappearance of the eruption on the 14th day of disease —recovery.

Bartholomew H., aged 17.—The brother of J. H. (see Case III.). A moderately stout, fair, well-made youth, by trade a baker, was admitted into the London Fever Hospital under the care of Dr. Tweedie, Nov. 3, 1848. He always enjoyed health till his present illness, but had been subject to very frequent attacks of epistaxis. Having passed a good night, Thursday, October 26th, he awoke on the morning of the 27th with headache, pain in the limbs, slight rigors, and sense of chilliness, followed by heat and sweating; the rigors, etc., were repeated frequently up to the date of his admission; his bowels acted regularly from the outset, and there was no vomiting. He had taken some aperient medicine before he entered the hospital; he kept his bed from the first day; his nose had bled two or three times.

The following note of his condition was taken November 4th, i.e. the ninth day of disease :—Severe general headache; the pain being occasionally of a shooting character; little sleep; very restless at night; expression heavy; mental powers dull; no delirium; muddy hue of face; no flush; some dusky-red mottling of the face; pupils normal; conjunctivæ slightly more vascular than natural; humming noise in the ears, and unpleasant taste in the mouth; no affection of vision; vertigo in the erect position. He can leave his bed unassisted, so as to reach a close stool adjoining, but with considerable difficulty; lips dry; sordes on the teeth; tongue dry, pale brown centre, red border; three watery stools; slight tenderness at the epigastrium; no fulness nor increased resonance of abdomen; pulse 120; no abnormal physical chest signs; no cough; skin hot, dry, spotted; spots numerous, dusky pink, irregular in shape; the majority with ill-defined outline; some round; the large majority not elevated; fade only on pressure; a few, slightly elevated, disappear on pressure; a few spots on the face; no miliary vesicles.

The spots, which on admission disappeared on pressure, faded only on pressure on the 11th day of disease; the eruption grew more dusky in hue on the 12th; on the 13th it was unchanged in character, and began to grow paler on the 14th day. The tongue continued brown and dry till the 13th day, when it was noted to be moist and loaded, yet there was a little desire for food on the 12th day. The pulse gradually fell from the date of his admission; thus, on the 11th and 12th days it was 100; on the 13th and 14th days, 96; and on the 15th day, when the next and last note was taken, it was only 72. With the exception of mental dulness, some want of sleep till the 11th day, and then trifling somnolence for twenty-four hours, there were no symptoms referable to the head.

The epistaxis had probably no relation to the fever, as the lad frequently suffered when in ordinary health from bleeding from the nose.

The youth who formed the subject of this case was the brother of J. H. (see Case III.). The identity of the eruption in the two is obvious. They both had well-marked mulberry rash; the disease in both was tolerably severe and uncomplicated; its duration was nearly the same in the two cases, viz. thirteen and fourteen days. These two brothers had probably been exposed to the same specific cause.

CASE XIX.—Sudden headache, vertigo, and sense of weakness—trifling rigors—confined bowels—mulberry rash—quick pulse—loss of sleep—fall in the pulse—delirium—somnolence—recovery.

John M., aged 24, a man of sober habits, who before his present attack had suffered much from want, slept in union-house, etc., by trade a type-founder, was admitted into the London Fever Hospital under the care of Dr. Tweedie, May 8th, 1848.   His previous health had been, with the exception of occasional catarrhs, good. On 2nd of May he was seized with a sense of general weakness, frontal headache, and vertigo.   On the 5th he took to his bed in consequence of increased sense of weakness; slight shivering occurred on the 6th and 7th.   He lost his appetite, suffered from thirst and confined bowels from the outset.

On the 9th of May, *i.e.* the 8th day of disease, the following particulars were noted :—He slept well last night ; there is no headache ; slight heaviness of expression ; injection of conjunctivæ ; occasional singing in the ears ; other senses normal ; mind unaffected.

Though weak, he is able to leave his bed to reach the close stool without assistance ; movements and position in bed unconstrained.

Tongue moist, furred posteriorly ; no appetite ; some thirst ; five stools ; some gurgling in the right iliac fossa ; no abnormal fulness nor tenderness of the abdomen.

Pulse 108 ; heart and breath sounds healthy.

Skin hot and dry ; trunk and extremities covered with eruption ; the spots are irregular in outline, of a dusky red colour, darker on the posterior surface of the trunk than on the anterior ; some fade only, others disappear on pressure ; no sudamina.

During the night he became very delirious, left his bed several times to wander about ; had no sleep.   On the following day he was still delirious ; his conjunctivæ were injected, and he complained spontaneously of headache.   The tongue, though moist, was brown ; his bowels acted twice, and he vomited frequently and copiously some green fluid ; there was no tenderness of the abdomen ; the pulse was 120 ; the eruption little changed in appearance.   His head was now shaved, and cold applied.   Some simple saline effervescing mixture, with four drops of hydrocyanic acid was administered every six hours, and 4 oz. of wine ordered to be given in divided doses during the succeeding 24 hours.

On the next day, that is, the 10th of disease, he was reported to have slept some hours at the early part of the evening.   After waking, he attempted frequently to quit his bed.   He was delirious at the time of the visit. ,He asserted that he had no headache. His conjunctivæ were still injected.   The vomiting ceased the evening before ; in other respects he was as on the 9th day ; the spots, which disappeared on pressure when he first came under observation, *now only faded* ; that is, grew paler on pressure.   On the 11th day somnolence commenced.   He was still delirious when awake, but made no effort to leave his bed.   On the 12th day his state was nearly the same; the pulse continued 120 and weak; the wine was increased to 6 oz. in the 24 hours.

From this time his pulse began to fall. On the 13th day it was 108; the 14th, 100; the 15th, 84; the 16th, 80; 18th, 66; 20th, 60. His tongue became moist on the 19th day; the bowels were regular or confined. On the 16th day there was slight deafness. The spots were much paler on the 17th day than they had been before that date. Delirium continued till the 19th day; the somnolence, which had disappeared, increased on the 18th day; and on the 19th he slept almost constantly night and day. His appetite began to return on the 21st day, and at the same time his pulse rose to 72.

This was a well-marked case of rather severe typhus fever. Some of the spots still disappeared on pressure, when J. M. was first seen, *i.e.* on the 9th day of disease; but, in the course of the disease, they passed into what I have previously described as their second stage. They began to grow paler on the 18th day of disease. There were two symptoms, usually termed 'head symptoms,' present in this case, which call for remark.

1st. The continuance of the headache complained of spontaneously, after the commencement of delirium. This combination of symptoms is generally of very important and grave import, indicative of increased vascular action within the cranium. It serves to separate meningitis from fever with symptomatic headache. In this case, however, the continuance of the headache appeared to be sympathetic, or dependent on the state of the stomach and liver. It disappeared when the vomiting ceased. The cessation of the vomiting, and the consequent disappearance of the headache, was probably due rather to the wine than to the hydrocyanic acid. Vomiting in typhus fever, unaccompanied by tenderness at the epigastrium, often ceases at once on the administration of stimulants. Louis, speaking of headache in typhoid fever, says that its cessation, when delirium or somnolence supervened, could not be attributed, in all cases, to the imperfect perception of the patients, because they often complained of pain in other parts of the body when they declared they had no headache. This is also true of typhus fever, and, I may remark, that, on the first commencement of the delirium, the patient, while declaring he had at that moment no pain in the head, will add, but ' I have had terrible headache.' The truth of Louis's remark is confirmed by the fact that in meningitis the patient will complain bitterly of headache while talking in other respects most incoherently.

2nd. The continuance of the delirium after the fall in the pulse, and general improvement in other respects. This symptom is not a very frequent one. When present the delirium generally disappears after a profound sleep. Like some of the cases previously detailed, this man became deaf about the termination of the second week.

CASE XX.—Trifling sense of illness for a fortnight—sudden debility—rigors on 5th day—headache—disturbance of mental functions, at first confusion only, then delirium—mulberry-rash on 7th day — somnolence — heaviness of expression—muddy hue of face—tongue dry, brown, and finally black—confined bowels—fulness and tenderness of abdomen—rapid pulse—extreme prostration—death on the 20th day—non-granular consolidation of the most depending part of the lungs—increased vascularity of the lining membrane of the urinary bladder—other organs normal.

Mary H., aged 44. A stout, dark-complexioned woman; a widow, the mother of three children, the youngest 12 years old, all living. Her mother died when very young; her father aged 70 'of old age;' a native of London; of sober habits; night-nurse at the London Fever Hospital.

Previous Health.—She stated that, although not very strong, she generally enjoyed health; ceased to menstruate at forty-two. She was once, many years since, confined to her bed, in consequence of an injury to her back, and once since that time from 'lumbago.' The other nurses stated, that she had, during her residence in the Hospital, frequently complained of pain in the back, and was in the habit of sleeping with a pillow under her loins. Seven years since was cupped in consequence of headache, to which she is subject. She suffers more or less constantly from cough, accompanied with expectoration.

Present Attack.—On the evening of August 22, 1849, she was exposed to wet; from that time she felt slightly unwell, though unable to state any particular symptoms. Her bowels were regular, and she had no headache. On Monday, September 6, she felt decidedly worse, and during the night was too ill to assist the patients even to a little water, although she still sat up. At this time she had neither headache, vertigo, singing in the ears, nor epistaxis, her bowels were confined. On September 7th she took to her bed, on the 8th had an emetic of ipecacuanha, which produced copious vomiting of bitter fluid, and acted on her bowels. On the 11th she had some rigors, for the first time. In addition to the emetic, she had taken before I saw her, some simple saline effervescing mixture, *i.e.* sodæ sesquicarb. and acid. tart. When she came under observation, September 12th, *i.e.* the *seventh day of disease*, the symptoms were as follows:—Decumbency dorsal, unconstrained; twice during the night of the 11th she left her bed unassisted, but was, at the time these notes were taken, quite unable to assist herself on to the close stool, or even to sit up in bed unsupported. There had been no delirium, and she answered questions rationally, but her memory was rather defective, and her mind generally rather dull. She had had some sleep the preceding night, undisturbed by dreams. There was a little frontal headache; the conjunctivæ were slightly injected, the pupils normal in appearance; there was no deafness, singing in the ears, nor vertigo; the cheeks were flushed; the expression was slightly anxious; the tongue, dry and cracked in the centre, was moist at the edges; the abdomen was full and resonant, there was no tenderness nor gurgling; there had been two or three relaxed stools during the preceding twenty-four hours, from a dose of castor oil; there was no appetite, some thirst.

The pulse was 110, and possessed some power; the respiration was 40 in the minute, quick and short; there was a little cough, and some sonorous and sibilous rales over the whole chest; the percussion note was normal, and there were no abnormal heart sounds.

The skin was hot, dry, and spotted; the spots were rather numerous, of a dull pink hue; on the abdomen and chest were many, a fourth of an inch in diameter, slightly elevated, but flat on the surface; their shape was somewhat irregular; they were effaceable on pressure, but resumed their previous appearance when the pressure was removed; on the arms were some very small, half a line in diameter, and not elevated; there was no eruption to be seen yesterday.

On the 9th *day of disease*, the slight anxiety in the expression, observable on the 7th, had disappeared, and was replaced by a dull, heavy aspect. The conjunctivæ were still more injected, and the eruption, which disappeared under the finger on the 7th day, now only faded on pressure; that is to say, the spots grew paler, but could not be effaced; 5 grains of sesquicarbonate of ammonia every six hours were substituted for the tartrate of soda. In the evening she became very delirious, and continued so at intervals till the termination of the disease. On the 10th *day* the headache had disappeared, nor did it return ; the flush of the cheeks was purplish. The debility was so great that she could not turn in bed, and had to be lifted out when the bed was made. On the parieties of the abdomen were two bright purple spots, round, not elevated, and unaffected by pressure, i.e. petechiæ. The pulse was now 130; the bowels relaxed, i.e. three or four relaxed stools were passed daily. On the 11*th* *day* somnolence commenced, and for the first time there was slight tenderness of the abdomen, and the following note respecting the spots was made :—' The centres of some spots are unaffected by pressure the circumferences of which fade, i.e. grow paler on pressure. Other spots are less affected by pressure than before.' On the next day the urine and stools were passed into bed unconsciously. The prostration became extreme ; her conjunctivæ still more injected ; she dozed almost constantly ; the dusky or muddy hue of the face grew daily more intense; the tenderness of the abdomen more decided, and especially marked in the hypogastric region. From the 16th day of disease till her death on the 20th day the urine had to be removed by catheter ; its quantity varied from two to three pints daily ; it was acid, and contained a few crystals of uric acid ; its specific gravity was 1·016.

On the 16th day she lay on her back immovable, constantly sleeping (when roused, she said that she felt much better) ; her mouth open ; cheeks sunken ; tongue dry, baked, black ; her bowels were confined, and she took 3 drs. of castor-oil. On the 18th day there was muttering delirium when aroused, and she generally lay in a semi-comatose state. The pulse had risen to 150, and was very feeble. There was abundant mucous rale over the anterior surface of the chest. She was too prostrate to be raised for the purpose of examining the back.

She died on the 20th day of the disease.

4 oz. of wine were given on the 11th day and increased to 6 oz. on the 14th day. A pint of porter was added on the 15th day. On the 16th, 2 pints of porter, 8 oz. of wine, and 1 oz. of brandy were administered.

The examination of the body of M. H. was made 50½ hours after death ; the weather was cool ; cadaveric rigidity was well marked ; there was no appearance of decomposition, and no emaciation. There was 1½ inches of fat on the abdominal parietes. On the anterior surface of the trunk, the spots marked during life by ink, to indicate that they faded or grew paler, without being obliterated on pressure, were still visible as pale reddish-brown stains ; of those marked in such a manner as to indicate that the circumference faded, while the centre was unaffected by pressure, the latter part retained the appearance it presented during life ; the former resembled the pale reddish-brown stains above described; while the spots which during life were entirely unaffected by pressure, *i.e.* the petechiæ, preserved the characters described as belonging to them before death. The traces of the spots were much more distinct on the inferior than the superior portion of the lateral regions of the trunk; while on the back they were of a deep purple colour.

Head.—There was a little colourless serosity at the base of the brain, and in the lateral ventricles; slight congestion of the vessels of the *pia mater*; and a few more red points than usual in the *white substance.* The consistence of the organ was normal throughout.

The *larynx and trachea* were healthy in all particulars.

Right lung.—There were no adhesions and no fluid in the pleura. The most depending part of the posterior portion of the organ was dark red, flabby; contained much thick dark bloody serosity, and little air; sank in water; broke down rather too readily under the finger. This abnormal condition extended about 1 inch into the substance of the lung.

Left lung.—The pulmonary and costal pleura were firmly united throughout their whole extent by old adhesions. The morbid appearances resembled those described in the opposite lung, but were rather more extensive.

The *bronchial tubes* contained much frothy mucus, and their lining membrane was rather more vascular than usual.

The *pericardium*, which contained about 1 oz. of transparent yellow serosity, was healthy.

The *heart* was somewhat flabby, but otherwise normal. It contained a little semi-fluid dark blood, frothy from the admixture of air, probably introduced in the act of opening the organ; large dark coagula in both auricles and in the large veins at the root of the heart, and large fibrinous coagula extending from the ventricles into the aorta and pulmonary artery. The descending aorta contained much fluid and dark semi-coagulated blood.

The *pharynx* and *œsophagus* were healthy.

The *stomach* was normal in all particulars, excepting some minute injection of the cardiac extremity. The *large* and *small intestines* contained much flatus. Their mucous membrane was pale throughout; its consistence and thickness being perfectly natural. *Peyer's patches* were found with difficulty.

There was no enlargement of the *mesenteric glands.*

The *liver* was flabby, and somewhat softer than natural; otherwise normal.

The *gall-bladder* contained from 2 to 3 oz. of pale thin bile, and a large number of small gall-stones (cholesterine with nuclei of inspissated bile); its lining membrane was normal.

Pancreas healthy.

The *spleen* weighed only 5¾ oz. It was flabby, but did not break down with abnormal facility ; its colour was natural.

The *kidneys* were large but healthy.

Urinary bladder.—There was minute capillary injection of the whole lining of this organ, especially intense on its anterior surface.

The *uterus* and *ovaries* were not removed ; they appeared as seen *in situ* healthy.

The reader's attention is especially directed to the progress of the spots in this case ; their three stages : the continuance of the same spot, from its first appearance till the termination of the disease in death ; and, finally, the persistence of the spots after death.   In order to direct attention to the same spot during its varying phases before and after death, a circle of ink thus ○ was placed around several when first seen, *i.e.* when they disappeared on pressure ; this mark was changed into a diamond thus ◇ when the spots faded only on pressure ; this diamond was surrounded by a square, thus ◈ when the centre was unaffected by pressure, and the circumference faded ; while a simple square, thus □ indicated the spots unaffected by pressure.   Without some such contrivance it is impossible to feel confident, that the same spot is observed on succeeding days, or that particular spots persist after death.   The tenderness of the hypogastric region was explained by the condition of the bladder.   The abnormal vascularity of that organ could not have been due to the retention of urine, because that symptom did not appear till the 15th or 16th day of disease, while the tenderness was first noted on the 11th day.   The urine, it may be remarked, was, as it usually is in typhus fever, quite as abundant as in health, and acid.   Its specific gravity was rather, but not abnormally, low.   The presence of a deposit of uric acid is worthy of note.   The sonorous and sibilous rales were probably proper to the chronic bronchitis from which this woman appeared to have suffered before her attack of fever. Peyer's patches and the mesenteric glands were, as they *always are* in fever accompanied by the mulberry rash, perfectly healthy, and the whole gastro-intestinal mucous membrane in a state that completely excluded the idea of this having been, in any sense of the word, a case of gastro-enteritis. It is not usual for the cadaveric rigidity to be well marked so many hours after death from typhus fever.

The lesion of the lungs was that which is so frequently found after death from typhus fever, *i.e.* non-granular consolidation of their most depending parts. That accidental position is the determining cause of the consolidation appears to be proved by the fact, that the solidification, unless it involves some depth of the pulmonary tissue, is limited to the most depending part of the inferior lobe; the extreme apex, base, and root of the lung still remaining crepitant; *i.e.* the consolidated part lies in the hollow formed by the fourth, fifth, and sixth ribs, between their tubercles and angles; that it is not due to cadaveric congestion is proved by the frequency with which physical signs indicative of its existence can be detected during life.

Death in this case could not be ascribed to the condition of the lungs; the lesion of those organs was too slight, and of too small an extent, to account for the fatal termination. In fact, there was no lesion revealed by the scalpel which could be regarded as the cause of death. It is not common for patients to survive till the 20th day of typhus fever, and then exhibit so little local morbid change after death.

The lengthened duration of the disease, conjoined with the total absence of anything approaching to a lesion of Peyer's patches is important, for certain German writers have asserted, that the cause of Peyer's patches being unaffected in typhus fever with exanthematous rash, is the early period of the disease at which such cases prove fatal— signifying that time sufficient for the deposit in those organs does not elapse between the commencement of the disease and death. Now, as I have said, this case did not prove fatal till the 20th day of disease (Cases v., VIII., and XXI. survived the 20th day), and there was no deposit in the glands, while I shall have hereafter to refer to a case of typhoid fever in which the deposit was very abundant on the fourth day of disease, and others which proved fatal, with very extensive ulceration, long before the termination of the third week. These cases in conjunction with the one I am here considering, and Cases v., VIII., and XXI., which survived the 20th day of disease, appear to me conclusive against the argument adduced in support of the identity of typhus and typhoid fevers, founded on the assumption that nature does not allow time enough before death for the deposit to take place in the agminated and mesenteric glands in the latter disease.

CASE XXI.—Imperfect history—delirium—prostration—deafness—loss of sleep—absence of abdominal signs—quick pulse—mulberry rash—erysipelatous inflammation of nose, pharynx, and larynx—dulness of right side of chest—friction right pleura—brain healthy—slough on arytæno-epiglottidean fold—post pharyngeal diffused abscess—fluid and recent lymph in right pleura—consolidation right lung—no lesion of gastro-enteric membrane.

Mary W., aged 42, a native of London, mother of several children: the wife of George W. (Case II.), and received into the hospital at the same time.

A thin woman, with light hair and eyes and dark complexion. She states that she has often been ill before the present attack,— the nature and severity of the illnesses were not ascertained. Never had rheumatism nor fever; not subject to cough. Affirms that her habits are temperate.

Present illness began on or *about* August 2nd. Her bowels had been regular from the first; she had been very delirious some days before her admission. Her husband, from whom the above particulars were obtained, assured me that ' it all lay in the head.' No further history could be learned. On her admission under the care of Dr. Tweedie, the following notes were made :—

August 10th, *i.e.* about the 15th day of disease, she was very delirious and slept but little during the night; the little sleep she had was disturbed and she moaned much. Has not closed her eyes to-day; the mind is now dull and confused, the memory very defective, the expression heavy and dull, the complexion thick; there is much vertigo, but no headache as she lies quiet; but when disturbed, as by loud talking, she suffers pain in the head. She occasionally grinds her teeth and knits her brow. She is slightly deaf, and affirms that she has a ' stupid ' noise in her ears; the conjunctivæ are scarcely more injected than natural, the pupils normal. The nurse states that, occasionally, the whole face is covered with a dusky flush. She lies ordinarily on her back, but can turn in bed unassisted, though she is unable to leave it without aid. The tongue is pale brown and dry: she has passed two stools into the close pan and one into bed; much thirst; no appetite. There is neither fulness, resonance, tenderness, nor gurgling of the abdomen. The pulse is 108—very weak; the respirations 28; trifling cough. There is a little sonorous rale on deep inspiration.

The surface is cool, the hands cold, the feet warm since a hot bottle has been applied to them. The skin is spotted; the spots are dusky red, not elevated, fade on pressure; more abundant and darker on the posterior than the anterior surface of the trunk; the subcuticular rash is very pale anteriorly; the whole dorsum has a somewhat purplish hue from congestion. Mist. am. acet. 6ta q.q. hora; vin. alb. 3i. 4ta q.q. hora.

The following day somnolence set in, and continued, with the exception of the night of the 18th day, when she was very delirious, singing, etc., till the 20th day, when she was much more intelligent and wakeful. The prostration increased rapidly from her entrance, so that on the next, i.e. 16th day of disease, she lay constantly on her back, was quite unable to turn in bed, and permitted her limbs to lie as they were placed. The stools and urine were, at the same time, passed into the bed unconsciously. On the 17th day, when told to show her tongue, she opened her mouth, but made no effort to protrude the organ. The bowels continued relaxed till the 20th day, from three to five dark liquid stools being passed daily. Some redness at the bottom of the spine was noted on the 18th day.

On the 20th day the pulse, which had never exceeded 108, fell to 96, the spots had almost disappeared, and she appeared on the verge of convalescence; but on the 21st day erysipelas set in, affecting the tip of the nose, but chiefly the pharynx and larynx.

The following note was then made:—Pulse, 120, very soft; nose slightly red, and swollen at the tip; makes a noise in the nose in breathing; no cough; expiration prolonged; respiration, 30; a little tenderness of the larynx; no swelling of the throat externally; swallows with difficulty, some fluid returns back into the glass; *uvula, velum pend. palat.* and pharynx very red. Tongue only partially and slowly protruded, red, dry, and glazed; one copious stool in close pan.

On the morning of the 23rd day she appeared in every respect better: the pulse had fallen to 100; the expression was improved; she swallowed with much less difficulty; the tongue was more freely protruded; all redness of nose and tenderness of larynx had disappeared; but there was a little vomiting of yellowish fluid. On the evening of the same day the breathing again became noisy; a mustard poultice was applied to the throat.

On the 24th day, at noon, the pulse had risen to 126; the breathing was noisy and laryngeal; expiration prolonged; the voice whispering and guttural, and there was tenderness, on firm pressure, over the larynx; the tonsils, uvula, and velum were red, swollen, and covered with mucus; fluids remained some time in the mouth, and then were swallowed with difficulty.

I did not see her on the 25th, 26th, and 27th days; but there appears, from the hospital records, to have been little change in the general or local state.

. On the morning of the 28th day of disease, I made the following notes:—

Pulse very rapid and weak, more than 150; respiration 44, chiefly abdominal, the right side of the abdomen moving much more than the left.   There is absolute dulness to about two inches above the angle of the right scapula; comparative dulness to the spine of the same bone; no breath sound, and diminished vocal fremitus over the absolutely dull portion; above that, friction and slightly increased vocal fremitus, anteriorly dulness to upper border of third rib, excepting about a hand's-breadth next sternum; some friction over the same part; no obliteration of the inter-costal spaces; the laryngeal symptoms had disappeared; there was trifling cough; the conjunctivæ were pale, the pupils large; there was occasional delirium; profuse sweats broke out about 8 P.M., and continued till death at a quarter to 4 A.M., on the 29th day of disease.   During the last twenty-four hours she did not speak. For two hours before death, she rolled her head from side to side. There was no other struggle or convulsive movement.

On the 18th day 3 oz. of gin were given, in addition to the wine ordered on the 16th day, and carbonate of ammonia, in five-grain doses, substituted for the acetate.   A blister was applied at the same time to the forehead.   On the 25th day, 1 grain of disulphate of quinine was given, instead of the carbonate of ammonia, and the quantity of wine was reduced to 4 oz., and the gin increased to 4 oz.

Examination, August 31st, 1849, of the body of Mary W., 19¼ hours after death.

Some Emaciation.—Cadaveric rigidity well marked.   Numerous miliary vesicles along the sides of the trunk; a few on the anterior surface.   No discoloration in the course of the veins.   Very little congestion of the posterior surface of the body.

Head.—The dura mater was somewhat thicker than usual. There was no marked increase in the vascularity of the pia mater. The membranes separated from the surface of the convolutions with normal facility.   There was very little serosity in the meshes of the pia mater.   The plexus choroidea was pale.   About ½ oz. of transparent serosity was found at the base of the brain. The substance of the encephalon and the central parts of the brain were of normal consistence.

The *tongue* was dry and brown.   Much purulent-looking fluid was infiltrated between the muscles as far as the left great cornu of the os hyoides and thyrohyoid membrane. Numerous minute collections of a fluid, resembling pus to the unassisted eye, were found beneath the *lining membrane of the pharynx*. A slough about ¾ inch in length, and ¼ inch in breadth occupied the free border and the pharnygeal surface of the *right arytæno-epiglottidean* fold. This slough was of a dirty brown colour, tough, totally disorganised; the margin of mucous membrane around was brightish red ; the slough was detached with facility, leaving an ulcerated surface covered with purulent-looking fluid exposed. The tonsils were rather large and firm ; the anterior and posterior surfaces of the velum and uvula pale. On the under surface of the *epiglottis*, near its root, was a vivid red patch about half an inch in length. The mucous membrane of the larynx above the chordæ vocales was thickened and roughened; below the chords pale and healthy, as in the trachea.

There was no fluid in the *left pleural cavity*, and only a few old adhesions at the apex of the lung.

The *left lung* was healthy and crepitant throughout.

The r*ight lung* adhered to the pericardium by quite recent yellow lymph ; the free edge of the organ was fringed by similar matter.

The right pleura contained about 6 oz. or 8 oz. of slightly turbid serosity, floating through which was a considerable quantity of yellow lympho-purulent substance. Examined by a quarter-inch glass, this substance was found to consist of lymph, containing in its meshes much finely granular matter, and numerous non-nucle-ated granular corpuscles, about the size of pus globules.

The right lung itself was pale anteriorly, and of a dusky reddish violet posteriorly, especially the inferior portion of the inferior lobe. On section, the posterior portion of the inferior lobe, from base to apex, was of a brownish red colour, flabby, tough, non-crepitant, sank in water, and gave exit to some pale reddish serosity. The posterior part of the superior lobe was crepitant, of a dusky red colour, and contained but little excess of serosity.

The anterior portion of the lung was crepitant for nearly four inches from its margin ; the anterior part of the inferior lobe was coated with recent lymph. On removing the lymph from the pleura, that membrane was seen to be dull white and opaque, the hue varying from mere milkiness to absolute opacity.

There was a similar condition of the posterior part of the inferior lobe.

The *bronchial tubes* contained a moderate amount of aerated mucus ; their lining membrane was pale. There was no enlarge-ment of the *bronchial glands*.

The *pericardium* was healthy in appearance, and contained

about 6 drs. of transparent serosity. The substance and valves of the *heart* were healthy; its consistence good. Much dark loosely-coagulated blood escaped from the venæ cavæ and pulmonary veins on section. The right auricle contained a large fibrinous clot; the right auricle a small fibrinous clot, interlaced among the *columnæ carneæ*. The latter clot was continuous with one in the pulmonary artery. The left auricle contained a small black and fibrinous clot; the *conus arteriosus* of the ventricle a fibrinous clot, extending into the aorta, where it was moulded to the sigmoid valves. The endocardium was *unstained*.

The *œsophagus* was pale, covered for three inches from the pharynx by a dense white layer of epithelium; lower down the lining membrane was smooth and shining. The cellular tissue at the back of the pharynx and œsophagus as low as the first dorsal vertebra was infiltrated with a purulent-looking fluid. From this part to the inferior portion of the third dorsal vertebra, the organs contained in the posterior mediastinum, *i.e.* the thoracic duct, etc., were closely matted together by dense false membrane and lymph.

Examined by the microscope, this purulent-looking fluid presented the following elements :—

a. Fat globules.

b. Finely granular matter.

c. Granular corpuscles about the size of pus globules.

Acetic acid dissolved or rendered transparent the chief part of the granular matter; but brought no nuclei into view.

Stomach.—The colour and consistence of the lining membrane of this organ was natural; it was mammillated from near the pylorus to within about four inches of the cardiac extremity.

The *cæcum* and *colon* were distended with flatus; the latter contained a large tapeworm. The large and small *intestines* were healthy in colour, thickness, and consistence throughout, with the exception of a little increased vascularity of the sigmoid flexure of the colon. *Peyer's patches* were indistinctly seen.

The *mesenteric glands* were healthy.

The *liver* was perfectly normal in appearance. The *gall bladder* was moderately distended with thin orange bile. Its lining membrane was healthy.

The *pancreas* was pale and normal in appearance.

The *spleen* weighed 5¼ ozs.; it was pale, much corrugated, moderately tough, and flabby.

The *kidneys* were healthy in appearance, except that there were about twenty small cysts on the surface and in the substance of the left. The lining membrane of the urinary bladder was congested, its rugæ being dull red.

The *uterus* and *ovaries* were healthy.

This woman survived till the 29th day of disease. Her case offers a good illustration of the impropriety of confounding the duration of the typhus fever with the duration of the illness. The fever, properly so called, had terminated just before the 20th day of disease. Erysipelas supervened on the 22nd day. Doubtless the pleuritic disease was of the same nature as the erysipelatous inflammation of the skin of the nose and of the mucous membrane of the pharynx and larynx. It has been supposed that erysipelas of the head and face invariably has its starting-point from some minute abrasion of the surface. In fever it very frequently, as in this case, appears to commence in the pharynx, and thence extend, by the mucous membrane of the nose, outwards to the skin, and downwards to the larynx. Occasionally, however, it will commence in the pharynx, and a few hours after show itself on the ridge of the nose near the eyes. In such a case, the erysipelas takes its start from two distinct centres, one for the mucous membrane and one for the skin. The dry, red, and swollen mucous membrane of the pharynx was visible during life. The noisy, prolonged expiration, the whispering guttural voice, and the tenderness of the larynx, sufficiently indicated the condition of its lining membrane. The presence of the large slough found after death on the arytæno-epiglottidean fold did not prevent the more prominent laryngeal symptoms disappearing during life. The return of fluids from the mouth into the glass, and the holding of fluids in the mouth for some time before making an effort to swallow, were symptoms which indicated serious lesion of the pharyngeal mucous membrane, and rendered ulceration or sloughing of its surface, or purulent infiltration of the submucous tissue highly probable. The pharyngeal preceded the laryngeal disease in this case, as is the rule. It will be observed that no pus corpuscles were discovered in the post-pharyngeal abscess. The fluid presented the microscopic appearances generally discovered in similar cases; the distinctive nucleated corpuscles being rarely if ever present, however closely the fluid may, to the unaided eye, present characters of true pus. The miliary vesicles, or sudamina, were preceded by profuse sweating. This eruption is very infrequent on patients more than 40 years of age, and is rarely, if ever, seen after 50.

To sum up :—Cases I., X., XII., and XIV. presented no lesion after death ; they proved fatal before the 16th day of disease.

Cases II., XI., XIII., and XX. offered lesions too slight to account for the fatal termination ; these four terminated before the 21st day.

Cases V., VIII., and XXI. proved fatal after the 21st day ; examination of the internal organs sufficed to explain the death of these three patients.

Cases III., IV., XVIII., and XIX. recovered from the fever ; the rash in these cases began to fade respectively on the 13th, 15th, 14th, and 18th days.

Cases VI. and VII., in which no rash appeared, were convalescent on the 12th and 13th days respectively.

Taken conjointly, all these cases illustrated the facts—1st, that the ordinary duration of typhus fever is from 14 to 21 days ; 2nd, that uncomplicated typhus fever may terminate the life of the patient at any period before the 21st day ; 3rd, that after the 21st day, local lesions, sufficient to account for death, are, as a rule, discoverable.

It will be observed that 13 of the 21 cases detailed in these papers were part of as many families, more than one member of which suffered from the *same* disease.

The close resemblance of the disease in the brothers J. and B. H., Cases III. and XVIII., and in the man and wife, George and Mary W., Cases II. and XXI., must strike the most careless observer. I have previously alluded to this fact ; I will not here repeat.

Although I have stated the duration of typhus fever to be from 14 to 21 days—and I believe that the disease never exceeds 21 days in duration—it not unfrequently, in very mild cases, terminates before the 14th day, if the fading of the eruption be taken to be the index of the termination of the disease. The general symptoms in these cases are invariably exceedingly mild. There is nothing anomalous in this short duration of a specific disease which ordinarily lasts a longer period. In scarlet fever we occasionally see cases in which the eruption disappears in a day or two after its first appearance, the patient experiencing scarcely a single symptom of general illness.

§ 4. TYPICAL CASES OF TYPHOID FEVER.

CASE XXII.—Without known cause—frontal headache—pain in the abdomen—vertigo—debility—dry red tongue—diarrhœa—heaviness of expression—somnolence—delirium—flushing of cheeks—mucous rale—rose spots—symptoms of laryngitis—death on the 33rd day.

Forty-one and a half hours after death :—Ulcers of the pharynx—extensive ulceration of Peyer's patches—enlargement of the mesenteric glands—redness and thickening of lining membrane of larynx—imperfect consolidation of posterior part of left lung—redness and softening of mucous membrane of bronchial tubes.

Jane T., aged 32, a servant in a public-house, was admitted into the London Fever Hospital under the care of Dr. Tweedie, November 11th, 1847. She had resided in London about four or five years ; had never suffered want of food or clothing ; unmarried, but the mother of two children. She was of temperate habits ; her previous health had been excellent.

On Sunday, October 31st, she suffered from headache and pain in the abdomen, followed the next day by pains in the limbs and back. On Monday night she had rigors, which were repeated the three or four succeeding nights. At this time the bowels were relaxed, and they continued so till the 6th November, when, without having taken any aperient medicine, they became much relaxed. For the first two or three days of her illness she suffered from vertigo. During the course of her illness she has had a sense of unpleasant taste and smell with nausea, but no vomiting, and no epistaxis. She quitted her work on October 31st, but did not take to her bed till the 3rd of November.

The following notes of her condition were made, November 12th, i.e. the 13th day of disease :—' She slept but little last night ; intellect unaffected ; the expression natural ; a little frontal headache; vertigo in the erect position ; slight singing in the ears ; she is able to leave her bed unassisted, but with difficulty ; she complains of pain in the back ; the tongue is slightly furred—dry, smooth, and red; she has passed during the last twenty-four hours one scanty stool. There is no appetite, but much thirst; she complains spontaneously of pain in the abdomen, which is full and resonant. There is some tenderness on firm pressure in the right iliac fossa. The pulse is 120 ; there is no cough; with the exception of a little sonorous rale on deep inspiration, the chest signs are normal. The skin is warm and dry. A few—about twenty—slightly elevated rose-coloured circular spots, which

Q

disappear under pressure, are seen on the abdomen and thorax. There are no sudamina.'

She died on the 33rd day of disease. The following changes in her condition were noted between the 12th and 33rd days :—

The pulse 120 on the 12th day, fell on the 13th to 100, rose again to 120 on the 14th day, was 100 only on the 15th day, 110 on the 17th day, but only 96 on the 19th. It again rose to 120 on the 21st day. From the 22nd to the 30th it ranged between 126 and 130. On the 30th, however, it reached 160, which rate it maintained till her death.

The tongue became moist and clean two days after admission ; i.e. on the 14th day of disease, and continued so till the 17th day, when it became dry and fissured in the centre; at the same time it continued clean. On the 21st it became dry over its whole surface, and at the same time was covered with a pale yellow fur, cracked across at various parts; this fur commenced to separate on the 23rd day in large scales; the cracks in it communicating, and the edges of the scales curling up. On the following day the yellow fur assumed a brownish hue, which continued without change till death. Sordes appeared on the teeth for the first time on the 30th day.

The slight tenderness of the abdomen observed on her admission disappeared on the following day, and neither pain, tenderness, gurgling, fulness, nor resonance were observed from the 12th day till her death. At the same time the stools continued relaxed ; i.e. of thin pulpy consistence. On the 24th and 30th days they were absolutely watery; on the 25th and 29th days she had no stool ; with these exceptions, their number varied from two to three daily.

Some heaviness of expression was observed on the 19th, and it had increased considerably by the 24th day ; at the latter date, too, somnolence commenced, and she was noted to doze much night and day. This condition continued till the 29th day, when she slept less, and on the 30th was decidedly more wakeful; on the 31st the somnolence had disappeared. There was no delirium till the erysipelatous redness of the nose showed itself on the last day of life.

Deafness was first observed on the 22nd day of disease; it became more marked on the 24th day, and continued till death. The general strength was markedly impaired, yet she continued to leave her bed without the aid of a nurse ; i.e. to assist herself on to the close stool till the 24th day of disease; but from the 24th till her death she was quite unable, although even on the 31st she supported herself in bed without assistance, when raised by the nurse. On the 30th and 33rd days she passed one stool into bed, apparently unconscious of the act.

Flushing of the cheeks was frequently observed, but was not constantly present.

The cough trifling on the 19th day; was much more troublesome on the 30th day; it continued till her death. The sonorous rale remained with little change; but, on the 29th, subcrepitant rale was heard over the posterior part of the chest. There was no dulness.

The spots observed on admission were very pale on the 15th day of disease; at the same time, a few fresh ones were noted to be present. These, too, were paler on the 17th day; and, on the 21st day, all those previously observed had disappeared, but three or four fresh spots, of the same character as those first described, were marked. These spots, also, had nearly disappeared on the 23rd. No fresh spots had made their appearance on the 24th day. I failed to make any further note with reference to the presence or absence of spots. The skin was dry from the outset, and no miliary vesicles were observed.

On the 31st day, she complained, for the first time, of sore throat; the velum pendulum palati and tonsils were red, dry, and slightly swollen.

The following notes of her condition were made on the 33rd day of disease, about 2 P.M. :—'She passed a very restless night, wanting to leave her bed while delirious. Her mind is now wandering a little. The cheeks are free from flush. There is a faint red erysipelatous blush covering the nose and upper lip. The redness is somewhat darker over the lower than the upper half of the nose. She swallows with difficulty. She has lost her voice. The breathing is tracheal. There is slight tenderness on pressure over the upper part of the larynx. On listening over the trachea, the inspiratory sound is short and harsh; expiratory, prolonged and snoring. A little mucous rale is heard over both sides of the chest anteriorly.

She swallows with some difficulty; the tongue is dry and brown; she has passed two stools, one of them in bed; the expression of prostration is much more marked than before; she is unable to support herself in the least degree in bed.

She died at 9 P.M., without a struggle.

The treatment, at the first, was simply expectant. On the 21st day a blister was applied to the chest. On the 24th, 6 ozs. of white wine were ordered. The quantity of wine was increased to 8 ozs. on the 32nd day. At the same date a blister was applied to the side of the neck, and calomel and opium pills administered every three hours.

The body of J. T. was examined 41½ hours after death, and the following appearances noted :—

Cadaveric rigidity was well marked in all the joints; a moderate amount of fat on the surface. The spots marked during life had left no trace of their existence.

Head.—The larger vessels of the pia mater were slightly congested; a little transparent colourless serosity was found in the cavity of the arachnoid. There was also a little similar fluid in the meshes of the pia mater, by which the arachnoid was slightly elevated over the anfractuosities; it was not raised from the surface of the convolutions. There was no opacity of the arachnoid. The pia mater separated with normal facility from the surface of the brain. About 6 drms. of serosity escaped from the ventricles. The consistence and colour of the cerebral substance was natural.

The lining membrane of the *pharynx* was congested, and covered with thick muce-purulent matter. The mucous membrane covering the uvula was destroyed by an ulcer, which extended up the posterior surface of the velum pendulum palati for about two lines. It was about 4 or 5 lines in breadth in the latter situation; the edges of the ulcer were bright red; its floor, formed of submucous cellular tissues, was dull red; the edges of the ulcer were not thickened; it was quite superficial. A similar but smaller ulcer was seated on the hard palate.

Larynx.—The arytæno-epiglottidean folds were considerably thickened; a large mass of tough mucus filled the opening into the larynx; the rima glottidis was very narrow, in consequence of thickening of the chordæ vocales. The whole mucous membrane of the larynx was congested, and covered with purulent-looking fluid.

The *bronchial tubes* of both lungs were nearly filled with muco-purulent fluid. The mucous membrane of the larger tubes was minutely injected and soft, being readily removeable by a light scraping. The minute tubes were filled with purulent-looking fluid, which issued from the cut surface of the lung in drops.

Lungs.—There was no fluid in either pleura. The left lung was free. A few firm adhesions united the posterior inferior part of the left lung to the costal pleura.

Right lung weighed 15¼ ozs. It was crepitant throughout, but felt more solid posteriorly than anteriorly. The posterior part of the lung was of a deep dirty red colour. Portion cut from any part of the lung floated in water.

Left lung weighed 15½ ozs. The most depending part was of a deep violet colour, felt more solid than natural, contained but little air, broke down rather too readily on pressure, and after firm pressure sank in water.

The *pericardium* contained 1 oz. of yellow serosity. It was healthy in all respects.

The *heart* weighed 8 ozs. Its substance and valves were

healthy. The right auricle and ventricle contained a large firm yellow fibrinous clot continuous with a similar clot in the pulmonary artery. In the left auricle and ventricle there was a smaller similar clot extending into the aorta.

The *mesentery* was loaded with fat.

The *mesenteric glands* appeared numerous ; they were about the size of peas, of a reddish colour, and soft.

On the peritoneal surface of the lower part of the ileum were several oval patches of a purplish colour from minute injection. The small intestines were moderately distended with flatus. There was a little fæculent matter in the large and small intestines.

The *œsophagus*, the *stomach*, *duodenum*, and *jejunum* were carefully examined, and appeared healthy.

Ileum.—About three feet above the ileo-cæcal valve was one of Peyer's patches, finely injected, but scarcely thicker than natural ; on its upper part was an ulcer, 1 line in diameter, its floor formed of sub-mucous cellular tissue ; its edges not elevated. About 6 inches below the above described patch was a circular ulcer, about 3 lines in diameter, the margin of which was considerably thickened ; its floor was formed of sub-mucous tissue. From this ulcer to the ileo-cæcal valve, every Peyer's patch was more or less destroyed by ulceration. Some of the ulcers were circular, some oval, others irregularly oval. On some of the patches were two ulcers, separated by a narrow slip of undestroyed mucous membrane. There was no thickening of any of the patches. The floors of a majority of the ulcers were formed by the exposed and slightly enlarged transverse muscular fibres of a deep red colour. The margins of the ulcers were of a deep grey colour. Their diameters varied from 3 lines to an inch. Immediately above the ileo-cæcal valve the mucous membrane of the whole circumference of the intestine was more or less completely destroyed, here and there the ulcerated surface being divided or partially divided by narrow lines of mucous membrane of a deep grey colour. At some places the floor of this large ulcer was formed by transverse muscular fibres, at others, of the sub-mucous tissue.

The mucous membrane of the ileum, between the ulcerated agminated glands, was healthy in colour, consistence, and thickness.

The patches of injection, described as seen on the peritoneal surface of the small intestines, were found to correspond to the ulcerated Peyer's patches.

The *large intestines* were healthy in colour and consistence.

The *pancreas* was natural in appearance.

The liver.—The branches of the vena portæ and vena hepatica contained much dark fluid blood. The division between the lobules was indistinctly marked. There was some faint yellowish mottling of the surface and substance. The fracture and consistence was normal.

The *gall bladder* contained 1½ ozs. of rather pale yellowish bile. Its lining membrane was healthy.

The *spleen* measured 4½ inches by 3 ; *i.e.* it was small. Its external surface was corrugated. It was normal in colour and consistence.

The kidneys, urinary bladder, and uterus appeared in every respect healthy.

CASE XXIII.—Without known cause — debility — diarrhœa—noisy delirium—pink flush of the cheeks—rose spots —cough—sonorous rale—rapid pulse—great difficulty in swallowing—tension, resonance, and tenderness of abdomen —dry brown tongue—extreme prostration—*death* on about the 23rd day.

Twenty-two hours after death : loss of cadaveric rigidity —ulceration of pharynx—extensive ulceration of Peyer's patches—enlargement and softening of the mesenteric gland —enlargement of the spleen—recent adhesion of pleura— non-granular lobular pneumonia.

Fanny P., aged 16, a stout, fair, brown-haired girl, a domestic servant, was admitted into the London Fever Hospital, under the care of Dr. Tweedie, November 27th, 1848.

Her previous health was said to have been very good. She was in a situation, and not in want of any of the necessaries of life. She was born in London.

The following history only of her present illness could be obtained. She left her situation on the 16th November, and took to her bed the same day. Her bowels were said to have been confined till after she had aperient medicine, but this was doubtful. For a night or two preceding her admission she had been delirious, and had complained about as long of her throat. She appeared to those around her to have some difficulty in swallowing. Epistaxis, to a slight amount, took place directly after her entrance into the hospital. On the day after her admission the following notes were made :—

November 28th, *i.e.* 13th day after taking to bed.—She had no sleep till towards morning, and then very little. She was very noisy, frequently attempting to leave her bed, but unable. Mind very dull. Memory defective. Knows where she is, but has no idea how long she has been in the hospital. The expression of face is somewhat heavy ; the complexion is clear ; the right cheek is flushed, of a pink colour ; the conjunctivæ slightly injected ; the pupils natural. There is no headache.

She can lie in any position, but moves heavily and slowly, and is quite unable to leave her bed unaided by the nurse. The muscular movements are very unsteady; there is an ulcerated surface over the spine, just above the scapulæ, evidently the result of the application of a blister. There is no sloughing or discoloration over the sacrum.

The upper lip appears slightly swollen; it is pale; both lips are dry; the teeth are covered with black sordes; the tongue is dry and brown; the breath very offensive. She has passed since admission three watery stools, two of them into the bed. The abdomen is full and resonant, and somewhat tender, *i.e.* generally. She has great difficulty in swallowing, and appears to suffer when pressure is made behind the angles of the lower jaw. The pulse is 120, very weak; heart's impulse very feeble; there is slight cough; respiration 36. Much sonorous rale is heard over the whole chest; a little submucous rale at the base of the left lung posteriorly.

Skin coarse and dry; about twenty rose spots on the back, and about as many on the anterior surface of abdomen and thorax.

She died on the 12th day of her stay in the hospital, and on about the 23rd of her illness.

The following was the course of particular symptoms:—

The pulse rose to 144 on the 15th day, and continued at that rate till the 18th day, when it fell to 132; on the following day it rose again to 150; it was 160 on the 19th day, and the morning of her death it was too rapid to count. It continued to grow daily weaker till the last. The respiration was 48 on the 15th day, and 66 on the day of her death.

Slight cough and abundant sonorous rale continued till death. There was little change in the appearance of the tongue till the 17th day, when it became slightly moist at the edges. On the 20th day it was decidedly moister and cleaner, at the same time it was rather red. On the 21st and 22nd days it was much cleaner and moist at the edges.

The breath continued very offensive till she died. There was no difficulty in swallowing after the 16th day. There was no alteration in the appearance of the upper lip.

She passed one watery stool daily till the 21st, when my notes state, ' she has passed during the last twenty-four hours one scanty *solid* stool.' On the 22nd she had two scanty hard stools, and on the day of her death two stools of pulpy consistence. She passed about one pint of urine daily. The abdomen, which on admission was, as I have said, full, resonant, and generally tender, became on the following day still fuller and more resonant; the tub-shape well marked. The belly was yet more distended on the 15th

day, and the tenderness more decided. There was no change in
the condition of the abdomen from the 15th day till her death.

On the 14th day the expression was dull and stupid. The
sleepless delirium was replaced by somnolence, and both cheeks
were flushed. She still moved in bed unassisted. On the 15th
day she lost a few drops of blood from the nose. The somnolence
was constant, and she was aroused with difficulty; the conjunctivæ were somewhat more injected than on admission; the pupils
were rather large; the cheeks continued flushed; the expression
duller; the prostration had markedly increased; she did not
move in bed voluntarily, but lay exactly as she was placed on her
sides or back; somnolence continued till death. On the 17th day
the right cheek was flushed. She talked much in her sleep, and
when aroused uttered a few incoherent sentences. At the same
date she lay constantly on her back, with her knees drawn up.
Subsultus tendinum was observed on the 19th day, and at the
same time she sank towards the bottom of the bed.

On the 14th day the spots first noted were much paler, and
several fresh rose spots were observed. Eight or ten others
appeared on the abdomen and thorax on the 15th day, and several
on the back. All those previously marked had disappeared on
the 17th day; at the same time there were several fresh rose spots.
On the 18th day the following note was made:—'There is no
trace of some of the spots marked on the 16th day; those noted
yesterday are paler. There are about eight fresh spots on the
thorax and abdomen.' On the 20th day I wrote of the spots
noted on the 17th and 18th days, 'part of both dates have disappeared; the others are paler. There are no new rose spots.'

The following note was taken on the 23rd day, some three
hours before her death:—

Pulse very rapid and very weak; respiration 66; slight
cough; sonorous and mucous rale over both sides of the chest
anteriorly; no dulness of the same part (she was too prostrate to
be raised in bed); somnolence constant; extreme prostration.
Decumbency dorsal, knees elevated. Abdomen full, resonant,
rounded; two stools relaxed; no spots; breath still most offensive. Urine, 1½ pint.' She died at half-past four P.M. on the
23rd day of the disease. At 3 P.M. she vomited a considerable
quantity of dark, almost black, fluid; the vomiting was repeated
several times before death; she also passed, during the last hour
of life, two black liquid stools into bed. After the vomiting she
turned on to her face; and though twice placed on her side, she
replaced herself on to her face. She did not know her sister
at 3 P.M. She died quietly; there were no convulsions. 6
ozs. of white wine were given daily, in divided doses, till the
15th day; the quantity was then increased to 8 ozs. On

the morning of her death 3 ozs. of brandy were added. Opiate enemata were administered to check the purging. A mustard poultice was applied to the throat on the day of admission. Nitro-muriatic acid was given the last few hours of life.

Examination of the body of Fanny P., December 9th, 1848, twenty-two and a half hours after death. The weather warm for the season.

There was no cadaveric rigidity; some purple discoloration of the face, forehead, neck, and upper arms; there was no trace of the spots noted during life; the abdomen was moderately distended; about ½ inch of fat covered the abdominal parietes.

Head.—There was a little colourless serosity beneath the arachnoid; the pia mater was more congested than natural; a very small quantity of colourless, transparent fluid was found in the ventricles; the substance of the organ was firm throughout.

The *tongue* was covered with thick brown mucus; an ulcer about ¼ inch in diameter was seen on the left side of the organ, near the root of the anterior pillar of the velum; the base of this ulcer was formed of muscular fibres; its edges were pale and slightly elevated.

The *tonsils* were unaffected.

On the back of the *pharynx* was situated a large, irregularly-shaped ulcer, at one part ¾ inch in diameter; the floor of this ulcer was formed of dark-coloured muscular fibres; its edges were slightly elevated and sharp; around and beneath it were two or three similar but smaller ulcers; the mucous membrane of the pharynx generally was dusky red—around the ulcers dark purple.

The *œsophagus* pale; no trace of ulceration; its epithelium was still attached.

The mucous membrane of the *stomach* was pale and mammillated throughout, coated at places with thick mucus; its consistence and thickness was natural.

The *duodenum* and *jejunum* appeared perfectly healthy.

Ileum.—About 3 feet above the ileo-cæcal valve was a perfectly healthy Peyer's patch, without a trace of thickening or softening of its mucous membrane. About 4 inches lower was another patch, on the upper part of which was an ulcer a fourth of an inch in diameter; its edges thickened, and of a dusky red colour; its floor formed of submucous tissue, also of a dark red colour; the mucous membrane in the vicinity of this ulcer was slightly softened and considerably injected; the vessels running towards it were large, and filled with blood; the lower part of this patch was pale; its mucous membrane softened and slightly thickened. The next patch, in descending towards the cæcum, was a small one; its mucous membrane was vascular, softened, and slightly thickened. A small ulcer was seated near its lower extremity. From this spot downwards every patch was more or less extensively destroyed by ulceration, three, four, or more ulcers being seated on each patch. The floors of the ulcers were, in part or altogether, formed of transverse muscular fibres; their edges were considerably elevated, of a deep crimson, or of a slate colour; the latter hue was more marked in the vicinity of the cæcum than above.

Those portions of the agminated glands undestroyed by ulceration were slightly thickened; the thickening being due chiefly to a swollen state of the mucous membrane, but partly to a similar condition of the submucous tissue. There was no appearance of any deposit beneath or around the ulcers. At their edges the submucous tissue was highly vascular. Among these large ulcers were several—five or six—small and circular ulcers apparently having their origin in the solitary glands; and also many slightly enlarged but yet non-ulcerated solitary glands. The mucous membrane generally was of normal consistence and colour to within two feet of the valve; at this point it was finely injected, but neither thickened nor softened. The last eight inches of the gut were pale.

Large intestines pale and healthy in appearance throughout. There was no enlargement of the solitary glands.

Peritoneum.—There was a little injection of the serous membrane corresponding to the deepest ulcers in the ileum, but no deposit of lymph, and no opacity or thickening. There were about 5 or 6 ozs. of transparent yellow serosity in the peritoneal cavity.

The *mesentery* contained in its substance a considerable quantity of fat. The *mesenteric glands* were of a dark purple colour and soft. Their size varied from a pea to a large bean. The largest and softest being seated near the lower part of the ileum.

The *liver* was flabby. Its substance appeared healthy. The *gall bladder* was distended with thin orange-green bile. Its lining membrane appeared healthy.

The *spleen* large; weighed 11 ozs. It was flabby and rather soft.

The *pancreas* was pale and firm.

The *kidneys* were somewhat congested but firm. The *urinary bladder* contracted.

Larynx and *trachea.*—These organs were in all respects normal in appearance.

There were about 12 ozs. of transparent yellow serosity in either pleura. There were a few recent adhesions at the posterior part of the right lung.

The *left lung* weighed 16 ozs. It was of a dark purplish violet colour anteriorly: its posterior being scarcely darker than its anterior surface. Over the whole surface, from base to apex, were scattered at irregular intervals patches of variable size, of a deep purplish violet colour. The majority of these patches were distinct, bounded by interlobular septa. The number of lobules included in each patch varied from one to eight or ten. On section the darkest coloured of these patches were found to be non-crepitant, and saturated with opaque bloody fluid; the cut surface was nearly uniform. Portions cut from these patches sunk in water. The less dark patches contained some air, the amount of air and fluid being in fact in an inverse ratio to the depth of colour. The whole lung contained an abnormal amount of frothy serosity, and scarcely less anteriorly than posteriorly.

The *right lung* weighed 21¾ ozs. It resembled, in general appearance, the left; but none of the patches were free from air; every part floated in water.

The *bronchial tubes* were filled with a thin froth mucus. The bronchial mucous membrane was intensely congested, of a dusky red colour, the redness being in streaks, specks, and patches.

The *bronchial glands* were rather large and dark. One contained a mass of cretaceous matter the size of a large pea.

CASE XXIV.—Without exposure to any known source of contagion—diarrhœa—loss of appetite—rigors—headache—debility—epistaxis—pain in the abdomen—gurgling in the right iliac fossa—enlargement of the spleen—rose spots—miliary vesicles—emaciation—tedious recovery—convalescent on about the 28th day.

R. P. R., aged 18, a plasterer, was admitted into the London Fever Hospital, June 7th, 1849. He was a thin lad, fair skin, light hair and eyes. He stated, that his general health had always been good; that he had small-pox when a child. He had not suffered from want. He was a native of London. There was no source of contagion traceable. On Sunday, May 27th, he took some sulphate of magnesia, not because he felt ill, but to relieve a constipated state of the bowels. Some few hours after he washed his head in cold water. From that day his bowels have been relaxed. On the Monday and Tuesday he lay down on the grass in the open air, after considerable muscular exertion. He dated his present illness from the 31st of May. He said, that, while working in a cellar beneath the South-Eastern Counties Railway Office, Regent Circus, he observed a most offensive odour. In the afternoon of that day he had slight rigors, but continued his work. His bowels were then more relaxed than on the preceding days, and he experienced griping pains in the abdomen. On Saturday, June 2nd, he began to suffer from frontal headache. On Saturday evening, by the advice of a medical man, he took two aperient pills, and two more on Sunday. He was told these pills would work it all off. His appetite failed him on the 31st. On the 4th of June he lost a little blood from the nose. The epistaxis was repeated two or three times on the 5th; on the whole, about a tea-cupful of blood escaped. He is not subject to epistaxis. He vomited some green fluid on the 4th. The diarrhœa and pain in the abdomen continued till admission.

The following were the first notes of this case :—

June 9th, i.e. the 14th day, reckoning from the commencement of diarrhœa. 'He slept well last night, but talked in his sleep. The cheeks are slightly flushed; the expression of countenance is nearly natural; the mind is unaffected; the memory is good; there is no vertigo, no affection of the special senses; the conjunctivæ are pale, the pupils natural, the complexion clear.

He feels weak, but can walk across the ward unassisted. The tongue is red and glazed, dry in the centre and very slightly furred posteriorly. There is complete loss of appetite, no sore throat, and no marked thirst. During the last twenty-four hours he has passed three stools of pulpy consistence. He suffers occasional griping pains about the umbilicus. There is a little gurgling in the right iliac fossa. The superficial veins over the right iliac fossa are larger than those over the left. There is no tenderness, abnormal fulness, nor resonance of the abdomen. The splenic dulness is extensive, about 6 fingers' breadth; it does not extend below the false ribs. The pulse 84, soft; respiration, 24. No cough. A few sonorous and sibilous rales on deep inspiration. The skin is hot and dry. He says he sweated freely in the night. There are no miliary vesicles. When I saw him yesterday afternoon, I marked about a dozen rose spots on the abdomen, thorax, and back. Those spots are now much paler than they were, and several fresh spots, of similar character, i.e. bright rose colour, circular, slightly elevated, disappearing on pressure and returning when the pressure is removed, have appeared.

On the following day the tongue was dry, glazed, and fissured over the greater part of its extent; he had passed three relaxed stools; in other respects his state was as before described. On the 21st day, reckoning from the date when he took the Epsom salts, the following notes were made:—'Pulse 96; skin hot and dry; several fresh rose spots; those previously marked have either disappeared or they are much paler; the tongue is the same as on the 15th day; he has passed three relaxed stools; there is no abdominal tenderness nor pain; gurgling continued in the right iliac fossa, and the belly is very resonant. The mind is unaffected; he can leave or sit up in bed with facility; he sleeps well, but talks much in his sleep. On the next day more spots had disappeared, and fresh ones continued to make their appearance. A few miliary vesicles were observed for the first time; they were seated above and beneath the clavicles. He stated that he had sweated a good deal about two hours before the visit, but that he had often sweated as much since his admission; he had passed no stool for twenty-four hours. The miliary vesicles or sudamina had disappeared on the 17th day; in other respects he was the same.

On the 18th day the pulse was 96; the skin dry; an abundant crop of minute miliary vesicles covered the chest and abdomen; he stated that he had sweated during the night freely and a little this morning; he talked much in his sleep; the expression of countenance was less lively and slightly anxious; the general strength was much more impaired, so that he left his bed with difficulty. The tongue was cleaner, but fissured; he had passed one solid stool; on the next day the pulse had risen to 108; the skin was hot, harsh, and dry; the cheeks covered with a pink flush; the physical chest signs as on admission; the miliary vesicles continued abundant, though many had shrunk up; he passed two formed solid stools; in two days I noticed that his abdomen was fuller and more resonant, and he passed two loose stools; several fresh spots had appeared on the back. He grew thinner daily. In two days more, however, his pulse had fallen to 72; there was less heat of the skin; his tongue was cleaner; he ate a little bread; no fresh spots appeared, yet he was long in gaining his strength, and appeared to emaciate, even after all trace of the febrile symptoms had disappeared. This lad had a very tedious convalescence.

The treatment was expectant, with two small doses of grey and Dover's powders.

CASE XXV.—After exposure to contagion, or the same cause which had produced typhoid fever in others—ensued gradually—loss of appetite—debility—diarrhœa—headache—quick pulse—fulness and resonance of abdomen—rose spots—convalescence on about the twenty-fourth day.

Charles B., aged 11, a spare-made, fair child, was admitted into the London Fever Hospital, under the care of Dr. Tweedie, Saturday, October 28th, 1848. His mother informed me that his previous health had been very good,—that he had never been ill before. His present illness began very gradually, about a fortnight before his admission, with loss of appetite, sense of fatigue, and faintness and pains in the limbs. He complained occasionally of chilliness and retched several times. His mother gave him a dose of aperient medicine, and after that his bowels were relaxed. What their condition was before he took medicine was doubtful. He continued up the greater part of the day, and even walked out of doors daily till the day preceding his admission, when, for the first time, he had distinct rigors and headache. He then took to his bed.

This boy's sister was admitted into the hospital at the same time, suffering from typhoid fever. I went to the home of these children, in a court leading out of Great Tower Street. It was a wretched abode. The house was dark, filthy, and offensive. The people begged hard for me to speak to 'somebody,' that its condition might be seen into; that the landlord might be compelled to whitewash the dingy walls and cleanse the offensive sewer. I found that death had visited their house,—the youngest child had died of brain fever with severe diarrhœa, and another child had suffered from fever, during which blood had passed in quantity from its bowels. I saw the surgeon, and learned from him particulars which convinced me that these two children, like the other two—Charles B. and his sister—had suffered from typhoid fever. Surely, while England tolerates the existence of these nurseries of disease, it is a mockery—a very cant—to appoint days of national fasting and humiliation, in the hope of staying the progress of epidemic scourges! As well might the drunkard, indulging in gin daily, pray God to spare him the miseries of diseased liver and its attendant dropsy.

On the 29th of October the following particulars were observed :—

He has had little sleep since his admission; his mind was unaffected. There was occasionally a little pain in the temples. The expression of countenance was natural; the complexion clear. There were no pains in the limbs, no rigors, no affection of the special senses.

He was able to walk with assistance, but he felt very weak. The tongue was moist, thinly furred—white. He had passed four relaxed stools during the preceding twenty-four hours. There was much thirst, no desire for food, neither abnormal fulness, resonance, tenderness, nor gurgling of the abdomen.

The pulse was 108, soft. There was trifling cough, a little sonorous rale. The skin was hot and dry. One imperfectly marked rose spot was noted on the back.

On the following day, the spot first observed had all but disappeared, and three fresh well-marked rose spots had come out. He complained spontaneously of frontal headache, and the abdomen was observed to be much fuller, and abnormally resonant,

His pulse rose the next day to 120, and preserved that rate for four days, it then fell to 108. Fresh rose spots continued to make their appearance every day or two till the 9th day after his admission; the number, however, present at one time never exceeding a dozen. The bowels, on the 5th day after his admission, became, without known exciting cause, very much relaxed. He passed five watery stools in twenty-four hours. The tongue continued moist throughout.

On the 10th day after admission, his pulse was 96. He slept well; the tongue was moist and clean; the appetite good, and he passed, in twenty-four hours, one solid stool.

With the exception of a little mist. cret. co., when the diarrhœa became severe, this case required nothing but fresh air, cleanliness, and restricted diet. The absurdity of active treatment in such cases as these is too manifest to require pointing out.

The reader's attention is particularly requested to the following points :—

1st. Those patients were all young.

2nd. In one instance only was contagion a probable exciting cause.

3rd. These cases agree with each other in the presence of the diagnostic symptom, i.e. a succession of rose spots. The brother and sister who had the disease from exposure to the same cause, offered the same succession of rose spots. The two cases which proved fatal presented the anatomical character of typhoid fever, i.e. lesion of Peyer's patches and enlargement of the mesenteric glands.

4th. The duration of disease in these four cases varied between 23 and 43 days.

5th. The case which proved fatal after the 13th day, did so from laryngeal disease, secondary to the primary affection, i.e. the typhoid fever.

§ 5. GENERAL DESCRIPTION OF THE SYMPTOMS AND PATHOLOGICAL APPEARNCES OBSERVED IN TYPHOID FEVER.

I propose now to give a general description of the symptoms and lesions of typhoid fever; and in so doing I shall endeavour, as I did when describing typhus fever generally, to avoid all unnecessary detail—giving a mere sketch, not a finished portrait of the disease. The minute details shall be filled in when narrating the cases selected to illustrate particular circumstances, symptoms, or lesions.

Symptoms.—Typhoid fever rarely affects persons more than 50 years of age. I have seen but one exception to this rule, and that was in a female aged 55 years. It is common in young children, being one of the many different diseases confounded together and described as 'infantile remittent fever.' In a large majority of cases, however, typhoid fever occurs in persons between 15 and 30 years of age, and it is not very common in persons more than 40 years of age.

It affects both sexes, and, so far as is known, in about equal proportion.

The duration of the disease is from 21 to 28 or 30 days.

Typhoid fever usually commences more or less gradually, so that the patient is often unable to fix the date of its outset. All he can say is, that his illness began about such a day.

The first symptoms are loss of appetite, pains in the limbs, frontal headache, chilliness, and frequently abdominal pains, or diarrhœa. The patient continues to keep about, although feeling very weak. Lies down, perhaps, a part of the day. After a few days, four, five, or six, he takes entirely to his bed, the diarrhœa increases, or, if not previously present, commences, the increase in the severity of the diarrhœa being frequently referred to the use of a purgative.[1] The countenance is indicative of anxiety and want of strength, or, perhaps, of apathy; the mind is clear; the conjunctivæ pale, slightly injected; the pupils normal; the cheeks, perhaps, somewhat flushed, sometimes one, sometimes both, being so affected. There is frequently loss of sleep from the first, or the sleep is disturbed; the patient now and then fancying that he has not slept a wink, when he has been dozing for hours.[2] Vertigo, especially in the erect position,

[1] 'Take a pill and draught,' says the druggist to the sufferer from typhoid fever, who crawls to his counter to receive gratuitous advice and buy physic; 'that can do you no harm.' Hemorrhage and perforation, with their attendants, suffering and death, prove the TRUTH (?) of the aphorism.

[2] The coma vigil of Chomel.

singing in the ears, an unpleasant, undefinable taste, are pretty constant symptoms at the outset, and epistaxis, varying in amount from a few drops to many ounces, is very often one of the earliest symptoms. The latter is sometimes repeated more than once during the first week; occasionally there is dimness, or even loss of vision. The belly is usually somewhat distended, its shape being peculiar, viz., rounded from side to side rather than 'pot'-shaped, *i.e.* enlarged from above downwards, as in mesenteric disease. It is resonant on percussion. Gurgling, on firm pressure, may commonly be detected in the right iliac fossa, and there is often tenderness in the same situation. The urine is usually at this period rather scanty, and somewhat high-coloured. The skin is hot and dry, though occasionally perspiration follows the heat of the skin which succeeds to the rigors or chilliness. Such are the symptoms present during the first week or ten days of the majority of cases of typhoid fever.

From the 8th to the 12th day a new and characteristic symptom appears, viz., an eruption on the skin. The spots constituting the eruption are scattered irregularly at various and often considerable distances from each other; few in number; confined, in a majority of cases, to the anterior and posterior surface of the trunk; now and then, however, existing on the extremities. Each spot is of a delicate rose-colour; circular; the hue gradually passing into that of the surrounding cuticle without any well-defined margin or outline; when the finger is passed over them gently they are found to be very slightly elevated; if firmly pressed by the finger they disappear entirely, but resume their colour and elevation when the pressure is withdrawn. Each spot varies in diameter, from half a line to a line and a half. The number of spots ranges from two or three to several hundreds; from six to fifty may be considered the most usual. Each spot continues visible about three days, fresh spots continuing to appear every day or two till the termination of the disease. In some cases, however, there is no eruption present. The headache continues till about the 6th to the 12th day confined to the forehead, and without any definite character. At the time that the headache ceases delirium commences, at first only observed

R

at night, but subsequently more or less constant. The
character of the delirium varies, being, however, in a majority
of cases, somewhat active. The patient is noisy, or he leaves
his bed to roam about.

The *tinnitus aurium* commonly disappears about the
end of the first week. The delirium continues till the death
or recovery of the patient, interrupted, however, as the
disease advances, by somnolence. The latter symptom
ordinarily commences about from the 12th to the 21st day,
and terminates only with the general affection. At first the
patient is said by the nurse to sleep a good deal; then he not
only sleeps much, but heavily; and finally, it may be, he is
aroused with some difficulty.

As the diseases progresses the strength of the patient
diminishes, so that by the commencement of the third week
he is often unable to walk alone, and, by the 21st day, even
to reach the close stool without some assistance. He lies
now pretty constantly on his back, with his arms across his
chest or abdomen. The cheeks are usually flushed by this
time, if not before. The flush is pink and circumscribed,
sometimes one, sometimes both cheeks being affected at the
same moment. The flush appears and disappears frequently,
many times in the day; as a rule, perhaps, it is more marked
towards evening. Sudamina beneath the clavicles, in the
groins, at the epigastrium, or even covering the whole surface, .
are frequently present.

The tongue, which at the outset was white, soon grows
red at the tip and edges, then becomes dry in the centre;
finally quite dry; at the same time it appears contracted,
small, its edge and tip often continue red, while its dorsum
is covered with a smooth, pale, yellowish brown fur. This
fur is fissured, split across longitudinally, and transversely;
the tissue seen between the fissures being deep red; ultimately
the fur may become dark brown, and at the same time sordes
may form on the teeth. In rare cases the patient, as the
disease advances, is unable even to protrude the organ.
Difficulty of swallowing, fluids being rejected by the mouth
or nose,[1] is an occasional symptom during the third or fourth

[1] Chomel says, this symptom may arise from feebleness of the muscles of
deglutition. He does not give any case to prove the assertion. In every

week. The abdomen becomes more distended; the diarrhœa increases; the stools, often amounting to five, six, or even eight or ten in the day; they are liquid, pale, brownish yellow, with flocculi of an opaque whitish yellow floating through them, like coarse bran. As the patient loses his strength they are passed involuntarily. Pain in the abdomen, unless perforation occurs before extreme somnolence or coma has set in, is rarely complained of. Hemorrhage from the bowel is an occasional symptom during the third or fourth week. The urine is usually tolerably abundant.

The pulse, frequent from the outset, often attains the rate of 120 during the second and third weeks; at the same time, the frequency is found to vary much from day to day, without any appreciable alteration in the general or local symptoms coinciding therewith, thus, to-day 96, to-morrow it may be 110, and the next again 96, to be on the succeeding day or two 120, and again to fall to 100, without, as I say, any alteration in the condition of the patient for the better when it falls, or for the worse when it rises. There is some cough and a good deal of sonorous rale present from the commencement to the termination of the disease. Mucous rale is sometimes observed in the later stages. These signs now and then lead to the disease being mistaken for some chest affection, and it is only as it progresses that it is said to pass into 'typhus.'[1] Death, in a majority of cases, occurs towards the end of the third week; frequently during the fourth; more rarely before the termination of the second. Sloughs often form at the lower part of the sacrum during the third or fourth week; now and then they occur over the hips, when the patient has lain long on his side; and in exceptional cases they are found on the heels, the inner aspects of the knees, the ankles, and every part exposed to pressure.

case of the kind which I have examined after death, there has been some local,—pharyngeal, œsophageal, or epiglottidean,—physical lesion to account for the symptoms.

[1] This is an absurd expression. One specific disease is never converted into another specific disease. A local inflammation is never converted into a specific disease. Pneumonia can never pass into typhus fever, any more than it can pass into scarlet fever; the one fever, like the other, having its distinct cause, its definite course, and its peculiar symptoms.

Death may be the result of the general disease, or it may ensue from some local complication. Of these, ulceration of the intestinal mucous membrane, leading to hemorrhage, or to perforation of the peritoneal covering of the gut is the most common. When resulting from the general disease, the fatal termination always occurs before the 30th day. Local lesion of sufficient moment to account for death is always found after that date, proving the natural duration of the general disease to·be about four weeks, that is, from 28 to 30 days. When recovery ensues, the change from disease to health is very gradual. The improvement begins about the end of the fourth week. The tongue grows moist, the skin soft, the pulse falls in frequency, somnolence disappears, and the appetite returns. The diarrhœa ceases. A remarkable fatuity remains, in some cases, long after recovery: and in the majority of cases I think there is some diminution of intellectual power for some little while after convalescence is established. I have seen many cases in which a childishness of mind remained for more than a month after, in other respects, restoration to health.

Although the foregoing is a description of the ordinary form of severe typhoid fever, yet there are certain deviations from that form which require notice; firstly, because cases of this description very frequently occur, and, I think, are little understood; and, secondly, because they occasionally prove fatal before any idea of their serious nature has crossed the mind of the practitioner. The patient, unable to fix on any particular day as that on which his illness commenced, feels ill, weak, languid, chilly, loses his appetite, and suffers from slight frontal headache. He feels 'done up,' 'ennuyé,' listless, unapt for the cares of life, sits about, perhaps lies down on his bed for a part of the day, and then, feeling a little better, tries voluntarily, or by the persuasion of his friends, to exert himself; he leaves the house to walk for a while; is soon, however, too tired to continue exertion, returns again, lies down on his bed; night comes, and generally with it an increase in those symptoms denominated febrile; the pulse, which was rather high ·during the day, rises to 100 or 112, or even more; the skin is hot; occasionally, however, the patient sweats a little, but experiences no permanent relief. He is restless and uneasy.

Some days, perhaps, he thinks he feels better, and the medical man hopes all will soon be well; he can discover no local lesion; at most a little cough, with occasional sonorous rale, leads to the opinion that the patient has catarrh; or it may be that slight diarrhœa, some griping pain in the abdomen, and a little tenderness in the same region, favour the idea that he is suffering from trifling gastro-intestinal irritation. The invalid himself declares that it is 'all weakness,' that 'what he wants is strength,' and his friends fully believe *him*. They can but note his tremulous movements; they hear him loudly complain of weakness, they see him emaciate daily, for loss of flesh is generally a prominent symptom. Stimulants and strong meats are administered, the medical attendant fancies that he sees in this injudicious diet, persisted in openly or covertly, by the friends, in spite of his protestations, the cause of all the trouble, and so the case hangs on hand from day to day, from week to week, the relatives anxious and dissatisfied, the physician at fault, and *consequently* worried. Such a case may terminate in two ways: slowly, after the expiration of about a month or five weeks from the outset, the abdominal symptoms, perhaps all along very trivial, disappear; the patient gradually, but daily, regains his flesh and strength, and all goes well.[1] But in other cases the event is far different; the patient, while at the close stool, faints, the utensil is found half filled with blood, hemorrhage returns, and ultimately he sinks. Or he is suddenly seized with intense pain in the abdomen and vomiting, and the surface is cold, the features sunk, the whole expression anxious and depressed. Distension and extreme hardness of the belly soon follow, and death quickly closes the scene.

An examination of the subject reveals in such cases ulceration, generally *very extensive*, of the agminated glands at the lower part of the ileum, and enlargement of the mesenteric

---

[1] Every man who has seen much private practice must have witnessed this kind of case times and often, and, I may add, if not perfectly familiar with the varying phases of the diseases I am describing, have been baffled, foiled, worried. Perhaps, too, after two or three weeks' attendance, he may have had the annoyance of losing his patient's confidence, and of seeing another called in to reap the credit of a cure, because at the expiration of about four weeks the disease terminates naturally.

glands. In the last supposed case, the floor of one ulcer has given way, and peritonitis supervened. Cases to illustrate these important varieties, I shall detail hereafter.

Cadaveric appearances.—Subjects dead from typhoid fever are usually much emaciated. The cadaveric rigidity continues marked in all the limbs for more than twenty-four hours after death. The cadaveric congestion of the posterior surface of the trunk and extremities is not particularly deep, and extends but little up the side of the trunk. Signs of decomposition do not, as a rule, appear very rapidly. Miliary vesicles, if noted just before death, are still seen. *There is no trace of the spots noted during life.*

The quantity of serosity in the cavity of the arachnoid, beneath that membrane, and in the lateral ventricles, differs but little from that found in health. The colour and consistence of the brain are usually natural. The mucous membrane of the bronchial tubes is very frequently vividly injected and filled with frothy mucus. The congestion of the most depending part of the lung is not extreme. Lobular consolidation of the pulmonary tissue is present in a large majority of cases.

This lobular consolidation occurs in two distinct forms,—non-granular and granular.[1]

Occasionally there is, in addition to lobular, extensive lobar-pneumonic solidification. In about one-third of the cases, signs of recent pleuritis are observed. The pericardium appears healthy. The heart in about one-third of the cases is softer and more flabby than it is usually found after death from other diseases. The earlier death occurs in the disease, the more likely is the heart to be soft and flabby. The lining membrane is rarely much discoloured from imbibition, unless a considerable time has elapsed between the fatal termination and the examination of the body. The blood is fluid in a few cases, but in the majority tolerably firmly coagulated in the auricles and ventricles.

The spleen is considerably enlarged and softened. The

[1] For a particular description of these two forms, as seen in the lungs of subjects dead from typhoid and typhus fevers, I must refer the reader to my papers on those diseases in the *Monthly Journal of Medical Science.* (See *ante*, p. 112 *et seq.*)

liver is occasionally flabby. Signs of peritonitis, that disease being the consequence of the lesion presently to be described (perforation) are not infrequent. The kidneys are generally healthy. The above structural changes are only occasionally found after death.

Enlargement of the lymphatic glands and ulceration of the mucous membranes are constant phenomena.

Of the latter, ulceration of the pharyngeal mucous membrane occurs in about one-fifth of the cases. Ulceration of the larynx occurs occasionally, but less frequently than ulceration of the pharynx. The œsophagus is similarly affected in about the same proportion of the cases as the larynx. Occasionally, yet rarely, ulcers are found in the mucous membrane of the stomach, still more rarely in the duodenum.

The *diagnostic lesion* is found in the ileum, viz. enlargement of Peyer's patches followed by ulceration. The patches next the ileo-cæcal valve are the largest and the most extensively ulcerated—the thickening and the ulceration of these bodies diminishing as they recede from that situation.

Two varieties in the affection of these glands are observed. In the *first*, the mucous and submucous tissue is thickened, so that the whole patch stands considerably above the level of the adjacent membrane. The mucous membrane of the patches farthest removed from the ileo-cæcal valve is rugose, as it were pitted all over. On the whole, perhaps, to say they offer a miniature representation of that condition of the mucous membrane of the stomach which has been termed mammillation conveys the best idea of their aspect. At the same time that it is thickened, the mucous membrane of the patch is softened and redder than natural. The submucous cellular tissue, also, presents a pinkish hue. The ulceration in the patch is the more marked as the latter is situated nearer to the cæcum. At a variable distance above that viscus the agminated glands are found ulcerated, the ulcers increasing in depth and extent as they approach the termination of the small intestine. In the *second* form, the thickening of the patch appears due chiefly to a deposit of yellowish white substance in the submucous cellular tissue, splitting that, as it were, into two layers. The patches sometimes stand as much as a third of an inch above the surrounding mucous membrane. Ulceration follows also this form of thickening. The solitary glands at the lower part of the ileum are frequently enlarged and ulcerated.

Ulceration of the mucous membrane of the large intestine, generally of the cæcum and colon adjacent, is present in about one-third of the cases. The mucous membrane of the gall-bladder, the urinary bladder, and the vagina are occasionally, but rarely, the seat of ulceration.

Of the lymphatic glands, those constantly affected are the mesenteric. And of the mesenteric glands themselves the most extensively diseased are those seated next the termination of the ileum.

The mesenteric glands are invariably enlarged, reddened, and softened. Sometimes they are the seat of a deposit of a yellowish white friable matter, and occasionally of a collection of purulent-looking fluid. The size these glands may attain varies from a bean to a pigeon's egg.

The mesocolic glands are sometimes large, red, and soft. Occasionally the bronchial glands, the lumbar glands, the glands in the vicinity of the cystic duct, of the œsophagus, of the small curvature of the stomach, and in the cervical region, are enlarged and redder than natural.

The modifications produced in the lesions by the duration of the disease, as well as more particular descriptions of the lesions themselves, will be given with the cases to be hereafter detailed.

§ 6. EXAMINATION OF THE CONDITIONS, SYMPTOMS, AND COMPLICATIONS ON THE VARIATIONS IN WHICH THE DIFFERENCES OBSERVED IN INDIVIDUAL CASES OF TYPHOID FEVER DEPEND.

Hemorrhage from the Bowels.

There is no single symptom observed in the course of typhoid fever more alarming to the patient or his friends than the escape of blood per anum. It occurs most frequently during the third and fourth weeks of the disease, i.e. about the period when the sloughs, so frequently formed in the small intestines, are in the act of separating. Sometimes hemorrhage takes place after the fourth week, and, in very rare cases, before the termination of the first week. The quantity of blood varies from sufficient only to stain the fæcal matters to a very considerable quantity. It is often of a red colour; sometimes in clots. The alkaline reaction of the stools, in typhoid fever, shown by my colleague, Dr. Parkes, and also the rapidity with which the blood is expelled from the intestine, may account for the absence of the black tint commonly assumed by blood before its escape from the intestine.

Hemorrhage from the bowels is a very grave symptom, but is by no means necessarily fatal; of Chomel's seven cases, six died; of seven detailed by Louis, three were fatal. My own experience leads me to regard Louis's as the nearer approximation to the truth. Intestinal hemorrhage may cause death directly or indirectly: 1stly, by producing fainting from which the patient never rallies,—perhaps he dies in an instant—of this form, Case xxvii. is an example; 2ndly, by reducing the strength of the patient, and so rendering him unable to bear up against the secondary local diseases that so often complicate typhoid fever.

The gravity of the prognosis is increased by the knowledge that, in a large majority of cases, the vessel from which the blood escapes is laid open by the detachment of a slough, and that consequently, it is highly probable that extensive local disease exists whenever blood in any quantity escapes from the intestinal mucous membrane. I shall hereafter adduce one or two cases to illustrate the fact, that the symptom under consideration is by no means necessarily fatal.

Case XXVI.—Without known cause, in a man, aged 27, gradual accession of illness. On the 13th day, defect of memory—tremulous muscular movements—loss of appetite —diarrhœa—hoarseness—rose spots, followed by tenderness and gurgling in the iliac fossa—enlargement of the spleen—hemorrhage from the bowels—quick pulse. On the 21st day, severe rigors, followed by signs of pleuro-pneumonia—rapid pulse — delirium — sloughing of cutis over sacrum—extreme prostration, and death on the 27th day.

Sixteen hours after death: ulcers in the larynx, œsophagus,

ileum, and urinary bladder—enlargement and softening of the mesenteric glands—abnormal injection of the peritoneum—fibrinous effusion into the cavity of the peritoneum —enlargement of the spleen—lymph and serosity in the pleuræ—lobular consolidation of the lungs.

James W., aged 27, a stout man, with fair skin and light hair and eyes, employed as a labourer on a railroad, was admitted into the London Fever Hospital under the care of Dr. Tweedie, May 11th, 1849.   His previous health had been good ; he never spat blood, but was subject, on catching cold, to trifling cough ; he was of temperate habits ; had resided in London ten years, and was not in want ; no cause could be assigned for the present attack. After ailing for a week from 'cold' and cough, he quitted work May 6th, but continued to leave his bed daily till his admission into the hospital.   During the course of his illness he had taken several doses of Epsom salts, hoping 'to work off' the disease.

The first notes of his case were taken May 12th, *i.e.* the 7th day after leaving his work, and about the 13th from the first symptom of illness.   His memory was then very defective ; he thought he had been in the hospital three days ; still he answered questions rationally ; he had passed a restless night, and slept but little ; there had been no delirium ; the conjunctivæ were slightly injected, the pupils rather large ; he complained of an unpleasant taste, and some dimness of vision ; the expression of the countenance was somewhat heavy ; there was no headache, and no vertigo.   He was able to walk up the ward without assistance, and, although his muscular movements were unsteady, he did not feel very weak.

The lips were dry ; the tongue moist, loaded, and tremulous ; there was no pain nor tenderness of the abdomen ; no gurgling in the iliac fossa ; the abdomen retained its normal shape ; the thirst was considerable, but the man had no appetite.   He had passed during the twenty-four hours subsequent to his admission four watery stools.

The pulse was 96 and soft.   He suffered from a rather troublesome cough ; there was a little sonorous rale on both sides of the chest ; the voice was markedly hoarse.

The skin was warm and dry, and over the surface of the trunk were scattered a few imperfectly-formed rose spots.

My notes show but little change on the following day, excepting that there was gurgling and some tenderness in the right iliac fossa ; the skin was hot and dry, and two or three of the rose spots marked the preceding day had disappeared, others were much paler, and several fresh ones had appeared ; the characters of the latter were perfect. On this day he passed three stools of pulpy consistence.

On the 15th day of disease several fresh rose spots were observed, and some of those present on the 14th day had grown paler. He was reported to have passed a restless night; to have had very little sleep; there was no delirium. The skin at the time of the visit was warm and covered with perspiration; there were no miliary vesicles; the cheeks were flushed; the muscular movements unsteady, although he still left his bed unassisted with facility; the tongue was moist, loaded, and tremulous; there was extensive dulness over the region of the spleen; the abdomen generally was full and resonant, there was slight tenderness, but no gurgling in the right iliac fossa; he had passed three liquid stools; but in one was a small solid mass of fæces. *All the stools were tinged throughout with blood*. There was slight cough, and a little sonorous rale was audible over the entire chest.

For the next five days there was little change; fresh spots appeared occasionally, those previously noted disappearing; although he sweated occasionally, the absence of miliary vesicles was recorded; the tenderness in the right iliac fossa continued; the hoarseness was as on admission. On the 18th day he vomited a little yellow fluid. He passed two liquid stools, containing very little blood, on the 16th day; on the 17th day four watery stools, of a reddish brown colour, and *very offensive* odour; on the 18th two liquid stools, of a decided crimson colour, but containing no clots of blood. On the 19th day he had no stool. The general powers had by this time considerably diminished; so that, although still able to leave his bed unassisted, it was with considerable difficulty. The pulse had risen to 120; it was noted to be full and soft. A little mucous rale was heard on the 20th day over the anterior part of the chest.

On the 21st day the following notes were made:—The nurse reports, that about 1 A.M. he had a very severe attack of rigors, which lasted a quarter of an hour. In the middle of it, he appeared to the nurse to lose his senses for two or three minutes; his skin, while the rigors were on, felt hot, and he did not complain of any sense of cold, nor has he appeared chilly since. He began to sweat about 12 last night, and continued to sweat profusely for two hours; he sweated while shivering.

He has had very little sleep, and no delirium. At the time of the visit, the pulse was 120, small and weak; the respiration 36, and he was suffering from troublesome cough. He was lying on his back; though still able to quit his bed alone, it was with extreme difficulty, and the muscular movements generally were very unsteady. There was a little fine crepitation at the base of the left lung posteriorly. The raw surfaces left by the blisters

applied to the chest and side on the 15th and 17th days were
very sore. The tongue was moist, covered with a white fur,
and very tremulous. He had passed during the twenty-four
hours preceding my visit, three stools, in all two pints, of dirty red
fluid, of watery consistence, containing several clots of dark blood
of considerable size. The abdomen was full and resonant, and
there was some tenderness in the right iliac fossa. There were no
miliary vesicles. Orders were given that on *no consideration*
should he be allowed to quit the horizontal position. He was to
use a bed-pan. During the night, however, he became, for the
first time, very delirious, and, while so, left his bed.

From this time till his death, on the 27th day from the first
commencement of illness, the pulse continued to rise, so that, on
the 25th and 26th days, it reached 150; at the same time it was
very feeble. The respirations increased in frequency, and became
chiefly abdominal.

On account of the prostration, and the severity and nature of
the abdominal symptoms, the chest was examined only so far as
to ascertain the existence of the physical signs of pleuro-pneumonia,
i.e. friction, crepitation, dulness. At no time was there any
expectoration. No fresh spots were observed after the 20th
day—no miliary vesicles at any time. The delirium continued,
but without violence. Generally wakeful, he dozed frequently on
the 25th, but was then readily aroused. The blistered surfaces
continued very sore; the cheeks flushed occasionally; the conjunctivæ very pale. On the 23rd day a purple spot, from which
the cuticle had partially separated, was observed over the sacrum,
and two smaller purple spots, one on either buttock. At this
time the tongue became brown in the centre—it was still moist.
He was often observed, during the night of the 24th day, picking
the bed-clothes. He attempted to protrude his tongue when told,
on the 25th day, but its movements were too unsteady for him to
accomplish his object.

He passed no stool on the 23rd; on the 24th day, one liquid
stool of a reddish colour, with lumps of dark solid stool floating in
it. The bowels were confined on the 25th day, but on the 26th
he had one solid stool, without any trace of blood.

On the 23rd, it was noted that he continued 'very hoarse,'
and 'that his voice was reduced to little more than a whisper.'
On the night of the 25th, while delirious, he left his bed unassisted.
On the 26th day he was so prostrate as to be scarcely able to raise
his arm from the bed. On the morning of the 27th day, reckoning from the first symptom of illness, or the 21st, counting from
the day he left his work, I noted as follows:—

'Pulse 132, irregular in frequency; respirations 36; expression still more cadaverous than yesterday. Last night the nurse
reports that he was very delirious, and attempted to quit his bed;

POST-MORTEM EXAMINATION

tongue dry and brown; no stool; much less fulness, but slight tenderness of abdomen; no sleep night nor day; no coma vigil.'

He *died* at a quarter to nine the same evening.

An examination of the body of James W. was made *sixteen hours after death*, the weather being warm and dry.

There was no appearance of decomposition. Cadaveric rigidity was well marked. There was some purplish discoloration of the most depending part of the body. The loose cellular tissue superficial to the *recti abdominis* was infiltrated with blood; there was no distinct clot.[1]

Head.—The pia mater was somewhat more vascular than natural. There was a little serosity beneath the arachnoid. The grey matter of the brain had a pinkish hue and the red points in the white substance were more numerous than usual. The consistence of every part of the brain was normal. The plexus choroides was pale; a little colourless transparent serosity was found in the lateral ventricles, and at the base of the brain.

The *pericardium* was healthy.

Heart.—Tolerably firm, and large clots were found in the cavities of the heart. The substance of the organ and its valves were perfectly healthy; it was slightly hypertrophied.

Larynx.—The chordæ vocales were decidedly thicker than natural, and on the left chorda were three small superficial ulcers, with pale edges. The mucous membrane of the larynx generally was pale, and of normal consistence.

Lungs.—Lymph and serosity in the pleuræ proved the existence of inflammation of that membrane during life. There was pretty extensive granular and non-granular lobular consolidation, especially affecting the posterior parts of the inferior lobes. There was no trace of tubercles.

The *bronchial glands* were large and dark.

The lining membrane of the *bronchial tubes* was of a deep red colour.

The *pharynx* was pale and healthy in aspect.

In the *œsophagus*, about two inches below the pharynx, were four ulcers, each from 2 or 3 lines in length; they were quite superficial; their edges and floors pale.

The *stomach* was contracted; its mucous membrane was very rugose. There was much punctiform redness of the mucous membrane near the cardiac orifice, and at the red parts it was softer than elsewhere. The pyloric half (excluding two inches next the pylorus) was mammillated. There was no trace of ulceration of its lining membrane.

[1] Dr. John Reid observed only four examples of effusion of blood into the cellular tissue, without external violence, out of 500 bodies he examined. He regarded the fact of importance in a medico-legal point of view. See *Phys., Patholog., and Anat. Researches*, by Dr. J. Reid, p. 510.

Small intestines.—The mucous membrane of the jejunum and ileum was somewhat softer than natural. The free margins of the *valvulæ conniventes* were thickly studded with red *puncta.*

From the upper portion of the ileum shreds of mucous membrane half an inch in length were obtainable with facility.

About seven feet above the ileo-cæcal valve, on one of Peyer's patches, was a thickened spot, the thickening being confined to the mucous and submucous tissues. The centre of this spot was occupied by an ulcer 3 lines in diameter; the edges of the ulcer were red; its floor was formed of transverse muscular fibres. About fourteen inches lower in the gut was another and similar ulcer; and, from that point downwards, every Peyer's patch was very extensively destroyed by ulceration. The edges of the ulcers overlapped the floors, the latter being covered with a tough, thick, amorphous, sloughy-looking substance, or it was formed by the naked transverse muscular fibres. In one or two of the ulcers the centre of the floor was formed by longitudinal muscular fibres, and in two the peritoneum was exposed. The ulcers increased in size as they approached the ileo-cæcal valve. High up the intestine the edges of the ulcers were bright red; next the cæcum they were deep grey.

Between these oval ulcers were many smaller circular ulcers, the latter varying in size from a pin-head to half an inch in diameter. As the larger oval ulcers were evidently seated on Peyer's patches, so these smaller circular ulcers appeared to occupy the situation of the solitary glands. Thickly scattered over the lower four feet of the ileum were minute elevated white points; they were about the size of small pin-heads, and were evidently due to some change in or beneath the glands. The mucous membrane of the last twelve inches was decidedly softened; higher up it retained its normal consistence.

The *large intestines* were healthy in all particulars.

The *mesenteric glands* were large, varying in size from a pea to a large nut,—soft, friable, and of a pale yellowish red colour. The largest were those in the vicinity of the ileo-cæcal valve.

There was no enlargement of the *lumbar or mesocolic glands.*

The *peritoneal cavity* contained about twelve ounces of transparent yellow serosity, in which floated a transparent, yellowish, jelly-like mass of considerable size. By pressure it was converted into an opaque, stringy, elastic substance, much smaller than the original mass.

The serous membrane lining the abdominal parietes was more opaque than natural, and through it could be seen much capillary injection. The vessels of the peritoneum corresponding to the ulcers in the ileum were also finely injected with blood.

The *liver* was pale and flabby; its acute margin was overlapped by the transverse arch of the colon. The *gall bladder* distended with thin greenish-yellow bile; its lining membrane healthy in all respects.

The *pancreas* was pale and firm.

The *spleen* weighed 10½ oz.; its vertical diameter was 7½ inches; its antero-posterior, 4 inches. It was dark and firm.

The *kidneys* were congested, but appeared otherwise healthy. Their pelves were somewhat more injected than usual. The *ureters* were pale and healthy.

The *bladder* was contracted, and contained very little transparent yellow urine. Its lining membrane was minutely injected: on its anterior surface were numerous minute scarlet points; its posterior surface had a purplish hue. Scattered over the anterior and posterior surface were numerous patches, of a dirty yellow colour, distinctly elevated above the level of the adjacent mucous membrane. At some places the yellow substance, by the effusion of which these patches were formed, was removable without injury to the subjacent membrane; at others it appeared to be incorporated with the latter. The mucous membrane immediately around these yellow patches was of a vivid scarlet or of a deep purple colour, gradually shading off. Here and there the surface of the mucous membrane was destroyed by minute superficial ulcers. The aspect of the whole mucous membrane was identical with that of the large intestine in some forms of dysentery.

The *ganglia of the solar plexus* were carefully dissected out, and appeared perfectly healthy.

This case illustrates certain facts common in typhoid fever: 1st, the gradual accession of the illness. J. W. felt unwell a week before quitting his work. He continued to move about the house, more or less, for a week after he quitted his work, and was able during the fourth week to reach the close stool without aid. As a rule, it is better to date the onset of the disease from the first sense of illness. Men of the age and in the rank of life of J. W. continue their employment as long as they are able, taking but little heed of that which others might consider serious ailment. In estimating the period of any two given diseases at which persons affected with either take to their beds, it is essential that persons in the same rank of life only, as near as may be, should be counted.

2nd, His memory was defective. He thought time prolonged; thus, after having resided in the hospital twenty-four hours, he stated he had been there three days. At the same time there was no delirium.

3rd, The pupils were fully as large as natural.

4th, The stools were numerous and watery.

5th, Sonorous rale was heard over the whole chest.

6th, There were rose spots on the trunk when he first came under observation. These spots ran their ordinary course, *i.e.* they remained for two or three days and then disappeared—fresh spots making their appearance every day or two, without relation to those which preceded them.

7th, Flushing of the cheeks; a transient but frequently recurring circumscribed pink flush on one or both cheeks is one of the most constant symptoms in typhoid fever.

8th, The splenic dulness was extensive.

9th, The shape of the abdomen and its resonance and the gurgling, were all signs common in well-marked cases of typhoid fever.

It is important to observe that perspiration pretty copious in quantity occurred repeatedly, without any relief to the symptoms. Louis pointed out the tendency of blistered surfaces to ulcerate in typhoid fever. This case illustrates the fact.

With reference to the hemorrhage, it may be remarked that this man had, before his admission, taken repeated doses of an irritating purgative.

Blood was first observed in the stools on the 15th day. The colour of the stools was, as is usual in typhoid fever, more or less red. The reddish brown colour and peculiarly *offensive* odour noted on the 17th day are very common characters of typhoid stools, containing a moderate quantity of blood. The clots, on the following day, indicated that the blood had been poured out rapidly, and, therefore, probably from a vessel of some size; blood is never poured out from the general surface of the intestine in typhoid fever, its escape is invariably due to destruction of tissue of appreciable magnitude—ordinarily, as I have before said, in consequence of the separation of a slough of some size laying open one or more veins or arteries. The condition of the bowels and the character of the stools during the last four days of his life are interesting. The bowels were confined, or he passed only a small quantity of solid stool, in which there was no trace of blood. This man did not then die, as the next case did, from the hemorrhage directly but indirectly; the loss of blood perhaps might have tended to bring about the fatal termination. The hemorrhage occurred at that period of the disease when he was the least able to bear it. Although he had just lost a considerable quantity of blood, inflammation of the lung and pleura set in early on the morning of the twenty-first day. The blood-letting did not prevent the supervention of the pleuro-pneumonia.

The attack was ushered in by severe rigors. Louis regards the occurrence of rigors in the progress of typhoid fever as invariably indicating the establishment of local inflammation. This case illustrates and supports his position. It affords an example of serous inflammation being set up in the course of typhoid fever. The *frequency with which the pleura becomes the seat of inflammatory action*, and of the effusion of lymph, will be abundantly evident from the cases here related. Recent adhesions were found in the pleura of Fanny P., Case XXIII.; and I shall have occasion to point out the same lesion in several other cases. The tremor of the tongue and limbs, out of all proportion to the mental aberration, were important signs, as indicative of extensive intestinal disease. I shall advert to this fact when commenting on the next case. The delirium, when it did occur, was of the character common in typhoid fever: the patient frequently left his bed—it was active. The occurrence of carphology—a dry, brown tongue—extreme prostration—sloughing of the sacrum, and the continuance of active delirium, taken together, showed how deeply the nervous system had at last become involved.

The recorded particulars of the examination after death of the body of J. W. very clearly prove that typhoid fever is *not* an inflammation of the brain. The ulcer on the chorda vocalis, and the thickening of the substance of both chordæ, afford a ready explanation of the hoarseness. No symptoms during life had indicated the ulcers in the œsophagus. The gastric mucous membrane, although not healthy over its entire surface, was too slightly affected for us to consider its lesion to have been the cause of the grave symptoms from which James W. suffered.

S

The ileum offered a good example of one form of the anatomical character of typhoid fever,—the *plaques molles* of Louis. The ulcers were seated on Peyer's patches; they increased in extent as they approached the ileo-cæcal valve. The floors of the ulcers were formed, according to the depth of the ulcers, by submucous cellular tissue, transverse or longitudinal muscular fibres, or peritoneum. It is rare to find the *longitudinal* muscular fibres forming the floor of an ulcer; the *transverse* are constantly exposed. Perforation must shortly have followed. The thickening of the patches was due—as in Case XXIII.—to increased thickness of the mucous and submucous coats, and not, as in the next case— Case XXVII.—to a deposit in the substance of the submucous cellular tissue—*i.e.* the *plaques dures* of Louis. The solitary glands were affected in the same manner as the agminated. The softened condition of the mucous membrane of the lower twelve inches was of secondary moment. The presence of a fibrinous clot in the peritoneal cavity is interesting. Was it the result of inflammatory action set up in the peritoneum corresponding to the ulcers of Peyer's patches? That portion of the peritoneum is often covered by recently formed false membrane—an attempt on the part of Nature to guard the peritoneum from perforation. I have before adverted to the condition of the bile in typhoid fever. It presented in this case the characters ordinarily observed in the affection referred to in contradistinction to those presented by it in typhus fever—*i.e.* thickness of consistence and darkness of colour. The urinary bladder had evidently been the seat of inflammatory action during life. The dirty yellow elevated patches, and the ulcers on its mucous membrane bore evidence of the extent it had partaken of the general disease.

The reader's attention is requested to the condition of the abdominal portion of the sympathetic nerve. Rokitansky and some other German observers have stated that nerve to be invariably diseased in typhoid fever. In this case, as well as in some others I have examined—in one examination I was assisted by my friend Dr. Beck, than whom no one can be better able to give an opinion as to the healthy structure of the sympathetic—the great abdominal ganglia and plexuses offered in all particulars the characters of health. This remark applies to cases of typhus and typhoid fever.

Taken as a whole, the most striking circumstance revealed by the examination of the body of J. W. was the number of organs that had during life been the seat of ulceration—larynx, œsophagus, ileum, colon, and urinary bladder; and of those that had suffered from inflammation,—pleura, lungs, peritoneum, etc., etc.

Disseminated inflammations, disseminated ulcerations, these are the two features eminently characteristic of typhoid fever.

CASE XXVII.—Without known exposure to contagion—in a male, aged 23: headache—trifling rigors—confined bowels—nausea—slight increase in frequency of pulse—loaded, moist, tremulous tongue—finally, loss of appetite—little sleep—muscular movements tremulous—one rose spot—hemorrhage from the bowels, and death from fainting on the 25th day of disease.

Thirty-six hours after death.—Marked cadaveric rigidity—thickening and ulceration of Peyer's patches, and of the solitary glands, of the large and small intestines—enlargement and softening of the mesenteric glands—enlargement and softening of the spleen.

Peter A., aged 23, 5 feet 3 inches in height, moderately stout, fair skin, dark hair and eyes, by trade a carpenter, was admitted into the London Fever Hospital, August 28th, 1847. He was a man of temperate habits; he had lived in London sixteen months only; he attributed his present illness to exposure to damp and cold. The first symptoms were headache, slight rigors, pain at the epigastrium, and nausea. He had epistaxis the day before his admission. His bowels were confined from the outset. I saw him for the first time the day after his admission—*i.e.* on August 29th, the 11th day of illness. At this time the man appeared to ail very little. He slept well; his mind was perfectly collected, his memory good. There was a little headache, and some vertigo when he stood erect.

There was no marked loss of strength, he left his bed unassisted with perfect facility, and could walk without aid; nor did he complain of any particular sense of weakness.

His tongue, loaded with yellowish fur, was tremulous; yet he had some appetite, and there was no thirst. There was no abnormal fulness of the abdomen, but he made slight complaint when it was pressed firmly. His bowels were confined. The pulse was 80, regular, soft; there was no cough, with the exception of a faint soft murmur with the first sound of the heart heard at the base only; there were no abnormal physical chest-signs.

The skin was warm; there were no spots.

Half-an-ounce of castor oil was ordered to be given directly, and a little simple saline medicine every six hours.

On the following day the tongue was cleaner; the castor-oil had acted three times; he said he had slept well.

September 1st, *i.e.* the 14th day of disease.—Pulse 80; tongue cleaning; two stools.

September 4th, *i.e.* the 17th day.—Pulse 80; no stool; tongue still furred posteriorly; appetite returning.

September 7th, *i.e.* the 20th day.—Pulse 84; tongue furred and tremulous; two stools; a little appetite.

On the 22nd day his pulse had risen to 96. He complained of want of sleep; there was no headache; much thirst; a total loss of appetite; and not only was the tongue, which continued moist and furred, tremulous, but the whole of the muscular movements were unsteady, yet he sat up in bed quickly when bid, supported himself without aid, and with facility left his bed unassisted. One rose spot was observed on his back.

On the 24th day of his illness, about half-past one A.M., I made the following note: 'Pulse 96—slept but little—mind unaffected —tongue rather dry—a little pale brown fur in its centre—two stools the last twenty-four hours.'

In about half-an-hour I was recalled in haste to his bed.

He had placed himself on the close pan as soon as I had quitted the ward. The nurse observed him turn pale and assisted him on to the bed. The close-pan was half-full of a reddish fluid mixed with large dark clots of blood. There was no fæculent matter. His whole surface, although warm, was pallid. The abdomen was full and resonant—there was no tenderness.

Four discharges of blood, very large in quantity, followed; the last at 4 A.M., when he fainted, and died instantly.

Examination of the body of Peter A., thirty-six hours after death. —Weather cool. The cadaveric rigidity was well marked (even fifty hours after death)—the surface was markedly bloodless. There was no appearance of decomposition; very little fat on the abdominal or thoracic parietes.

Head.—The membranes and substance of the brain were very pale, and in all other particulars healthy.

The *pericardium* contained a little transparent yellow serosity.

Much dark fluid blood escaped on dividing the aorta, pulmonary artery, veins, and venæ cavæ. Cavities of the heart were empty.

Heart.—The substance was pale and flabby. There was a little thickening of the free edge of the aortic valves, and some beading of the free edge of the greater section of the mitral valve.

The *larynx, trachea, bronchial tubes,* and *lungs* were healthy, excepting a few old adhesions between pulmonary and costal pleura. The *bronchial glands* converted into putty-like and cretaceous matter.

The mucous membrane of the *pharynx* and *œsophagus* was pale and healthy; that of the stomach slightly rugose, pale, not mammillated, and of normal consistence.

The *mesenteric glands* were enlarged,—some were as big as filberts,—the largest corresponded to the lower part of the ileum. Their colour varied from pale purple to greyish yellow. In the centre of several was an opaque deposit of a yellowish white colour, and of a soft and friable consistence. About three and a half yards above the ileo-cæcal valve was one of Peyer's patches, opaque and thickened at intervals. On the next patch were two or three thickened spots, each three-eighths of an inch in diameter. The *deposit* to which the increase in thickness was due, was of a pink colour, and had its seat in the substance of the submucous tissue. The mucous membrane covering this patch was pale and softened. From this point to half a yard above the ileo-cæcal valve, every patch was more or less similarly affected. A few of the solitary glands between the patches were also enlarged.

Every patch in the last half yard of the ileum was ulcerated; the floors of some of the ulcers were covered with an opaque, yellow, and structureless mass; in others, the transverse muscular fibres were exposed, or covered merely by a thin layer of submucous cellular tissue.

Water thrown into the superior mesenteric artery, welled forth from the edge of one of the ulcers. The solitary glands between the patches were considerably larger than natural; the mucous membrane on their apices softer than natural.[1]

Large intestines.—The mucous membrane of the *cæcum* was of a deep grey colour, but normal in consistence and thickness; that of the colon bright red mottled with grey. Scattered over it were several round spots, about a line in diameter, considerably elevated; their centres white and opaque; their bases grey. In some places, the central white spot had partially separated, a line of ulceration having been set up around it. Here and there the little white slough had separated, and a small ulcer marked the spot it had formerly occupied.

The *liver* was pale, its consistence good.

---

[1] For a more minute description of the intestines in this case, see papers reprinted from the *Edinburgh Monthly Journal* (*supra*, p. 76).

The *spleen* was large, it weighed 13 ozs.; it was soft but not pulpy.

The *kidneys* and *urinary bladder* were in all respects normal.

This case is one of marked interest. It affords an illustration of what has been termed latent typhoid fever. The man, on his admission, appeared to be suffering from slight gastric disturbance: the foul moist tongue, the partial loss of appetite and absence of thirst, with slight tenderness of the abdomen, and pulse scarcely accelerated. A gentle purgative, rest, and abstinence, it was supposed, would soon restore Peter A. to health. The tremulous state of the tongue, however, awakened some suspicions, especially as the man affirmed that he was of temperate habits. Yet who can trust to the affirmation of hospital patients on this head?[1] The continuance of the tremulous condition of the tongue, on the 20th day of disease, and the 10th of his residence in the hospital, even though the tongue was cleaner than on admission, and he had a little appetite, was a very grave symptom. The general muscular unsteadiness, increase in the frequency of the pulse, want of sleep, and the rose spot, rendered the probability still higher, that the man had typhoid fever; but one cannot say that all doubt was dispelled till the occurrence of that symptom, which at once rendered the diagnosis certain, and the prognosis most grave. If the extent of the splenic dulness had been percussed out, less doubt would, perhaps, have been entertained as to the nature of the case. Three years' experience, since this case came under observation, has led me to attach extreme importance, in typhoid fever, to muscular tremor, when unaccompanied by mental disturbance of a grave character, as indicative of extensive ulceration, or, rather, of *deep* destruction, by ulceration or sloughing of the agminated glands. In these cases, hemorrhage and perforation are very common. Not long since, I ventured, from the muscular tremor being in a temperate man labouring under typhoid fever, out of all proportion to the mental abnormal phenomena, to write to a friend in daily attendance on the case, but who was unable to meet me, that he must beware of

[1] The majority of hospital patients should be asked not if they drink, but *when* they were drunk last.

hemorrhage or perforation. I visited the patient again in a week, and was met by the cry of the nurse, 'Oh, Sir, he has just passed such a quantity of blood!' and the same evening, on seeing the patient again, by 'Oh, Sir, he is in such pain—he has been screaming with agony!' Perforation had occurred.

The absence of diarrhœa—nay, the presence of constipation—is another symptom which may mislead the inexperienced; it is, however, by no means a very rare occurrence in typhoid fever. I shall have occasion to refer to more than one example. No more striking illustration of the absurdity of supposing prostration, a dry brown tongue, hot skin, and delirium, to be the essential symptoms of fever could be offered than that of the case of Peter A: no more striking proof of the imperfect character of the description of fever contained in English systematic works on medicine. Typhoid fever is a *very common* disease, especially in young persons; it is the endemic fever of London; but, from its latent character, *i.e.* from its being frequently unaccompanied by Cullen's diagnostic characters, it is misunderstood, and too often maltreated by the patient, his friends, or his medical advisers, *e.g.* my own case, referred to at the commencement of this essay, p. 167.

The examination after death proved that a small branch of the mesenteric artery had been opened by the detachment of a slough, illustrating my assertion, that hemorrhage from the bowels, in typhoid fever, has its origin in destruction, either in mass or molecular, of the intestinal coats.

The duration of typhoid fever is from twenty-one to thirty days. There was no attempt at reparation in this case; in fact, the fever had not run its full course. The lesion of the patches was that described by Louis as *plaques dures;* there was a deposit of a non-vascular material in the substance of the submucous coat, and to the presence of this deposit the thickened state of the patches was due. A similar material was found in the mesenteric glands. It appears probable, that by about the 30th day of disease the whole of this *almost* structureless deposit, acting as a foreign body, is thrown out by sloughing from Peyer's patches. Whether it is ever there metamorphosed and absorbed, as in some cases it unquestionably is from the mesenteric glands (an example of which I propose subsequently to describe), admits of doubt. The condition of the mucous membrane of the large intestine was interesting, as exhibiting one mode in which ulceration of that membrane commences. The spleen presented the characters it so often does in typhoid fever: it was considerably enlarged, and softer than natural. In these particulars it resembled the spleen of Fanny P., Case XXIII., who died, it may be remembered, on the 23rd day of disease, and that of James W., Case XXVI., who died on the 27th day. In Jane T., Case XXII., who survived till the 33rd day, the spleen was rather small, but then its corrugated surface rendered it probable that in her, too, at some earlier period of the disease, it had been enlarged. These observations accord with those made by Louis; he found that, in the forty-six fatal cases he analysed, it was between the 20th and 30th day of the disease that the organ in question attained its maximum size; and that, after the 30th day, it appeared gradually to return to its normal dimensions.

I shall now detail the particulars of a case, in which, although the quantity of blood lost was pretty considerable, yet the patient did well.

CASE XXVIII.—In a man, 35 years of age, after five months' residence in London—depression of spirits—cold chills—headache—loss of strength—violent delirium—a want of sleep—eruption of rose spots—diarrhœa—hemorrhage from the bowels—convalescence between the 20th and 30th day of disease.

James S., an ostler, aged 35, of temperate habits, was admitted, Saturday, July 20, 1850, into the London Fever Hospital, under the care of Dr. Tweedie. James S. was a thin man, with fair skin and red hair. His friends stated that he had always enjoyed health till his present attack; that six months before entering the hospital he left Cumberland to reside in London. About a month before his present illness he lost a sum of money; this loss caused him much depression of spirits. On the Tuesday preceding his entrance into the hospital he was seized with cold chills and headache. He took to his bed directly. His bowels were confined till after the administration of aperients. On the following night, Wednesday, July 13th, he became violently delirious; he was restrained in bed with some difficulty. Whether James S. had experienced any symptoms of illness before the day he took to his bed it was impossible to ascertain, in consequence of his previous state of mental depression.

On the 21st I made the following notes :—'Is reported to have slept well; no headache; mind confused and wandering; expression natural ; complexion clear ; colour of cheeks natural; no flush; no injection of conjunctivæ; no dislike to light; pupils normal; on the temples are the marks of eight or ten leech bites.

He leaves his bed unassisted, but with considerable difficulty ; tongue moist, anterior half red, posterior half slightly furred ; no stool; no gurgling, tenderness, nor abnormal fulness of the abdomen ; no thirst ; no appetite. Pulse 108, soft ; respiration quiet ; cough trifling; skin warm, dry, and clear.'

During the night he was delirious, and while so left his bed with the intention of dressing. Slept but little. On the following day he passed one relaxed stool ; gurgling was observed in the iliac fossa, and his tongue was dry and glazed. On the 23rd there was little change ; but on the 24th of July his mind was in its natural state. All delirium and confusion of intellect had disappeared ; his pulse was only 72 ; a few imperfectly marked rose spots were observed on the abdomen and thorax ; he passed two stools. On the morning of the 25th there was little change, excepting that the bowels were more relaxed ; five stools had been passed the preceding twenty-four hours.

July 26th, the following notes were made :—'Tongue dry, glazed, and tremulous. The nurse states that yesterday afternoon after the visit he had two copious evacuations from the bowels of pure blood. He has passed two stools to-day, and in both are clots of blood—the abdomen is slightly concave, there is neither tenderness nor gurgling in the abdomen—the rose spots noted on the abdomen are now well marked—the skin is hot and dry—the pulse is 80, soft.'

On the next day, July 27, the tongue became moist, and there was for the first time a little appetite ; his mind was normal in all respects ; the stools, one and two respectively, on this and the following day, were relaxed and very dark. On the 29th and 30th the bowels were confined. On the 31st he passed one copious relaxed stool ; an emollient clyster was administered in the evening of the same day, and 2 drms. of castor-oil on the morning of the 1st of August, but no stool was passed on the latter day. After this, however, his bowels acted daily by means of a small dose of castor-oil administered every morning. On the 28th of July two fresh rose spots were observed on the abdomen. On the 29th of July two new rose spots were again noted, and on the

31st several fresh ones. At this time the pulse was only 76, and he was gaining strength. On August 4th, *i.e.* probably between the 20th and 30th day of disease, when the last note of the case was made, his pulse was only 64—his appetite was good, tongue nearly clear—his bowels had acted twice the preceding twenty-four hours, the stools being formed, and natural in appearance. It was noted that he had evidently lost much flesh since his admission, and also that a blister applied to the nape of his neck before he came under observation had not healed: he was gaining strength daily. He left the hospital August 10th.

Experience has proved that those who have only recently taken up their abode in large cities are particularly liable to be attacked with typhoid fever. James S.'s case illustrates this fact. The exact date at which his illness began could not be fixed. The depression of spirits under which he had laboured for a month before he took to his bed not only rendered him more susceptible to the influence which excites the disease, be it contagious or not, but also prevented his friends appreciating that change in his appearance which, had he been in his ordinary mental state, would doubtless have been obvious. He was delirious at the time he was first seen by a medical man, so that no history of his past state could be obtained from the patient himself. The cessation of the delirium at the moment of the appearance of the eruption is a fact worthy of remark, especially when taken in conjunction with a like fact concerning a case hereafter to be recorded. The loss of blood from the bowels could not have been the cause of the improvement in the mental state, inasmuch as that improvement was manifested on the 24th, and the escape of blood from the intestine did not take place till the afternoon of the 25th. The rose spots ran that course which is natural to them. The points, however, on which I wish the reader to fix his attention, as illustrated by this case, are—1st, The recovery of the patient in spite of the copious hemorrhage from the bowels; 2nd, the cessation of the violent delirium consentaneously with the eruption of the rose spots; 3rd, the repeated eruption of fresh rose spots after the patient appeared in other respects convalescent. I shall refer to the last point, when speaking of the *duration* of typhoid fever. The raw surface left by the blister applied to the neck, before James S.'s admission, was not healed a fortnight after. The tendency in blistered surfaces to ulcerate, in persons affected with typhoid fever, was pointed out by Louis. I have before adverted to it.

Scarlet Rash.

A delicate scarlet tint of the whole surface of the cutis is now and then seen to precede for two or three days the eruption of the diagnostic rose spots. In such cases the disease may at first simulate scarlet fever, as in the following :—

CASE XXIX.—A man aged 19 years—pain in the abdomen—diarrhœa—rigors—headache—sore throat, followed by scarlet rash—subsequently rose spots—moderately quick pulse—sonorous rale—dry brown tongue—delirium—extreme prostration—somnolence—convulsions—their general improvement—deafness—convalescence.

Robert P., aged 19, a cellarman, of very temperate habits, dark brown hair and eyes—strong made—moderately stout—was admitted into the London Fever Hospital, July 12th, 1849. He stated that his general health had before his present illness been good—that in 1844 he had an attack of 'fever.' His mother died in a 'mad-house.' About a fortnight before his present illness began he had a slight attack of diarrhœa. It disappeared in a few days. On Sunday evening, July 8th, he was seized with pain in the abdomen and diarrhœa. He had slight rigors the same evening—the rigors were repeated several times before his admission into the hospital ; sore throat and headache were among the earliest symptoms. There was no vomiting nor nausea. Although, from the first, he lay about on the straw in the cellar or elsewhere, he did not take to the bed entirely till he entered the hospital. He lost about a tablespoonful of blood from the nose on the 4th day of disease. The day of his entrance into the hospital I made the following notes :—

July 12th, the 5th day of disease.—The mind is in all respects normal ; little sleep last night ; trifling frontal headache ; expression natural ; conjunctivæ pale ; pupils in all particulars natural ; no vertigo ; no affection of the special senses.

He can leave his bed unassisted with facility, but states that he feels he could *not walk* alone. Tongue moist, red at the tip, covered with a yellowish fur posteriorly ; papillæ large, red—some pain in deglutition—tonsils, *velum pend. palati*, *uvula*, and posterior wall of pharynx deep red; no tenderness behind the *rami* of the lower jaw; bowels much relaxed; he passed six or seven stools last night; abdomen resonant, gurgling limited to the right iliac fossa—pulse 96, full and soft; trifling cough; no abnormal physical chest signs—skin warm, moist, *covered with a delicate scarlet rash.*

On the following day the tongue was rather dry in the centre, and very red at the tip; in other respects—mind, rash, throat, and diarrhœa—he was as on the 12th. On the 7th day the rash was paler, and the throat was less sore; and on the 15th of July, *i.e.* the 8th day of disease, I noted :—' The nurse reports that he slept well last night—no headache; cheeks flushed; tongue moist, red, smooth, with large papillæ, covered with a yellowish fur posteriorly; stools relaxed; less sore throat than on admission; abdomen resonant; loud gurgling on pressure in the right iliac fossa; there is decided tenderness in the same situation. *Scarlet rash gone; four rose spots on the abdomen and thorax, and five on the back.*

From this time till the 15th day the disease pursued its ordinary course; the spots first seen disappeared in three or four days, fresh spots having in the meantime made their appearance, to be in like manner followed by others. On the 10th day he became delirious, and while so left his bed repeatedly to wander about. His bowels continued very much relaxed, and the stools of watery consistence. The cheeks were often flushed, sometimes one, sometimes both; the sore throat on the 14th day was very trifling, and at the same time he was so weak that with difficulty he turned in bed unassisted; his tongue was dry and brown, and his stools were chiefly passed into the bed unconsciously. His pulse was 108 and reduplicate; he slept much night and day.

On the 15th day he was reported to have dozed, with little interruption, from the time I saw him on the 14th day till 2 A.M. on the 15th, when he had an attack of convulsions. Both sides of his body and face were equally affected—his eyes, the nurse said, kept opening and shutting—there was no foaming at the mouth—the convulsive movements were so violent that the night nurse stated that she thought he would ' have been out of bed during the fit;' they lasted for a quarter of an hour. He appeared to those with him insensible at the time he was convulsed; the insensibility continued for about half an hour after the convulsions ceased. Before he recovered his consciousness he had an attack of rigors, and seemed, the night nurse said, ' like a person with ague.' The rigors were followed by profuse sweating, and it was while sweating that he recovered consciousness. He then complained of feeling very cold. At the time of my visit he was lying asleep on his back—cheeks flushed—pupils equal—

conjunctivæ somewhat more vascular than natural—slight deafness. There was no headache. He could now sit up in bed with a little assistance, and he turned unassisted more easily than on the preceding day. On the 16th day I found him asleep on his side; and on the 17th he was reading his Bible. He continued, however, delirious at night till the 19th day. On the 20th he was able to reach the close stool without aid. At the same time the back appeared about to slough, so that it was considered desirable to place him on a water-bed. No notes of spots were made after the 22nd day; still, on the 26th day, the skin was hot and dry, and the pulse 108.

From the 25th to the 27th.—Several small abscesses formed under the skin of the scalp. On the latter day his appetite was reported to be good. He passed one solid stool; his tongue was moist, and only slightly furred.

On the 29th day he was extremely deaf, but in all other respects improving. No note was made after this date.

Submucous rale was heard for the first time at the extreme posterior base of both lungs on the 13th day, and a day or two after, a little mucous rale was observed over the whole chest. At no subsequent period was any dulness detected.

A physician of eminence gave Robert P. a certificate, stating that he was labouring under scarlet fever; and certainly the symptoms, at the time of the man's admission, closely resembled those characteristic of that affection; but the fact that the disease began with diarrhœa, that epistaxis had occurred the day before Robert P. entered into the hospital, the co-existence, when he came under observation—a week from the outset of the illness—of diarrhœa and headache, and the presence of fulness and resonance of the abdomen generally, with gurgling in the right iliac fossa, and the sonorous rale heard over the whole chest, led me to think it highly probable that he was really suffering from typhoid fever. I had several times seen a scarlet rash precede the evolution of the rose spots; I thought it, therefore, probable that the rash was of that kind, and the sore throat an accidental complication. The patient had been ill only six days when he entered the hospital; on the eighth day of disease the appearance of rose spots removed all doubt. The subsequent course of the case would have rendered its nature evident even to the least experienced.

This man presented a striking exception to the rule, that

cases in which convulsions occur in the progress of typhoid fever are fatal. The day after the convulsions he was decidedly better than the day before. Severe rigors followed the convulsions, and yet there was no evidence that any local inflammation was being set up. Were the convulsions due to cerebral congestion or to inflammation? There is not in the notes of the case, or in the subsequent or antecedent history of the case, any evidence in favour of either view. That general morbid condition of the blood which is the cause of so many of the symptoms, was probably the cause of the convulsions. I have before referred to this when commenting on Case XII. (see page 218). It was, in the case now under consideration, as in many others, interesting to watch the progress of the spots, i.e. the repeated eruption of scanty crops, each spot remaining visible only a few days, the fresh spots appearing without any relation to the fading of those which preceded them. Just as *tinnitus aurium* is often present at the early stage, so deafness is a common symptom towards the termination of typhoid fever. I cannot say that either is a favourable or unfavourable symptom.

Mental Weakness sometimes a Sequela of Typhoid Fever.

CASE XXX.—In a lad aged 16—headache—epistaxis— diarrhœa—delirium—noise in the ears—loss of strength —enlarged spleen—dry, brown, glazed, and fissured tongue— confined bowels—solid stools—copious eruption of rose spots —convalescence about the 28th day—mental weakness for more than a fortnight after convalescence.

Thomas S., aged 16, a thin, fair-complexioned lad, with light hair and eyes, a native of London, by trade a plasterer, was admitted June 13th, 1849, into the London Fever Hospital, under the care of Dr. Tweedie. He states that six years ago he had a severe attack of fever, and that since that time his health has been good.

His present illness began Tuesday, June 8th, with pain in the head, general weakness, loss of appetite, trifling epistaxis, drowsi-ness, and diarrhœa. The epistaxis was repeated several times before, and the diarrhœa continued till his admission. Delirium began on the day he entered the hospital, i.e. the 8th day of disease, when the following notes were made:—

Some general headache, no vertigo — answers questions rationally, but thinks it is a fortnight since he left his work; yet he remembers correctly enough that the day of the week on which he left his work was Tuesday. Face pale—conjunctivæ very slightly injected—pupils natural—expression dull, vacant, stupid—complains of noise in the ears, compares it to children bellowing —other senses normal.

He can leave his bed unassisted, but is unable to walk. Tongue dry, centre covered with a thick, pale, yellowish-brown fur, fissured; abdomen resonant, a little pain about the umbilicus, no marked tenderness; no stool since admission, i.e. one hour—splenic dulness 7 inches by 5 inches.

Pulse 84, reduplicate, moderately full, soft; a little sonorous rale on deep inspiration; no cough.

Skin warm, dry—from one to two hundred rose spots scattered over abdomen, thorax, back, and upper and lower extremities—no miliary vesicles.

The rose spots, very numerous on the 9th day, were still more so on the 18th. At that time my notes state many hundreds were present; [1] and, also, that those marked on the 9th day had disappeared. Fresh rose spots were observed every day or two till the 24th day of disease. An abundant crop of miliary vesicles was noted on the 20th day. Although diarrhœa had been a prominent symptom before the boy's admission, the stools never exceeded two in the twenty-four hours after he came under observation, and were always solid and well-formed. On the 20th day he complained of want of food, and from that time ate some bread daily. On the same, i.e. the 20th day, his tongue, which up to that time had been dry, glazed, yellowish, brown, and fissured, became slightly moist and rather white. From his entrance till the 26th day he slept much, more than natural; and, till the 23rd day, he was delirious when awake. After that there was no distinct delirium, but he appeared to be silly—quite childish. He was considered to be convalescent some time between the 26th and 30th days, but the childishness of mind and manner continued till he left the hospital, near the end of July.

Rose spots, although ordinarily limited to the trunk, are now and then, as in this case, found on the extremities; far more rarely on the face. The spots were present on the 9th

---

[1] A cast of the spots was taken on the 12th day of disease. A wax model, prepared from that cast, is in University College Museum. A drawing from the model was made by Mr. George of Hatton Garden, and was published in the thirty-third volume of the *Transactions of the Medico-Chirurgical Society*. This plate is reproduced in the present volume, p. 144.

day of disease, when the boy was admitted; how long before could not be ascertained. Unless especially looked for, rose spots, even when numerous, as in this case, are apt to be passed by unnoticed. The course of the spots is of equal, if not more importance, with reference to their diagnostic value than their characters. The repeated eruption of fresh rose spots every day or two, without reference to the continuance or disappearance of the spots that preceded them, each spot lasting from three to five days, is not only a character of, but is absolutely peculiar to, typhoid fever. Fresh rose spots made their appearance after the tongue had begun to clean and the appetite was returning. An abundant crop of *sudamina* broke out at the end of the second week; the connection between this eruption and perspiration is as yet undetermined. At one time they were supposed to stand to each other in the relation of cause and effect, but Louis's observations have thrown doubt on this imagined connection. I have before adverted to the fact, that *sudamina* are rarely seen on individuals more than forty years of age, and still more rarely, if ever, on those more than fifty years old.

The peculiar condition of the mind, which leads an individual to suppose that a longer time has elapsed since any given event than has really passed away—that a given time has been prolonged, was observed in this case. The mind thus affected may recall particular events, while it prolongs the interval between the given event and the time of narration: thus, James S. thought he had been ill fourteen days instead of nine days; at the same time, he knew that it was on a Tuesday that his illness commenced. The state of mind here referred to was present in others of these cases. Its analogy with the mental state which constitutes dreaming is striking. How often, during a dream, do minutes seem hours or weeks! And when was the reverse, with reference to duration, ever dreamed?

Tinnitus aurium was, on the boy's admission, a marked symptom. He complained of it spontaneously, and used the emphatic expression, ' bellowing of children,' to indicate its annoying character. The whirl of the railway train, the waving of trees by the wind, the ringing of bells, and the roaring of the sea, are often referred to as descriptive of the noise in the ears which disturbs the patient labouring under fever. The stools were solid after the boy's admission although he had previously suffered from diarrhœa.

This case has been given especially to illustrate the fact that mental weakness occasionally follows typhoid fever. The loss of intellectual power is, however, only temporary. A few weeks ago (September 1850) I met this boy. He had grown stout and healthful, and his mind had regained its normal vigour.

PERFORATION OF THE INTESTINE.

Perforation of the intestine is by far the most fatal of the complications of typhoid fever. Rokitansky affirms that the adhesions which now and then form after perforation has occurred are never permanent; that a cure, consequently, is never effected. Louis refers only to fatal cases; Chomel the same. My own experience affords no example of recovery after this lesion. Perforation of the ileum takes place during the progress of only one acute disease, and that is typhoid fever, of only one chronic disease, and that is phthisis. One of Peyer's patches, in the lower part of the ileum, is the ordinary seat of the perforation. Chomel details one case in which it took place in the colon. In a majority of cases perforation occurs after the termination of the second week of the disease, very often after the fever properly so called, *i.e.* the specific blood disease—if the blood is the part primarily affected—has terminated, when the ulcers in the intestine have passed into a chronic form, constituting the 'atonic ulcers' of Rokitansky. Louis details eight cases of perforation; in one case, the lesion occurred on the 12th day of illness; in two on the 18th day; and in the five others between the 22nd and 42nd days inclusive.

Case XXXI.—In a man aged 37.—Diarrhœa—headache —chilliness—abdominal pains—early sense of severe illness, followed by slight deafness—fulness, resonance and tenderness of abdomen—abnormal extent of splenic dulness— rapid pulse—rose spots—restlessness—copious vomiting of green fluid—sudden death.

Twenty-two hours after death.—Lymph and turbid serosity,

mixed with a little fæculent matter in the peritoneal cavity—perforation of ileum eight inches above ileo-cæcal valve—extensive ulceration of Peyer's patches—pseudo-suppuration of one mesenteric gland—enlargement of spleen.

John P., aged 37, a moderately stout, fair-complexioned man, with light brown hair and eyes, a labourer, was admitted into the London Fever Hospital, April 15th, 1849. He was of temperate habits—had not suffered from want of food or clothing—had resided in London nine years. His previous health had been excellent. On first rising from bed at half-past six A.M., Tuesday, April 10th, he passed a watery stool; the day before, his bowels were regular, and he felt quite well. About two hours after the diarrhœa commenced, he began to suffer from severe frontal headache; at the same time he felt chilly. He left the fireside as little as possible, because he felt, when away from the fire, ' so shivering.' He left his work the day his illness began, but did not take to his bed till Thursday, April 12th. On the 11th he was, for the first time, troubled with aching, griping pains in the abdomen; these continued till his admission. The headache ceased on the 12th or 13th. He had no vertigo, noise in the ears, nor epistaxis.

On his admission, Sunday, April 15th, he walked unassisted from the door of the ward to his bed,—a distance of about 60 feet. He was seen by me for the first time, April 16th, i.e. the 8th day of disease. At that time there was no headache: his mind was clear; his memory good. With the exception of slight deafness, the special senses were unaffected; the complexion was clear; there was no vertigo—no flushing of the face—no pallor; in fact, the aspect of the man's face, and the expression of his countenance, were natural. He lay unconstrainedly on his back, with his legs extended, was able to leave his bed unassisted, but said he felt too weak to stand alone: at the same time he sat up in bed, for me to examine the back of his chest, readily and with facility. The tongue was of a pale yellowish brown colour, dry, glazed, with a deep fissure down the centre. He had passed, in the preceding twenty-four hours, two watery stools. He suffered from occasional pains in the belly, not limited to any particular part. The abdomen was full and resonant, and decidedly tender in the hypogastric and iliac regions. The splenic dulness was abnormally extensive.

The pulse, 140 in the minute, was small and weak; there was trifling cough.

The skin was hot and dry. About thirty rose spots were present on the chest and abdomen. There were no miliary vesicles.

An enema, composed of 20 drops of laudanum and 4 ozs. of starch-water, was ordered to be administered night and morning.

Late in the evening he complained to the nurse of nausea; passed a restless night; had but little sleep. On the morning of the 17th, i.e. the 9th day of disease, he left his bed unassisted, but with some slight difficulty. About 7 A.M., he vomited some green fluid. The vomiting was repeated several times in the course of the morning; altogether he ejected more than two pints of transparent dark-green fluid. About 9 A.M., the nurse, observing his feet were very cold, had a bottle of hot water placed in the bed. He did not complain at any time during the day of pain in the abdomen. Just before 3 P.M., the nurse, seeing his feet projecting from the bottom of the bed, requested he would draw them up; he did so, and spoke to her. He was then quite sensible, and did not complain of any pain. In a minute or two, the nurse, not having left the ward, heard him let fall a small vessel he had in his hand to receive the vomited matters. He struggled violently, threw up his arms, vomited an immense quantity of turbid green fluid, which soaked the bed-clothes, and ran in considerable quantities on to the floor. He died in two minutes from the moment the vessel fell from his hands.

I saw him three-quarters of an hour after death. At that time there was no trace of the rose spots so well marked on the day before.[1]

The body of John P., was examined twenty-two hours after death, and the following notes made:—

Height 5 feet 10 inches; cadaveric rigidity well marked; no sign of decomposition; very little fat on the abdominal parietes.

Head.—*Cerebrum and cerebellum, and their membranes,* perfectly normal.

Larynx.—Mucous membrane of larynx generally, especially the under surface of the epiglottis, somewhat redder than ordinary.

Bronchial tubes contain very little mucus; lining membrane deep purple, but of normal consistence.

No enlargement of *bronchial glands.*

Lungs.—Crepitant throughout; the most depending part of either lung contains a slight excess of dark fluid blood.

Pericardium healthy in all particulars; contains about ½ oz. of transparent yellow serosity.

Heart.—Right side moderately distended by a soft, dark, and tolerably firm pale fibrinous clot continuous with a similar clot in the pulmonary artery, moulded to the sigmoid valves; a similar

[1] This man's stools were analysed by my colleague Dr. Parkes, whose researches on this subject were detailed in a Clinical Lecture published in the *Medical Times.*

smaller clot in the left side of the heart continuous with a clot in
the aorta moulded to the sigmoid valves. Substance and valves
healthy. Weight 10 oz. Blood fluid in the veins of the
extremities.

Tongue dry; yellow.

Pharynx pale purplish red.

Œsophagus yellow; no trace of ulceration.

Abdominal cavity.—The parietal peritoneum is thickened, opaque,
dull white, finely streaked with delicate pink capillaries. It
adheres, by means of recent lymph, to the large omentum; the
lymph is dull yellow, readily breaks down on pressure, and contains much serosity in its substance. On raising the great
omentum the folds of the intestine are found in a great measure
covered by yellow lymph, most abundant in the angles formed by
adjacent folds of intestines. The small and large intestines are
distended with flatus. Several folds of small intestine are situated
in the pelvic cavity, adhering loosely to each other, and to the
upper surface of the bladder. One fold of the intestine is adherent
by its side to the mesentery; on breaking down this adhesion
three openings are exposed, leading into a cavity situated between
the folds of the mesentery, and near to the ileo-cæcal valve. The
cavity is filled with purulent-looking fluid, and appears to have
been formed by pseudo-suppuration of one of the mesenteric glands.

About eight inches above the ileo-cæcal valve is an opening,
one-third inch in diameter, leading into the interior of the ileum.
Attached by one point to the edge of the aperture, hangs some
deep yellow tough shaggy-looking tissue, apparently composed of
the remains of that portion of the peritoneum by the sloughing of
which the aperture was formed.

In the cavity of the pelvis is a considerable quantity of turbid
yellow fluid, with particles of fæculent matter diffused through it.

The convex surface of the liver is covered with a purulent-
looking matter, and adhesions, very readily broken down, have
here and there formed between the liver and the diaphragm; the
convex surface of the spleen is similarly affected; the peritoneal
surface of the stomach offers a beautiful specimen of redness of a
serous membrane, characteristic of inflammation.

The *mesenteric glands* are generally enlarged, purplish red, and
softened; the one which has been the seat of the pseudo-suppura-
tive process before referred to, is about the size of a walnut; the
portion of that gland undestroyed is soft and red.

The *mesocolic glands* are soft, friable, and palish purple.

Stomach partially distended, moderately rugose, mammillated,
with the exception of the great cul-de-sac, of a pale dusky grey
colour; consistence normal.

Intestines.—Vessels of *duodenum* rather more filled with blood than usual. The mucous membrane of the lower three feet of the *ileum* softened. About twenty-two inches above the ileo-cæcal valve is an ulcer measuring $\frac{1}{4}$ inch by $\frac{1}{4}$ inch; its edges slightly elevated and bright red; its floor pale, and formed of transverse muscular fibres, then follow three ulcers closely resembling the last described, except that the floors of the two first are bright red, and that of the third covered by a thick mass of sloughy-looking yellow matter. The ulcer in which the perforation has occurred is 1 inch in breadth and $1\frac{1}{2}$ inch in length; its long axis corresponding to the long axis of the intestine; its edges scarcely elevated above the adjacent mucous membrane, are speckled with bright red; its floor, deep red, is formed of transverse muscular fibres, and in its centre is the aperture seen externally, with the yellow slough attached at one point to its margin. There are two large ulcers between the one in which the perforation is seated and the ileo-cæcal valve; the floors of these ulcers, like the floors of those seated higher in the intestine, are formed of transverse muscular fibres. The mucous membrane of those folds of the intestine which have fallen into the pelvic cavity, is of a dusky reddish hue; it is in the lowest of these pelvic folds that the perforation has occurred; the mucous membrane of the last six inches of the ileum is quite pale.

With the exception of the lowest three feet of the ileum, the mucous membrane of the jejunum and ileum is pale, and of normal consistence.

The ulcers are all placed on that side of the ileum which is opposite to the mesentery, and are evidently seated on Peyer's patches. There is no enlargement of the patches above the first ulcer, but from that to the ileo-cæcal valve every patch is extensively destroyed.

The solitary glands at the lower part of the ileum are very distinct, and of a dull white colour.

Cæcum pale, and healthy in all particulars.

The *colon* was not examined.

The *liver* weighs 4 lb. 9 ozs. It is firm as in health, and moderately congested. The congestion is central.

The *gall bladder* contains a moderate quantity of bright orange-coloured bile. Its lining membrane is perfectly healthy in appearance.

Spleen 10 ozs. in weight; is slightly softened; not particularly dark.

The *pancreas* weighs 3 ozs. It appears healthy.

Kidney.—The right one is wanting; the left weighs 11 ozs. It is slightly congested, but in other respects healthy; its capsule separates readily; its surface is smooth. Lining membrane of the pelvis of the kidney pale.

Mucous membrane of the *urinary bladder* pale and healthy.

It is very rare for perforation to occur so early in the disease as the 9th day. Yet, in the case of John P., it must have taken place on or before that date. It is worthy of note that he lay with his legs extended till the last, that he never complained of pain in the abdomen, and that the nurse, an intelligent woman, observed nothing in his appearance to indicate approaching dissolution. How different from the symptoms occasionally present when perforation occurs! How different from the symptoms ordinarily assigned as those of perforation! The severe vomiting, then, was the only symptom to indicate the complication which so rapidly caused death. Yet John P. was neither somnolent nor delirious; the nurse had been repeatedly at his bedside during the day, on account of the incessant vomiting, and he spoke to her sensibly and collectedly not more than four minutes before he died. The slight but decided tenderness of the hypogastric region present, at the time of my visit on the 8th day, was probably due to localised inflammation of the peritoneum, the consequence of the softening and pseudo-suppuration of the mesenteric gland. It is evident that if the peritoneum had given way over that gland, all the symptoms of perforation of the intestine might have occurred, and yet that lesion not have been present. I shall hereafter adduce a case of this kind. Tenderness limited to one part of the abdomen, even though it follows sudden severe pain, and be accompanied by symptoms of collapse, is of no value as a diagnostic sign of perforation. The aperture in the intestine was formed by sloughing; the slough was yet attached at one point to the margin of the opening. This case illustrates one mode, then, by which perforation of the gut may be effected in typhoid fever. There are two others —namely, *by rupture*, the peritoneum is exposed by ulceration, and thus that delicate membrane, perhaps as Chomel supposes from distension by flatus, gives way at the most attenuated point; or the opening may be formed *by ulceration*,—i.e. molecular death. The aperture formed by rupture or by molecular death (ulceration) is small, sometimes not larger than a pin-point; if the consequence of sloughing, as in the case of John P., the aperture may be much larger. The pain experienced is by no means in proportion to the size of the perforation. I have before referred to a case in which the patient suffered acutely; after death the opening through the peritoneum was not larger than a small pin-head. In the case here detailed it was the size of a fourpenny piece; and yet no single word or look indicated that the man endured a pang. Be it observed, also, that the patient who suffered so acutely was delirious before the perforation occurred; and that John P., who suffered nothing, was in the possession of all his mental faculties—that his powers of perception were unimpaired up to four minutes before death.

It is far more common (as in this case) for the transverse than for the longitudinal muscular fibres to be laid bare; when exposed by ulceration they are ordinarily large and red.

The condition of the mesocolic glands renders it highly probable that the colon was the seat of ulceration; but, unfortunately, it escaped down the pipe of the sink into the cesspool before it was examined. The size of the spleen was indicated by the extent of dulness present during life. Its weight was considerable, considering the man had been ill for only nine days when he died; but then it must be borne in mind that the intestinal lesion was very extensive for the period of the disease at which John P. died. As bearing on the same point, i.e. the rapid course of the disease, it is interesting to note that this man was obliged to quit his work directly his illness began, and never left his bed after the second day of illness—facts indicating clearly the extensive injury the disease had inflicted on the system at large, even at that early period.

CASE XXXII.—In a female aged 36 years—gradual commencement of illness—repeated rigors followed by sweating —headache—loss of appetite—confined bowels—sense of weakness—moist slightly-furred tongue—repeated sudden pain in the abdomen followed by slight tenderness—marked emaciation—vomiting—tenesmus—*death* on about the 46th day of disease.

Forty-eight hours after death.—Lymph and serosity in left pleura—imperfect consolidation of inferior part of left lung—lymph and serosity in peritoneal cavity—perforation of the ileum—ulceration of the ileum—spleen rather large.

Jane H., aged 36, a servant, a large-made, thin, and rather dark woman, was admitted into the London Fever Hospital, under the care of Dr. Tweedie, September 5th, 1848. Her general health, before her present illness, had been tolerably good, but she had suffered occasionally, after eating, from pain at the epigastrium, and flatulence.

Jane H. had resided in London two years. She had lived in her present situation, 17 Albany Street, only three weeks. Her mistress stated that she had not appeared well from the moment she entered her service. Before that she had for some time suffered from privation of food.

The history the woman herself gave of her present illness was, that about a fortnight before her admission she was seized in the night with rigors; the rigors were repeated several nights in succession, and were on each occasion followed by sweating. At the same time she began to suffer from headache, loss of appetite, nausea, pain, and general soreness of the limbs. During the whole of this time her bowels were confined. She continued her household duties till the morning before her admission, though often obliged to lie down during the day.

On her admission I noted as follows :—

About 16*th day of disease.*—Little sleep last night, and that disturbed; no headache; mind quite unaffected; with the exception of an unpleasant taste, and imperfect sense of odours, the special senses normal; no increased vascularity of conjunctivæ; some heaviness of expression; complexion dusky; face pale.

Says she feels very weak, at the same time she can walk without assistance; tongue slightly furred, moist, large, red; one stool; no appetite; some thirst; no fulness, resonance, tenderness, nor gurgling in abdomen.

Pulse 108; no cough; no abnormal physical chest-signs.

Skin warm, perspiring freely; no spots.

From this date till the 15th of September there was little change in her condition. The bowels never, or very rarely, acted without the administration of castor-oil, three or four doses of which aperient were at different times administered. Rose spots, although repeatedly looked for, were never found. She generally passed restless nights. Her tongue continued as on admission. Her pulse varied from 96 to 108.

On the 18th September, *i.e. about the* 28*th day of disease,* ' Pulse 90; skin cool; she had slept well the preceding night, no restlessness; tongue clean and moist; one stool; no appetite.'

She was considered to be convalescent; but on the 26th and subsequent days I made the following notes :—

26th September.—Slept well last night; this morning early was *suddenly seized with severe pain in the abdomen*; altogether it lasted several hours, *alternately ceasing and returning.*   Is now lying on her back; legs extended; skin warm; tongue moist and furred; abdomen somewhat fuller than natural, and slightly tender; has passed three stools since the pain in the abdomen commenced; pulse 120.   Calomel 3 grains, opium ½ grain directly, castor oil ½ oz. in two hours.

Sept. 27th.—Pulse 120; skin hot and dry; little sleep; face flushed; tongue as yesterday; four stools; suffered from severe pain in the abdomen about 6 A.M.; no fulness of abdomen, slight tenderness.

Sept. 28th.—Pulse 108; skin hot and dry; some sleep; face flushed; occasional pain in the abdomen; tongue moist, furred, dirty white; two stools, solid and lumpy.   The calomel and opium pill was repeated at bed-time, and a senna draught prescribed for the morning.

Sept. 29th.—No note made.

Sept. 30th.—Pulse 120; very weak; skin cool, moist; hands cold; dozed occasionally during the night; about 8 o'clock severe pain in the abdomen, followed by vomiting of about 8 ozs. of dark green fluid; complains now of nausea; has passed four dark and lumpy stools during the last twenty-four hours; considerable tenderness in the region of the liver, and generally over the right side of the abdomen; tongue moist, covered with thick yellow fur.   Eight leeches were applied over the region of the liver, a blister to the same part, and a simple saline effervescing mixture was prescribed.

Oct. 1st.—Pulse 118; rather more power than yesterday; skin warm; dozed a little this morning; no return of severe pain; at the present time no pain in abdomen, a little tenderness; lost but little blood from leeches; blister rose but little; tongue red, dry in centre; bowels very much relaxed, stools watery, greenish; used bed-pan, felt too weak to leave bed; has emaciated considerably the last few days; no return of vomiting; no nausea; complexion clear; much thirst.   Omit the mixture.

Oct. 2nd.—Pulse 96, stronger; no sleep in consequence of noise in ward; complains of some pain in the left side of the abdomen; tongue moist; no vomiting; two stools; less thirst. Mustard-poultice to be applied to the left side of the abdomen.

Oct. 3rd.—Pulse 96; slept well; pain in left side of abdomen gone; tongue same; four stools, scanty, dark; much thirst; some nausea.   Mercury with chalk 4 grains at bed-time, castor-oil ½ oz. in the morning.

Oct. 4th.—Pulse 96; slept well; no pain in either side of abdomen; no fulness nor tenderness of abdomen; tongue rather cleaner; four stools, less dark; no nausea; no appetite; much thirst; face flushes occasionally.

Oct. 5th.—Pulse 90; little sleep last night in consequence of pain at the lower part of abdomen; some fulness and slight tenderness in the right iliac fossa; tongue the same; four or five stools, scanty; some tenesmus. Linseed poultice to be applied over the abdomen.

Oct. 6th, about the 46th day of disease.—Pulse 100; weak; little sleep; pain in lower part of abdomen the same; tongue cleaner, moist; five or six scanty stools, solid, dark; complains much of tenesmus; mind wanders a little, but she answers questions rationally. A simple enema to be administered to-night.

The enema was administered about 7 P.M.—it acted in fifteen minutes, bringing away some dark, lumpy stool. About 8 P.M. she became suddenly much worse; at 10 P.M. her skin was cool, and covered with perspiration; the countenance expressed collapse; the features seemed sunken; the breathing was very quick; the pulse rapid and weak; the abdomen rather tumid, and somewhat tender. She continued sensible to the last, and spoke to the nurse an hour before her death; at that time the surface of the body was cold; she dozed at intervals, and *died* without a struggle at half-past twelve at night.

The body of Jane H. was examined forty-eight hours after death. The body was greatly emaciated. Cadaveric rigidity well marked in the upper extremities, less so in the lower; the abdominal parietes had a greenish hue, excepting about the umbilicus, where they still retained their normal hue; numerous large *sudamina* studded the sides of the thorax and abdomen; a few very small ones were scattered over the anterior surface of the whole trunk. The *brain* and its *membranes* were in all respects normal. There was no enlargement of the cervical glands; the *larynx* and *trachea* were perfectly healthy in appearance. About 1½ oz. of serosity was found in the *right pleura*; the *right lung* was perfectly healthy.

In the *left pleura* was about 1½ oz. of serosity, with shreds of gelatinous-looking lymph floating in it. On the pleura covering the lower part of the inferior lobe of the left lung were a few shreds of soft yellow lymph; at places the thin layer of lymph could be stripped off. Numerous minute crimson points studded the pleural surface of the lower part of the inferior lobe. The vessels of the costal pleura for nearly its whole extent were finely injected with blood. The pulmonary tissue of the inferior portion of the lower lobe of the *left lung* was darker in hue, and contained less air than the other parts of the lung. Elsewhere the pulmonary tissue, with the exception of a small mass of soft, friable, cheesy-like material, of a dull yellowish colour, at the apex of the lower lobe, was healthy.

The *bronchial tubes* contained a little frothy colourless mucus; their lining membrane was pale and healthy.

The *bronchial glands* contained several cretaceous masses.

In the *pericardium* was about 1½ oz. of slightly turbid serosity;[1] the membrane itself was pale and transparent.

The substance of the *heart* was flabby, but in other respects it was healthy-looking. The valves appeared normal.

The *tongue* was slightly furred; the *pharynx* and *œsophagus* pale and healthy-looking.

On opening the abdomen the peritoneal surface of the intestines was found highly vascular; the redness was ramiform and capillary; it was most marked towards the inferior half of the abdomen. Several ounces of dirty sero-purulent-looking fluid, with large shreds of yellow lymph floating in it, were removed from the peritoneal cavity.

Near the lower part of the ileum was a fold of that intestine, the two portions constituting which were for a short distance closely adherent to each other. Just at the point where the two portions of the fold separated, and in the half next the cæcum, was a small round aperture, formed by perforation of all the coats of the intestine, from which a thin dirty gruelly-looking fluid, closely resembling that found in the abdominal cavity, could be pressed in considerable quantity. A knuckle of the ileum, situated about four inches above the ileo-cæcal valve, adhered, by tolerably firm and thick lymph, to the abdominal parietes of the right iliac fossa. Folds of the same intestine contained in the pelvic cavity, and situated just above it, adhered to each other, to the fundus of the uterus, and to both ovaries, by thick firm yellow lymph, evidently of recent formation. The fundus of the uterus and the peritoneum lining the post-uterine pouch were covered by a layer of tolerably firm yellow lymph, capable of being torn off in flakes or laminæ.

The *mesenteric glands*, especially in the vicinity of the lower part of the ileum, were large, and deep purple and soft.

The *pharynx* and *œsophagus* were pale and healthy.

The *stomach* was, with the exception of some linear white softening of its mucous membrane in the vicinity of the fundus, healthy in aspect.

The mucous membrane of the *duodenum* was stained of a yellow-colour; of the *jejunum and ileum* generally pale.

About three feet above the ileo-cæcal valve, at the inferior

[1] The serosity found in the pericardium after death may be turbid from the diffusion through it of the epithelium scales of the serous membrane detached by decomposition. The microscope reveals, in such a case, the cause of the turbidity.

portion of one of Peyer's patches, was a grey spot about ⅓ inch in diameter, the centre of which was pale, smooth, shining, and slightly depressed, evidently a healed ulcer. From this point downwards every Peyer's patch was of a more or less deep grey colour, and on every one were seated, superficial, or healed ulcers. Between the patches were several small round ulcers, with deep grey edges and pale floors. About nine inches above the ileo-cæcal valve was a perforation of the intestinal coats; the aperture, about three-eighths of an inch in diameter, was seated on one of Peyer's patches. Perforation of the intestinal coat had occurred through the next patch, but effusion of the contents of the bowel had been prevented by adhesion between intestine and the fundus of the uterus. On this same patch were two ulcers, the floors of which were formed of transverse muscular fibres. On the large patch next above the valve, were several small superficial ulcers, and smooth, slightly depressed, pale, shining spots, with grey margins,—evidently healed ulcers. The mucous membrane of the lower part of the ileum, between the Peyer's patches, was slightly softened, pale, and had an opaque aspect.

The mucous membrane of *cæcum* and *colon* was pale, and healthy in every respect.

The small intestines contained a large quantity of thin, dirty, gruelly-looking fluid; the large, some solid pale yellow fæces.

The *liver* was very flabby, and of a uniform dirty green colour, from the action of gases generated after death.

The *gall bladder* contained ½ oz. of bright yellow bile.

The *spleen* weighed 7¾ ozs.; it was pale and flabby, but not particularly soft.

The *pancreas* and *kidney* were flabby, but in other respects normal.

The uterus was covered by a thick layer of lymph, and the ovaries were imbedded in a similar substance.

This was one of the most marked examples of *latent* typhoid fever I ever witnessed. During the whole course of the fever, the mind was in *all* respects as in health. Loss of appetite, quick pulse, disturbed sleep, slightly furred tongue, and sense of weakness, were all the positive symptoms when Jane H. came into the hospital, on about the 16th day of disease. Nor had the symptoms been at any time before her admission more severe. Subsequently her bowels were con-fined—dose after dose of castor oil being administered, in order to procure one stool every day or two. Rose spots were carefully sought for daily, but not one could be detected.

On the 28th day of disease, with the exception of want of appetite, she appeared convalescent, and was allowed to leave her bed. The severe pain on the morning of the 25th of September (that is, of the 36th day), followed by slight tenderness of the abdomen, was probably the consequence of the first perforation, that which after death was found obliterated by adhesions. The intermittent character of the pain certainly misled me in appreciating the nature of the case. I was very particular in my inquiries on the point, and the woman was clear in her answers. Tenderness of the abdomen is not unfrequently observed after severe attacks of colic, without inflammation being present. It was curious to remark the way in which the pain recurred, at intervals of many hours, for three or four days, and then its extreme severity on the 40th day, followed by vomiting of dark green fluid, the passage of lumpy stools, and the limitation of the tenderness to half the abdomen; the latter rendered it improbable that effusion of the contents of the bowel into the peritoneal cavity had taken place. When the pain was felt in the left side of the abdomen the pulse had fallen to 96, and in all respects the patient appeared mending. Yet no very urgent symptom announced the occurrence of the lesion, nor did she appear so near her end as she really was at the time I saw her on the 46th day. Could it have been that the peritonitis, lymph, etc., was due to the first perforation; the sudden collapse, four and a half hours before she died, to the second perforation? On the whole, perhaps, this is the more rational explanation of the relation between the symptoms and lesions.

Constipation was a prominent symptom throughout; this is by no means a favourable symptom. I have seen other cases in which it was marked terminate in the same way, i.e. by perforation. Tenesmus is not often complained of in typhoid fever, even when the colon is the seat of ulceration. A large number of the ulcers in the ileum had healed, and many were healing, when this woman died, yet two or three had passed into chronic ulcers. These—the atonic ulcers of Rokitansky—are especially liable to lead to perforation. The fever had terminated by the 28th day, but two or three of the many ulcers, the consequence of the fever, continued to progress after the cessation of the primary disease, just as pneumonia or pleurisy, set up during the progress of the fever, may continue long after that has terminated, and ultimately may cause the death of the patient. There was no puckering of the intestinal coats towards the cicatrix of the ulcers. My experience is in accordance with Rokitansky's assertion, that contraction of the calibre of the intestine is not one of the sequences of typhoid fever. A smooth, shining, depressed, and not a puckered spot, indicates the previous site of the typhoid ulcer.

At what date did the pleura become inflamed? It seems probable that it was affected secondarily to the peritoneum, by extension, just as the pericardium sometimes becomes involved in the diseased action, when the pleura is the seat of inflammation. If this view be correct, then the pneumonia, still in its first stage, and small in extent, was secondary to the pleuritis, the pulmonary tissue being involved also by extension.

Was the slight turbidity of the serosity found in the pericardium due to particles of lymph or granular corpuscles? Or was it the consequence of the presence of detached epithelium scales? If the latter, the turbidity was the result of changes effected by incipient decomposition; if the former, of inflammation by extension.[1] The microscope could have determined the question in an instant. I omitted to apply that test.

SYMPTOMS SIMULATING THOSE OF PERFORATION OF THE INTESTINE WITHOUT THE EXISTENCE OF THAT LESION.

The two cases now to be detailed possess great interest, from the identity of the symptoms they presented with those laid down by the highest authority on the subject—Louis— as diagnostic of perforation of the intestine. With reference also to the second of the two cases here recorded this in addition may be observed, that, as the girl had been exposed to the contagion of typhus fever—had no examination of the

[1] Dr. John Taylor pointed out this as one of the causes of pericarditis, in his highly philosophical examination of the causes of that disease, published in the *Transactions of Royal Medico-Chirurgical Society*, vol. xxviii.

body been made, she might have been supposed to exhibit an exception to the law, that the contagion of typhus fever never produces typhoid fever.[1]

CASE XXXIII.—In a female aged 20.—Rigors—headache —diarrhœa—tenderness of abdomen—retching—loss of appetite—slightly furred tongue—greatly enlarged spleen— rose spots—convalescence between the 30th and 34th days— relapse on the 44th day; *i.e.* rapid pulse—diarrhœa—rose spots —tumour in right iliac fossa—second convalescence by 57th day. On 75th day, sudden pain in abdomen—collapse— vomiting—rigors—general tenderness of abdomen—constipation—commencing convalescence and erysipelas of face on 80th day—convulsions and *death* on 86th day.

Twenty and a half hours after death.—Fatty degeneration of mesenteric glands—recent adhesions of peritoneum— enlarged spleen—cicatrising ulcers on Peyer's patches.

Emma F., aged 20, a domestic servant, was admitted into the London Fever Hospital, August 20th, 1848. Her illness began Sunday, August 13th. The symptoms present before her admission were rigors and chilliness, alternating with sense of heat, headache, pain in the limbs, and loss of appetite. She vomited on the Thursday, after taking a dose of medicine. The bowels, confined at the outset of the illness, had been, before she came under observation, much relaxed. No cause could be assigned for her present illness.

From the date of her admission into the hospital till I saw her, the following symptoms were present:—Disturbed sleep ; trifling headache ; muscular tremors ; moist and nearly clean tongue ; little appetite ; diarrhœa ; fulness, resonance, and slight tenderness of the abdomen ; severe retching for a few hours on the evening of September 2nd.

September 4th, 24th day of disease.—Is reported by the nurse to have slept at intervals through the night, talking occasionally in her sleep; some deafness; face flushes occasionally; tongue moist, and slightly furred, not abnormally red : no appetite; has passed, during the last twenty-four hours, five pale, frothy, curdy-looking stools; abdomen full and resonant ; a tumour can be felt in the abdomen, the anterior margin of which is two fingers' breadth to the left of the umbilicus, its lower edge a little below

[1] See *Medico-Chirurgical Transactions,* vol. xxxiii., on the Identity or Non-Identity of the Cause of Typhus from Typhoid Fever and Relapsing Fever, by W. Jenner, M.D. (*Vide supra*, p. 133.)

the level of the umbilicus ; posteriorly, it is lost in the left lumbar region ; superiorly, it extends into the left hypochondriac region under the false ribs ; its anterior margin is acute and hard (this tumour was doubtless the enlarged spleen) ; liver dulness about two fingers' breadth below the cartilages of ribs on right side ; no tenderness of abdomen ; no trace of the rose spots previously noted, but several fresh rose spots have appeared since the last report. Pulse 90, weak.

On the 26th, four or five, and on the 27th day, two, fresh rose spots were observed.

By the 34th day she appeared convalescent ; her pulse was only 84. She had passed only two stools, her tongue was moist and clean and the appetite was returning ; the splenic dulness was much less extensive, and she seemed stronger. No fresh spots had appeared since the 27th day. She was, in fact, convalescent, the only symptom of illness being a little hysterical laughing, crying, and sense of choking on first waking in the morning.

On the 37th day I noted that there had been no return of the hysterical symptoms ; her appetite was good ; the tongue continued clean ; the splenic dulness was still less extensive than on the 34th day ; no fresh spots had appeared, and she had gained some strength ; she had passed during the preceding twenty-four hours two relaxed stools. She was considered convalescent.

On the 44th day the nurse reported that Emma F. had, the day before, refused her food, and, in the evening, had an attack of rigors. At the time of my visit on the 44th day I noted as follows :—

'Pulse 120, weak ; slept tolerably well last night ; some frontal headache ; no delirium ; spirits depressed ; expression rather anxious ; tongue moist, covered with thin white fur ; she passed three stools yesterday, none to-day ; very little appetite ; has retched frequently, but ejected nothing ; no fulness nor tenderness of the abdomen ; splenic dulness 5 inches by 3½ inches (i.e. although large, the spleen was much smaller than on admission). In the right iliac fossa is a round, firm tumour, about the size of a large walnut, perceptible on deep manipulation ; it is not tender. Skin cool, rough, and dry ; no spots.'

Between the 45th and 51st day she slept but little ; her mind occasionally wandered ; while asleep she often sweated freely. She complained frequently of attacks of sharp shooting pains, lasting for three or four minutes at a time ; in the intervals she was quite easy ; the pain did not precede the stools. During the seven days in question several fresh spots, at intervals of a day or two, made their appearance ; thus, one was noted on the 46th, one on the 47th, two on the 50th, and several on the 51st day. The splenic dulness, during the same period, again increased in extent.

On the 51st day the small tumour deep in the right iliac fossa was less defined than it had previously been. On the 61st day it could not be distinctly detected. By the 67th day the tongue had again cleaned; the appetite was good; the bowels regular, *i.e.* two solid stools were passed in twenty-four hours; the general powers were improving. She continued in this state—stools solid and appetite good—till the 75th day, when, having suffered from trifling griping pain in the abdomen for two or three hours, she was seized suddenly at a quarter past two P.M., *i.e.* about two hours after she had eaten her dinner, with severe pain in the abdomen; vomited what she had eaten at dinner; then left her bed and passed one copious, pale, nearly solid stool; she experienced no relief from the action of the bowels; on the contrary, the pain was increased in severity, so that she nearly fainted; her hands and feet became cold, and covered with clammy sweat. Being in the hospital at the time, I saw her about ten minutes from the commencement of the pain; the countenance then expressed anxiety, the surface was cool, the hands and feet cold and damp, the pain in the belly had in a great measure subsided; there was no marked fulness, but some slight tenderness of the abdomen. She described the acute pain she had experienced to have been seated chiefly about the umbilicus. Her pulse was extremely rapid and weak. I prescribed tinct. opii mxl., aq. ʒj., st. s., and gave strict orders that she should not be moved in the slightest degree; that *nothing* besides the medicine should be administered.

Twenty minutes to 5 P.M.—Has vomited three times since my last visit; ejecting, apparently, only half digested food; there has been no stool nor urine passed. At the present moment she is lying on her back, shoulders raised by pillows, legs drawn up to abdomen. Expression anxious, worn; tongue moist and nearly clean; abdomen slightly but distinctly tender, not very full; says that she is easier when her knees are drawn up towards her belly; pulse 88, extremely small and weak; surface of trunk warm, hands cold and damp, a little colour on the cheeks.

Pulv. opii, gr. i., 4ta qq. horâ sumend.: Foment. calid. abdom.

Urine to be removed if necessary by catheter. On no consideration is she to be removed from her bed (the necessity of absolute repose was impressed on the patient as well as on the nurse).

10 P.M.—Has had frequent rigors; tenderness of abdomen increased; is lying on right side, legs drawn up towards abdomen; in other respects as last report; pupils large, no drowsiness. About a pint of dark-coloured urine of strong odour just removed by catheter. Pulv. opii, gr. ij., st. s. Pulv. opii, gr. j., 4ta qq. horâ s.

On the following morning, *i.e.* the 76th day, I noted :—

U

Passed a restless night, dozed a little towards morning; her mind is in all respects natural; says that she is sometimes quite free from pain in the abdomen, but that every now and then the pain is very severe; abdomen full, resonant, and *very tender over its whole extent*; no stool, no urine; tongue moist, white, more thickly furred than at last report; feels constant nausea, and has vomited frequently, in all about 1½ pint of green, transparent, mucous-looking matter has been ejected from the stomach; she often retches without throwing up anything. Hands cold, trunk warm, face of good colour, countenance indicative of anxiety and depression. Frequent rigors, *no sense of chilliness*; on the contrary, she complains of feeling hot. Pulv. opii, gr. ij. statim sumend. Pulv.. opii, gr. j., 4ta qq. hora a.

On the next, *i.e.* the 77th day, she was evidently slightly under the influence of the opium. My notes state :—She dozed at intervals during the night and a little this morning; the pupils are small; expression much improved, anxiety almost gone; skin of trunk and extremities warm; no stool; abdomen full, resonant, and *very tender over its whole extent*; no pain in the belly except on pressure; position dorsal, legs drawn up; no return of rigors, no retching since last evening; pulse 120. Pulv. opii, gr. i., 4ta qq. hora a.

On the 78th day she was decidedly better; her abdomen was still full and resonant, but the tenderness was much less—trifling in fact, with the exception of the right iliac fossa. She lay on her back, but the knees were drawn up much less closely to the abdomen than they had previously been. No stool had been passed.

On the 79th day the pulse was only 100; at the same time it was fuller than before. The knees were still elevated, but there was scarcely any tenderness of the abdomen.

On the 80th day erysipelas of the face made its appearance, at first limited to the right side.

On the 81st day she complained of difficulty in deglutition, and the tonsils were red and swollen; there was considerable discharge from the nose. From this date till her death on the 86th day the erysipelas made progress; she became violently delirious; the difficulty of swallowing increased.

On the 85th day the erysipelatous inflammation of the pharynx had extended to the larynx; she spoke in a hoarse whisper, and inspiration was shrill and prolonged.

On the 86th day, about noon, she was seized with convulsions; the arms and legs being rigidly extended, the hands clenched; she frothed at the mouth; the breathing was stertorous, rapid, and occasionally convulsive; the pulse imperceptible. She died at half-past five P.M. Convulsive twitchings of the arms and frothing at the mouth continued till death.

The body of Emma F. was *examined twenty and a half hours after death.*

The peritoneal surface of the small intestines was finely injected; the lower three feet of the ileum were of a slate-grey hue, the colour increasing in depth as the ileo-cæcal valve was approached. There was an adhesion of the peritoneal surface of the jejunum, about eighteen inches from the duodenum to the peritoneum lining the right iliac fossa. Another fold of the jejunum, about two and a half feet from the duodenum, was also adherent to the same portion of the parietal peritoneum. The extent of peritoneum covered by the false membrane constituting the adhesions referred to was about ¾ of an inch; the two adhesions were about the same size; they were readily broken down, and were evidently of recent formation; the colour of the peritoneum around the base of the adhesion was dull red, *shading off into deep grey.*

One of the lower folds of the ileum adhered to the under surface of the meso-cæcum just adjacent to the ileo-cæcal valve. On breaking down this adhesion a soft yellow pulpy mass was exposed,[1] extending from beneath the cæcum between the folds of the mesentery. The long diameter of this pulpy mass was about 2 inches, the short diameter ¾ of an inch. The peritoneum over it was wanting for a space the size of a sixpence; the adherent fold of ileum had blocked up the aperture.

The mucous membrane of the *jejunum* was vivid red from minute injection; its consistence and thickness were normal. The adhesion at the lower part of the ileum was situated immediately adjacent to one of Peyer's patches, on which there was no trace of ulceration. The next patch, descending towards the ileo-cæcal valve, was of a deep grey colour. About eighteen inches above the ileo-cæcal valve was one of Peyer's patches, of a deep grey colour; near its centre was a smooth depressed spot, evidently a healed ulcer; there was no puckering of the tissue around. Every agminated gland from this spot to the ileo-cæcal valve was of a more or less deep grey colour. On each of the three patches immediately above the valve was an ulcer of considerable size, irregular in outline, its floor formed for the most part of submucous tissue; but at places the transverse muscular fibres were distinctly visible; the edges of the ulcers were here and there slightly elevated; at other places they were bevelled off, passing insensibly on to the floor.

The omentum was considerably injected; a little tolerably recent lymph covered the convex surface of the liver; the spleen

---

[1] Microscopical examination proved this mass to be composed chiefly of free fat globules.

was somewhat enlarged ; the peritoneal covering of the uterus and bladder was minutely injected. There was scarcely any fluid in the peritoneal cavity.

The mesenteric glands were enlarged, flabby, and of a deep grey colour. In the mesentery corresponding to the lower part of the ileum were two of the glands, of a purple colour externally, which internally consisted principally of a soft yellow pulpy matter, identical in all particulars with that found between the folds of the meso-cæcum, in the immediate vicinity of the ileo-cæcal valve.

The friends of this young woman resisted all the efforts made to induce them to permit a further examination of the body. In fact, it was only by stratagem that the above imperfect section was performed.

On her admission into the hospital Emma F. was evidently labouring under an attack of typhoid fever. Convalescent on the 34th day; her health improved during the ten subsequent days; she then had a true relapse—*a second attack of typhoid fever.* In about a fortnight she was again convalescent. Symptoms of perforation of the intestine occurred on the 75th day; convalescence from the attack of peritonitis and the commencement of erysipelas on the 80th day.

This case, then, may be divided into four stages :—

1st. That of the primary attack of typhoid fever.
2nd. That of the relapse.
3rd. That of sudden acute peritonitis.
4th. That of erysipelas.

1st. The *primary attack* of typhoid fever.—In this the most peculiar feature was the *very* large volume of the spleen. It was interesting to trace, by palpation and percussion, its gradual diminution in size as the woman advanced in convalescence. Fresh spots ceased to appear after the 27th day of the disease. Hysterical symptoms are not unfrequently observed in females during the early stage of convalescence, *i.e.* while the patient is suffering from extreme general debility.

2nd. *The relapse.*—If a patient, during convalescence from fever, suffers (suppose in consequence of error of diet) from hot skin and quick pulse, that patient is often said to be suffering from a relapse; but Emma F. had, on the 44th day of disease, *i.e.* ten days after convalescence, a return of typhoid fever. Not only was the pulse as frequent as during the primary attack, and the skin as hot, but the diarrhœa returned, *repeated scanty crops of rose spots reappeared, and the spleen again enlarged,* though it did not attain the size it reached during the primary attack. The small tumour felt deep in the right iliac fossa was evidently an enlarged mesenteric gland. Its size, the duration of the illness, and the general symptoms, rendered it probable that the gland was undergoing a process of pseudo-suppuration. The diminution in its size was probably the consequence of absorption of the more fluid portion of its substance, and also of the subsidence of vascular engorgement.

3rd. *Sudden symptoms of peritonitis.*—The sudden severe pain in the abdomen, accompanied by vomiting and symptoms of collapse, rendered it highly probable, from the moment I saw Emma F., at a quarter past two P.M. on the 75th day, that perforation of the ileum had taken place. This opinion was rendered still more probable when, returning to the ward, in less than three hours, I found that, although the patient had scarcely rallied from the collapse—for her hands were yet cold—all the symptoms of incipient peritonitis had supervened; and when, at 10 P.M., I found that rigors had occurred, and had been repeated several times, that the expression continued anxious, and that the symptoms of peritonitis were more marked than they had been at the time of my previous visit, I own I entertained no doubt as to the nature of the case.[1] I acted in accordance with the opinion I had formed, and treated Emma F. with full doses of opium, after the

[1] 'If in the course of a case of typhoid fever, whether severe or trifling, or even in unexpected circumstances, the disease having been up to that moment latent, there should supervene suddenly in a patient labouring under diarrhœa pain in the abdomen, greatly increased by pressure, accompanied by alteration in the features, and more or less quickly by nausea and vomiting, perforation of the small intestine should be diagnosed. The sudden appearance of violent pain in the abdomen, accompanied by change of expression, would be insufficient to make the same diagnosis with absolute certainty : the pain must be increased by pressure. . . . Not only is this increase in the pain (by pressure) necessary, but it is also necessary for the diagnosis to be made with certainty that the pain should extend with more or less rapidity to the whole abdomen.'—Louis's *Recherches sur la Maladie connue sous les Noms de Fièvre Typhoïde,* etc., 2d edit., vol. i. pp. 326, 332.

manner recommended by Dr. Stokes. The tenderness of the abdomen was general, not limited to any one part, so that it was evident the peritonitis was not localised. The tolerance of the opium showed the effect the peritonitis was exercising on the nervous system. On the third day from the outset of the peritonitis the abdomen was full, resonant, and very tender, but on the following day the tenderness had subsided, so far as concerned the abdomen generally, but was still marked in the right iliac fossa, pointing evidently to the spot where the lesion had occurred, on which the peritonitis depended. I was anticipating a successful termination of the case, when—

4th. *The erysipelas*, which terminated the life of the patient, commenced. In this case the erysipelatous inflammation probably extended by continuity of surface from the face to the pharynx, and then to the mucous membrane of the larynx. The erysipelatous inflammation of the pharynx often commences independent of the face, *i.e.* does not become involved by continuity of surface. I have elsewhere shown that the larynx is generally affected secondarily to the pharynx, *i.e.* chronologically considered.

The examination after death showed that I had committed an error in supposing the sudden supervention of the peritonitis to have been due to perforation of the intestine; it was evidently the consequence of the destruction of the peritoneum over a mesenteric gland in a state of pseudosuppuration; the substance primarily deposited in the glands had probably first softened, and then undergone fatty degeneration by a direct metamorphosis of its protein elements. The presence of the lymph on the convex surface of the liver, and the condition of the peritoneum covering the uterus and bladder, proved that the peritonitis had been, as was supposed during life, general; while the situation of the lesion on which the peritonitis depended, and the evidence of the greater intensity of the inflammation in that spot, sufficiently accounted for the continuance of the tenderness in the right iliac fossa after the abdomen generally was almost indolent. I need scarcely point to the grey colour of the mucous and serous membranes as indicating the chronicity of the inflammatory action.

Had this patient eventually recovered I certainly should have considered the case to have been one of peritonitis, the consequence of perforation of the intestine, cured by the free use of opium. The lesion really present was evidently far less likely to prove fatal than that I had diagnosed during life. The opium was doubtless highly beneficial, and to that, and the absolute repose enforced, perhaps it was that the patient did not die of peritonitis. This case is partienlarly interesting as teaching the danger that surrounds the attempt to judge of the value of remedies while our means of diagnosis are imperfect.

CASE XXXIV.—In a girl aged 16 years, the 5th day after the termination of typhus fever—sudden intense pain in the abdomen—collapse—rigors—vomiting—extreme tenderness of abdomen—diarrhœa—death. *After death*—abnormal vascularity of peritoneum—recently effused lymph on the surface of the peritoneum — enlarged spleen — abnormal development of the solitary glands of small and large intestines.

Emma T., aged 16, was admitted, under the care of Dr. Southwood Smith, into the London Fever Hospital at the latter end of February 1849. Her mother, aunt, brothers, and cousins were admitted about the same time—all were suffering from *typhus* fever. Emma was considered to be labouring under the same disease—her bowels were relaxed while she was under treatment in the hospital—she was considered convalescent on the 7th of March—I did not see her till the 12th. At the time I saw her she had just been led from the dinner-table to her bed—she had suffered a little pain in the abdomen all the morning, but while taking her dinner the pain became suddenly more severe, and in consequence, as I happened to be in the ward, the nurse requested me to see the patient. She was then lying on her back —skin cold and damp—her whole appearance indicating extreme collapse—she was quite sensible, and complained of pain in the belly. The abdomen was retracted, hard, and very tender— rigors, frequent vomiting of green fluid, and diarrhœa followed— she passed twelve stools during the night. On the following day her pulse was scarcely to be felt—the surface was cold, and she lay on her back—her whole appearance denoting extreme prostration. She died March the 14th.

The body of Emma Temple was examined March 16th.

There was no marked emaciation; the abdominal parietes were retracted, or they had fallen in; the peritoneum lining the anterior wall of the abdomen was more injected than natural—the small intestines were concealed by the great omentum—the minute vessels of which were abnormally loaded with blood, especially at its inferior or free margin; the anterior-peritoneal surface of the transverse arch of the colon was somewhat more vascular than natural—not so the peritoneal surface of the stomach. On turning up the omentum its posterior surface was found much more minutely injected than its anterior layer. The peritoneum covering the posterior surface of the transverse arch of the colon was vivid red from minute injection.

In the pelvic cavity were about 8 ozs. of turbid yellow serosity—the turbidity being in a great measure caused by minute particles of purulent-looking matter diffused through the fluid; on standing, the serosity let the larger of the particles fall to the bottom of the glass, where they formed a copious sediment.

Several folds of the small intestines lay in the pelvic cavity. The peritoneal surface of these folds was of a bright scarlet colour, the redness was punctiform or. uniform; the latter appearance being caused, apparently, by the juxta-position of puncta.

The folds of the small intestines situate below the umbilicus were evidently much more minutely injected, and much redder than those placed above the umbilicus. The whole of the peritoneum covering the small intestines and the posterior wall of the abdomen was coated by a thin layer of soft yellowish lymph. The quantity of the lymph was greatest at the angle formed by the separation of two adjacent folds of intestines.[1] There was *no enlargement of the mesenteric glands.*

The *small intestines* contained some dark green fluid, and shreds of dark green mucus adhered to the lining membrane; the latter membrane itself was pale—perhaps somewhat thicker than ordinary; its consistence was normal. P_{eyer's} patches were perfectly healthy in colour, thickness, and consistence. The solitary glands throughout the whole of the *ileum* and the lower part of the *jejunum* were enlarged, dull, white, and hard; they felt like little seeds scattered over the lining membrane of the gut. In no instance did they equal small pin-heads in size.

The *cæcum* was healthy in all particulars.

The *solitary glands* of the *colon* were abnormally distinct; from twenty to thirty could be counted on a square inch; they varied in size from a mere point to half a large pin-head. The mucous membrane was pale, and of normal consistence throughout.

---

[1] Redness of the peritoneum limited to these parts is *absolutely* diagnostic of the pre-existence of inflammation of that membrane.

The *gall bladder* was distended with dark-green bile.

The *liver, kidneys, pancreas, larynx, pharynx, stomach,* and *brain* and its membranes presented no appreciable deviation from their normal state.

The *spleen* weighed 7½ ozs.; *i.e.* it was heavier than natural; its size corresponded to its weight.

A small white patch on the anterior surface of the right ventricle was the only deviation from health in *heart* or *pericardium.*

Old adhesions united the right pulmonary and costal pleuræ. Both *lungs* were perfectly healthy in appearance; there was no puckering of their apices, and not the slightest trace of tubercle in either.

The *bronchial glands* were normal in all particulars.

The relatives of Emma T., admitted into the hospital, had well-marked *typhus* fever with *mulberry rush.* Her mother died, and after death her intestines were found in all respects healthy; there was no enlargement of the mesenterio glands, and no disease of Peyer's patches.

When called to see Emma T., it was evident that she was labouring under an attack of peritonitis, and that it had supervened during convalescence from an acute illness accompanied by relaxed bowels; sudden severe pain, compelling the patient to leave the table, and to beg assistance to enable her to reach her bed, accompanied, or immediately succeeded, by symptoms of collapse, and these again quickly followed by oft-repeated rigors, extreme tenderness of the *whole* abdomen, and frequent vomiting of green fluid, constitute that group of symptoms which are said by Louis to be diagnostic of perforation of the intestine.[1] An examination after death of Emma T. proved that the peritonitis was independent of any traumatic cause. It was an example of that rare affection, acute idiopathic peritonitis. My impression is that I have seen at least one other such case, *i.e.* a sudden attack of acute peritonitis with extreme collapse during convalescence from typhus fever, in which, of course, no ulceration of the intestine had occurred. At the present moment I cannot put my hand on the records of the case or cases to which I here refer. The condition of the solitary glands of the small and large intestines was a matter of interest. The appearance of the enlarged glands was equally as distinct

[1] See note, *ante*, p. 309.

from that they present in some cases of typhoid fever as from that they present when the seat of tubercular deposit. The glands seemed really hypertrophied. They did not appear to have been the seat of continued increased abnormal vascular action, for they were neither red nor grey. The girl, I am satisfied, had committed no error in diet; about 3 ozs. of boiled mutton and 8 ozs. of bread were all the food she could have taken in any twenty-four hours after she was convalescent.

The importance of this case, as bearing on the value of the symptoms which are said to indicate the existence of perforation of the intestine, appears to me considerable. In the case of Emma F.—Case XXXIII.—all the symptoms said to denote the occurrence of perforation of the intestine were present; but an examination of the body after death proved those symptoms had, in her case, arisen from a much less serious lesion; in the case of Emma Temple—Case XXXIV.— all the symptoms said to denote the occurrence of perforation of the intestine were also present, but, in her case, an examination of the body after death proved that those symptoms might be present without any traumatic lesion of the peritoneum, i.e. idiopathic inflammation of the peritoneum may supervene during convalescence from typhus fever.

§ 7. NATURE OF TYPHOID FEVER.

What is that deviation from normal structure or function which is essential to the existence of typhoid fever ? Peyer's patches are invariably found diseased after death; but then, as has been previously observed, their lesion may be the result—invariable, indeed, but *still the result*—of some general disease bearing only the same relation to the fever that the small-pox pustule does to the general disease or fever, termed small-pox—the latter is the essential, the primary affection; the former, i.e. the local lesion, an accident.

Now, some (as Cruveilhier) have considered the disease of the agminated glands as the essential or primary affection, and the general phenomena as being secondary to the local lesion.[1] This opinion rests chiefly on two grounds :—

[1] Louis has been incorrectly stated to hold this opinion.

1st. That the lesion is invariably present. To this argument the answer is, the identity in this particular between the small-pox pustule and the intestinal lesion of typhoid fever; and that, as in the former, the invariable sequence, *i.e.* the pustule, is not regarded as a cause; so in the latter the invariable co-existence of the lesion and the general symptoms does not prove that the general symptoms depend on the lesion.

2nd. That the abdominal symptoms are frequently those first developed; that pain in the belly is often the first symptom; and that, if a patient die ever so early in the disease, lesion of the agminated and mesenteric glands is constantly found. But to prove that lesion of function, or of structure of an organ, is even invariably the first of a series of morbid phenomena is by no means to prove that those which follow are the effect of the first.[1] Does the fact that lesion—inflammation?—of Peyer's patches occurs as the first symptom prove that typhoid fever is merely a species or variety of enteritis? Certainly not; for if the occurrence of sore throat anterior to the general symptoms of scarlet fever be not a proof that the general symptoms—including the eruption—of scarlet fever depend on the inflammatory affection of the throat, no more can the general symptoms, including the rose spots, of typhoid fever be considered, *i.e.* necessarily, to be dependent for their origin on the intestinal disease; and this argument has the greater force when we remember that sore throat precedes the general symptoms, rigors included, of scarlet fever *infinitely* more frequently than diarrhœa or abdominal pain precedes the general symptoms of typhoid fever.

It will be observed that I have not here used an argument drawn from analogy, a line of argument which has too often been the bane of medicine, to prove that typhoid fever is a general disease, but have only urged that the same mode of reasoning should be used in considering the relation supposed to exist between the local lesion and the general symptoms of two analogous diseases.

[1] The invariable antecedent of any given event is not necessarily its cause. Invariable antecedent and invariable consequent are not synonymous with cause and effect.

Now, as a positive argument against the view that the general symptoms of typhoid fever are dependent on the intestinal lesion, it may be urged that the former bear *no relation* in severity to the extent of the latter.[1]   The tongue may be moist and almost clean, the mind clear, the general strength comparatively little impaired, as in the case of Jane H. (p. 295) and Peter A. (p. 275), and yet the intestinal lesion be most extensive; or the intestinal lesion may be trifling, and every other organ healthy, so far as the scalpel enables one to determine their condition, and yet the tongue be dry and brown, the delirium constant, the prostration extreme (see the subjoined case of Walter B., p. 317). This want of relation between the local and general symptoms is sometimes observed in scarlet fever. Thus, I have seen a strong man die in scarlet fever when the throat affection was of the most trifling description, and the scalpel laid bare no serious lesions.

What I especially desire to impress on the reader is, that I do *not* argue, that because sore throat precedes the general symptoms of scarlet fever—and yet we allow that the latter are not dependent on the former—*therefore* the general symptoms of typhoid fever are not dependent on the intestinal disease; but what I *do* maintain is, that if the fact that the general symptoms of scarlet fever are preceded by the sore throat, *i.e.* by a local lesion, does not prove that the former depends on the latter, then the simple fact, that the

---

[1] I am quite aware that it has been argued that in some cases of pneumonia there is no relation between the extent of the local lesion and the severity of the general symptoms. There is, however, less force in this argument than might at first appear, and for this reason, that a man who has simply diagnosed the existence of pneumonia, and mapped out its extent, has done but little towards proving what is the disease under which his patient labours. Primary pneumonia must be separated from secondary pneumonia, idiopathic inflammation from that coincident with old-standing disease, as Bright's disease, and *from that set up during the progress of febricula.* In the latter case most severe general symptoms may have preceded the local lesion, and be out of all proportion to it; in the former case, the general symptoms, influenced doubtless by the condition of the blood, may be trifling, so that when cases *like* these are cut out from the list of pure pneumonias, then I suspect there will be found (if similar ages be alone considered, and similar forms of anatomical lesion) a general relation between the extent of the local lesion and the severity of the constitutional symptoms, at least no such discordance as unquestionably exists between the two in scarlet and typhoid fevers.

intestinal lesion precedes the general symptoms of typhoid fever, cannot be regarded as proof that the one depends on the other, that they stand in the relation to each other of cause and effect, and that, *moreover*, as the want of coincidence between the severity of the throat disease and the general symptoms of scarlet fever is held to be the cogent argument in favour of the non-relation of the two, so must the want of coincidence between the intestinal lesion and the general symptoms of typhoid fever be held to be an *equally* cogent argument in favour of the non-relation of those two.   I plead not that what is true of the one disease should be held to be true of the other; but that, in reasoning on the causative value of the chronological relations between the local lesion and the general symptoms, we should adopt the same line of argument in the two diseases.

My own impression is, then, that the intestinal disease bears the same relation to the general symptoms and to the essential deviation from function or structure in typhoid fever, that sore throat does to the general symptoms and to the essential deviation from function or structure in scarlet fever.   In both, the first notice of the poison having entered the system, or of the morbid condition of the blood, the vascular system, or nervous system (whichever it may please the reader to prefer) having been established, is manifested by that organ, which is the most susceptible to the influence of the diseased condition, or to the action of the poison ; that which determines whether headache, or diarrhœa, or sore throat shall be the first symptom, being the variation which exists in the degree of susceptibility of different organs in different individuals.

CASE XXXV.—In a man aged 22 years, after four months' residence in London.   Pain in the abdomen— frontal headache—rose spots—sonorous rale—epistaxis— delirium—dry, brown tongue—slightly relaxed bowels— sudden, intense pain in the abdomen—followed by rigors —chilliness—general abdominal tenderness—death on the 22nd day of disease.   *Twenty-two hours after death*—bronchial mucous membrane injected—extreme vascularity of peritoneum—recent adhesion of folds of ileum—turbid fluid in peritoneal cavity—perforation of ileum—ulceration of Peyer's patches—softening of mucous membrane of cæcum and colon—mesenteric glands enlarged—spleen large—other organs healthy.

Walter B., a strong, well-made man, 5 feet 11 inches in height, and measuring 16 inches across the shoulders, of fair complexion, light hair and eyes, aged 22, a policeman, was admitted into the London Fever Hospital, August 17th, 1850, under the care of Dr. Tweedie. His health, up to the date of the commencement of his present illness, had been very good. He had lived in London four months only, and resided during that time at Rotherhithe station-house. On Saturday, August 10th, he was seized with pain in the abdomen and frontal headache. His bowels were confined till he took an aperient. He left duty Wednesday, August 14th, and took to his bed the day before his admission. At no time since the outset had he had rigors.

A few hours after his admission I made the following notes :—

August 17th, 8th day of disease. No headache ; some vertigo ; mind clear ; expression nearly natural ; slept well last night ; pupils large ; conjunctivæ pale ; bad taste in the mouth ; states that any noise is offensive to him.

He rode this morning in an omnibus from Rotherhithe to King's Cross, and then walked from King's Cross to the hospital.

Tongue moist, large, red at edges, elsewhere covered with thick, dirty-white fur ; no stool to-day ; no appetite ; much thirst ; no fulness, resonance, tenderness, nor gurgling in abdomen. Pulse 84, soft ; trifling cough ; a little sonorous rale generally over the whole chest.

Skin warm and dry. About 100 rose spots on the anterior surface of the abdomen and thorax.

On the next day his tongue was nearly clean ; and although he had taken a teaspoonful of castor oil, his bowels only acted once. There was little alteration for the two following days, except that on both he sweated very freely, and passed two relaxed stools.

On the 23d of August, i.e. 14th day of disease, I noted :—

Pulse 96, soft ; *muscular movements* very tremulous ; sweated freely yesterday afternoon ; no miliary vesicles ; several fresh rose spots ; tongue moist, furred, white, *very tremulous* ; two relaxed stools ; gurgling in the right iliac fossa ; no tenderness, abnormal fulness, nor resonance of abdomen.

Although the muscular movements were very tremulous on the 24th of August, yet he sat up in bed, when bid, with facility. He continued to sweat occasionally. The pulse continued 96. In the evening he lost about 8 ozs. of blood from the nose, and subsequently became delirious.

On the 25th of August, the 16th day of disease, the delirium continued, the muscular tremor had increased, and his tongue was dry in the centre. He had no stool. On the following day I noted as follows, 17th day of disease :—

Pulse 96, soft ; face flushed ; tongue dry, brown, and very tremulous ; abdomen moderately full only ; no abnormal resonance, no gurgling ; characters of rose spots unequivocal ; position dorsal, legs freely extended ; slept better than the preceding night, but was delirious when awake ; did not attempt to quit his bed.

On the 18th day he continued in much the same state. He passed one stool only.

On the 29th of August, the 20th day of disease, his pulse was 120, weak ; he was reported to have slept much night and day, but was readily aroused ; had passed one relaxed stool.

On 30th of August, 21st day of disease, the following note was made :—

Pulse 108 ; mind confused, no idea how long he has been in the hospital ; conjunctivæ pale, pupils large ; general muscular tremor so great that he articulates imperfectly and with difficulty ; position dorsal, legs fully extended ; cheeks flushed ; tongue dry, brown, and fissured ; has passed two watery stools the last twenty-four hours. No fulness, abnormal resonance, nor tenderness of abdomen ; no gurgling ; skin hot, damp ; no miliary vesicles ; rose spots numerous and well marked ; some redness of the cutis covering the sacrum.

He lay quietly and appeared quite easy from the time of my visit until 11 P.M., when the nurse left him asleep. About half-past one A.M., the night-nurse reported, that he awoke complaining of violent pain at the lower part of the abdomen. She reported, that ' he cried dreadfully, and said the pain was so violent he did not know what he should do.' He then complained of sense of cold ; he shivered, and his skin felt considerably below the natural temperature to the nurse. He was at the same time covered with ' a cold sweat.' A blanket was placed on the bed, a hot bottle to the feet, and the abdomen fomented with hot water. From these he appeared to experience relief, and fell asleep about 5 A.M. At 7 A.M. he awoke ; and then complained of pain, and there was great tenderness of the abdomen. Hyd. chlorid. gr. j., pulv. opii, gr. ¼ in pill was given at 10 A.M., and repeated at noon. From 2 till 4 P.M. he slept quietly ; on waking, he left his bed to dress himself, fancying it was morning.

At 5 P.M. I saw him, and noted as follows :—

Pulse rapid and feeble ; was awake when I entered the ward,

ten minutes since—is now dozing, talking a little in his sleep; lies constantly on his back, with his legs fully extended; expression rather worn; face pale, conjunctivæ pale, pupils natural; tongue dry, covered with a thin, rough, yellowish fur, fissured, red at the tip and edges. He passed two stools while in much pain, early in the morning, and one about 10 o'clock; the last was liquid, consistence of the others not ascertained; no nausea; no vomiting; abdomen hard, parietes retracted, decidedly tender over its whole extent; tenderness greatest in the hypogastric region; a blister has formed spontaneously on the spine of the right ileum. Complains of pain in the abdomen when he coughs, but not as he lies quietly. No sense of chilliness; surface generally of normal temperature; hands rather livid and cool. Many well-marked rose spots on abdomen and thorax.

℞ Tinct. opii, ♏xx.; aqua ʒss.; M. ft. s.; pulv. opii, gr. j. 4tis q. hora s.

He died at 2 P.M., August 31st, i.e. the 22nd day of disease. I did not see him after making the foregoing notes. But from the nurse, an intelligent woman, I received the subjoined report. He slept from 7 P.M. till 10 P.M.; and during the night, at intervals, for half an hour; to-day he has dozed frequently, but not more than five minutes at one time. Although, to the very last, he answered questions rationally, yet every now and then his mind wandered. He never complained of pain in the belly, except once slightly this morning, just after drinking a little warm tea. He lay constantly till he died in the position in which I saw him, i.e. dorsal, with legs extended. His hands continued as yesterday, livid and cool and clammy, and to-day his face was rather purple. There was no return of the rigors, and he did not complain of feeling cold. But when, on one occasion, the nurse's hand touched him, he said, 'How cold your hand is.' Really it was not so. The nurse did not observe his belly to be swollen when she changed the poultices, application of which appeared to afford him satisfaction.

The body of Walter B. was examined twenty-two hours after death; the weather moderately warm. The following notes were made:—

Cadaveric rigidity strongly marked; moderate congestion of the posterior surface; abdomen full and resonant; very little fat on the abdominal or thoracic parietes; *brain* and *meninges* in every respect normal; a small non-adherent, colourless clot in the superior longitudinal sinus; arachnoid transparent; no abnormal vascularity of pia mater; rather more transparent colourless serosity beneath the arachnoid than usual, but not enough to raise that membrane from the gyri—the latter are rather narrow, and the anfractuosities rather broad; about half an ounce of colourless transparent serosity in the lateral ventricles, and as much at the base; the colour and consistence of the brain substance natural.

The *larynx, pharynx,* and *œsophagus* were not examined (the friends objected to the body being disfigured).

Pericardium contains very little fluid.

A firm yellow clot filled the right auricle and ventricle; a smaller one lay in the left cavities. The substance of the *heart* firm, healthy in appearance; valves normal.

No adhesions; no fluid in either *pleura. Lungs* models of health; pale and crepitant.

Bronchial Tubes.—Lining membrane considerably injected with blood. Opened to third divisions. *Bronchial glands* not visible.

Peritoneal Cavity.—External surface of stomach abnormally injected. Great omentum highly vascular, bright scarlet, especially its lower portion or free edge, and part adjacent, which latter are also covered with pulpy yellow lympho-purulent matter. About 13 ozs. of dark turbid dirty-looking fluid, with shreds of lymph in it, removed from the peritoneal cavity. Penetrating the coats of the ileum, about three inches above the ileo-cæcal valve, and through that portion of the intestine opposite to the mesentery, is an aperture about the size of a small pin-head; turbid, gruelly-looking fluid can be pressed from the intestinal canal through the opening referred to. Some soft lymph coats the peritoneal covering of the intestine, here and there in the vicinity of the aperture, but there are no adhesions around or adjoining it. Just above it, however, are three folds of the ileum, adherent to each other. These adhesions are readily broken down. There is no second perforation. [When the abdomen was opened, the portion of the intestine in which the aperture was found lay in the pelvic cavity.] The peritoneum covering the lower part of the ileum is either deep red or vivid scarlet. The redness, to the unassisted eye, is uniform at places, but even there a lens shows it to be really capillary. The vessels of the peritoneal surface of the bladder, and of the anterior wall of the abdomen, are finely injected with blood. The under surface of the great omentum is decidedly more vascular than the anterior surface.

Stomach moderately rugose. The mucous membrane is pale, excepting that of the fundus, which is of a deep yellowish-green colour; it is mammillated from the fundus to two inches from the pylorus. The consistence of the mucous membrane is good. Strips from ½ inch to ⅔ of an inch obtainable.

Duodenum.—Mucous membrane deep yellow; otherwise healthy.

Jejunum and Ileum.—The mucous membrane of the jejunum and upper part of ileum pale, of normal thickness and consistence. About forty-two inches above the ileo-cæcal valve, on one of Peyer's patches, are two ulcers one-fifth of an inch in diameter; their edges dull red; their floor, composed of the submucous tissue, pale, or faintly streaked with red. The whole patch is slightly thickened and opaque; there is no deposit in the submucous tissue of the gland. On the next patch, descending to the ileo-cæcal valve, is a pale, opaque, thickened spot, $\frac{1}{4}$ inch in diameter; then follow three patches, on each of which is an ulcer one-fifth of an inch in diameter, with deep red edges. Then comes the patch next save one to the ileo-cæcal valve, through which the perforation had occurred. On this large patch, which is over its whole extent somewhat thicker than usual, but offers no deposit in any part of its substance, are five small ulcers, their floors formed by transverse muscular fibre; the whole patch is rather redder than the surrounding membrane. The perforation has taken place through the centre of an ulcer seated on the centre of this Peyer's patch; the edges of the aperture are bounded by a few shreds of sloughy-looking yellowish-white substance. The ulcer through which the perforation has occurred is $\frac{1}{2}$ an inch in length and a $\frac{1}{4}$ of an inch in breadth; its floor is formed of transverse muscular fibres of a deep red colour; the perforation is as near as may be in the centre of this ulcer. The Peyer's patch immediately above the ileo-cæcal valve is thickened as in others, from the swollen state of the mucous and submucous coats, and not from any deposit in the latter. On it are three or four ulcers, neither exceeding one-fifth of an inch in diameter; their floors are formed of submucous cellular tissue. The lower six inches of the ileum are somewhat more injected than usual, the redness being capillary.

Cæcum and *Colon.*—Mucous membrane generally extremely soft, no strips obtainable; no ulceration; no enlargement of the solitary glands.

Mesenteric glands—corresponding to the whole length of the intestine—slightly enlarged; about the size of peas and beans, but flat; they are flabby and purple.

Pancreas pale and healthy.

Liver healthy in colour; flabby. *Gall bladder* moderately distended with thin yellow bile.

Spleen large, dark, soft, flabby.

Kidneys.—Capsules separate readily; healthy in all respects.

Urinary Bladder.—Mucous membrane pale; healthy.

Early in the morning of the 21st day, perforation of the ileum took place; in thirty-seven hours the man was dead. The symptoms were sufficiently well marked for the diagnosis to be made, and the prognosis given with confidence. This man, like John P., lay on his back, with his legs fully extended, although his peritoneum was intensely inflamed. Nor were the man's senses blunted to an extent sufficient to account for the slight pain he suffered.. He enjoyed the taste of the tea he drank on the morning of his death, telling the nurse that it was better than ordinary—a fact, as it was distinct from that of the other patients and stronger than usual. It is worthy of remark, that Walter B. walked on the 8th day of disease from King's Cross to the Liverpool Road, Islington, a distance of a mile—a most fatiguing walk, as he had to ascend the long and steep Pentonville hill. I never saw the same degree of muscular power in a severe case of typhus fever at the commencement of the second week. By the 16th day he was very delirious night and day; his tongue was dry and brown, and the prostration was extreme; yet, when he d'ed a week after, i.e. on the 22nd day of disease, the amount of intestinal or mesenteric disease was really trifling when compared with that present in Jane H. (Case XXXII.) or Peter A. (Case XXVI.). The ulcers were very small, quite insignificant, with the exception of the one through which the perforation occurred, and that would have been harmless but for its depth at one little spot.

Excepting the intestinal canal, mesenteric glands, and peritoneum, every organ was healthy. The peritonitis was of course set up subsequently to the occurrence of delirium, brown tongue, and prostration.

As to the softened state of the mucous membrane of the large intestine, I am inclined to consider that, in the case of Walter B., it was in a great measure cadaveric. The colour of the softened membrane was neither red nor grey, nor had it that granular appearance comparable to a mixture of flour and cold water, which characterises mucous membranes softened from inflammation. It is interesting to observe, that the delirium, etc., set in directly after he lost 8 ozs. of blood from the nose. Blood-letting is never required in fever because delirium occurs, however violent that may be. The large proportion of fibrine in, and the firmness of the clot found in the heart after death, was probably to be explained by the presence of the peritonitis. The spleen was enlarged.

§ 8. PREGNANCY—AGE—DURATION OF DISEASE.

Pregnancy.

Rokitansky says, ' Pregnancy offers an almost entire immunity from typhoid fever.' My experience is by no means in accordance with that of the celebrated Vienna pathological anatomist's, and I know others have repeatedly met with examples of women large with child suffering from typhoid fever. Pregnancy is a very serious complication. A *very* large proportion, I will not say all, of such cases die. Last winter (1849-50) I exhibited to the members of the Pathological Society the intestines of a woman who died on about the 12th day of typhoid fever. She was seven months gone with child.

Age.

When speaking of the influence of age on the prognosis in typhus fever, I stated that the mortality from that disease between the ages of 6 and 15 years was exceedingly small; this is far from true with respect to the mortality from typhoid fever; for about 25 per cent. of those suffering from the latter, whose ages lie between 6 and 15 years inclusive, die.

Of nearly 400 individuals suffering from typhoid fever received into the London Fever Hospital, three only have been more than 50 years of age; the ages of these three individuals were respectively 51, 55, and 55 years. Two of them were women, one a man. A brief account of the latter case is given below (Case xxxvi.) The fact that typhoid fever is very rarely observed after the age of 50, has been confirmed by every observer of the disease.

My impression is, that the rose spots of typhoid fever are more frequently absent from patients more than 30 years old than from those of less mature age. I should say they were rarely absent in young persons. This is, however, the reader must remember, merely a general impression. I have in an earlier part of this essay proved the reverse to be true with reference to typhus fever.

Case XXXVI.—John A., aged 55, a labourer, was admitted into the London Fever Hospital, June 1850, under the care of Dr. Southwood Smith. John A. was said to have been taken ill about ten days before his entrance into the hospital. He had been delirious for three days before he came under observation. His illness began with loss of appetite, pain in the abdomen, and diarrhœa; he had from five to six stools daily before entering the hospital. On admission all delirium had ceased; the expression of his countenance was natural; his tongue was dry, red, furred in the centre, and fissured; abdomen full and soft; his pulse was 84; sonorous rale was heard over the whole chest; the skin was cool; several rose spots were noted on the abdomen, and a few on the back. On the following day his mind was observed to be confused. He was convalescent by the 1st of July.

For these particulars of the case I am indebted to Mr. Birkett, M.B., Lond. I saw the man repeatedly, but did not take any notes of his case. The rose spots were exceedingly well marked; fresh spots appeared every few days. In themselves, when well marked in character and course, they are absolutely diagnostic of typhoid fever; but when conjoined, as in this case, with the delirium, followed by slight mental confusion, red and dry tongue, and diarrhœa, the most sceptical must admit the patient offering such a combination of symptoms to be labouring under typhoid fever.

CASE XXXVII.—Without known cause in a child aged 11 years.—Headache — delirium — weakness—vertigo — loss of sleep—flushing of cheeks—anorexia—diarrhœa—furred tongue—fulness, resonance, and slight tenderness of abdomen—a few rose spots—muscular tremors—general and physical signs of bronchitis and pneumonia—death on about the 30th day of disease. *Examination of the body about thirty-eight hours after death.*—Marked cadaveric rigidity—slight excess of serosity beneath arachnoid—some serosity beneath mucous membrane of arytæno-epiglottidean folds—ulceration of Peyer's patches in the last fourteen inches of the small intestines—slight enlargement of the mesenteric glands—spleen rather large—double lobular consolidation of lung—lymph on pleuræ.

Ellen H., aged 11 years, an inmate of the School of Discipline, was admitted into the London Fever Hospital, under the care of Dr. Tweedie, December 14th, 1847; a moderately stout, fair child, said to have had fever and small-pox three years before she came under observation; had enjoyed health for two and a half years.

Without having been exposed to contagion or other known exciting cause, E. H. was attacked with headache; gradually she grew decidedly ill, so that she took to her bed one week before admission into the hospital. Delirium was reported to have commenced on about the 11th day of her illness, i.e. 11th December. No further history could be obtained.

On the 15th day of disease the following notes were made:—Has slept but little since admission (i.e. twenty hours). General headache; vertigo; was very delirious and restless during the night, leaving her bed several times without purpose; memory defective; does not know how long she has been in the hospital; strabismus (natural); slight impediment in speech (natural); no flush; expression natural; no injection of conjunctivæ; she quits her bed (*i.e.* when not delirious) unassisted, but with some difficulty.

Tongue moist, furred, pale, large; much thirst; no appetite; swallows with ease; no stool (the bowels acted yesterday before admission); abdomen full, resonant; no tenderness of belly; no gurgling in iliac fossæ; pulse 120, weak; cough rather troublesome; no expectoration; sonorous rale over both sides of the chest, mixed with some mucous rale. The mucous rale is very abundant at the base posteriorly of both lungs; and, in that situation, the mucous rale is mixed with fine crepitation. The skin is hot and dry; there are two imperfectly marked rose spots on the abdomen.—A saline mixture every six hours.

On the following day the headache was more severe, and limited to the forehead. She had slept but little, and that little had been disturbed. A fresh rose spot had made its appearance; the vertigo had increased, and the child was unable to stand without assistance. The stools—three in number—were watery. The left cheek was flushed. Abundant sonorous and mucous rales were heard over the whole chest. The mucous rale was mixed with much fine crepitation from the extreme base of the right lung to a little above the inferior angle of the scapula. There was some want of resonance in the same situation. During the succeeding night she left her bed frequently; her mind at the time evidently wandering; she had but little sleep.

From this time, till her death, on about the 30th day of disease, her pulse varied from 120 to 130. On the 22nd day it was too feeble to count, and continued so the two following days; but, on the 25th, it was again perceptible—120; the 26th day it was 130; the 27th 120; and from that time, till her death, was too weak to be counted.

The delirium continued from the day of her admission till that of her death—its character unchanged. Thus, the day before her death, she was noisy, screamed violently, and, even on the day of her death, attempted to leave her bed. The want of sleep was marked even so late as the 27th day, at which time it was noted that she did not sleep more than five minutes at one time. On the 28th day somnolence commenced, and continued till her death, except when interrupted by delirium.

The spots, never very perfect in their character, continued to make their appearance till the 25th day.

The tongue moist, furred posteriorly, dirty white, large, and its mucous membrane, as seen at the edges, pale, on admission, was moist and nearly clean on the 25th and 26th days; very tremulous on the 27th; dry and slightly furred on the 28th; and, finally, dry and brown the last two days of life.

The stools, of which two or three were passed daily, were

watery. On the 22nd one was passed into the bed : and after the 26th, all the fæces and urine were passed unconsciously into the bed. The abdomen, from the first, was full and resonant. At no time was there any marked tenderess or gurgling. Prostration increased on the 27th; the muscular movements were very unsteady, and she was evidently much weaker than before. On the 28th, she lay on her back with her knees drawn up, and with a marked expression of prostration. A circumscribed pink flush was occasionally observed on the cheeks, one or both. The cough continued throughout. The re iration was counted on the 25th and 28th days only; it was the 36 in the minute. The abnormal physical signs became daily more marked and extensive, so that, on the 24th, mucous rale, mingled with fine crepitation, was audible over the whole right side of the chest; and there was some want of resonance, on percussion, over the same extent; the left side presented similar physical signs. On the 28th, the heart's sounds were inaudible, from the loud and abundant mucous rale emanating from the portion of lung overlapping that organ.

The chest was not examined the last two days of life.

No miliary vesicles were observed at any time.

She sank gradually, the breathing becoming more rapid and noisy, and the drowsiness more profound, and died at half-past seven P.M. on (about) the 30th day of disease.

The body of Helen H. was exar ned about thirty-eight hours after death; the weather was intensely cold and dry. The following notes were taken :—

Cadaveric rigidity well marked. No distension of abdomen.

Head.—Some colourless serosity beneath arachnoid—no marked injection of pia mater—most depending veins very full—arachnoid and pia mater removeable from surface of brain with tolerable facility—red points on cut surface of white matter rather numerous —substance of brain, including fornix and septum lucidum, normally firm—grey substance rather dark—very little serosity in the lateral ventricles—vessels of plexus choroides moderately filled with blood—base of the brain healthy in all particulars —cerebellum normal—about ½ oz. of serosity colourless and transparent in the cavity of the arachnoid at the base of the brain. Specific gravity of the white matter, 1·042; of the grey matter, 1·032.

Pericardium healthy; contains a little transparent yellow serosity. Much dark grumous and fluid blood escapes on dividing the large veins at the base of the heart.

Heart healthy; a large, firm, smooth, yellow clot in right auricle and ventricle.

Epiglottis and arytæno-epiglottidean folds thickened from effusion of serosity beneath the mucous membrane.

Larynx.—Mucous membrane pale and healthy in aspect; no fluid in either pleura.

Left Lung.—Weight, 9 ozs. The pleura covering the inferior lobe is thickened, dark red, and readily separable from the pulmonary tissue. A few old adhesions unite the lung to the costal pleura; a little recent yellowish lymph fringes the base of the lower lobe. The lung is pale anteriorly; dark pinkish violet posteriorly—the latter hue gradually passing into the former. The inferior three-fourths of the *superior lobe* are emphysematous; the line separating the emphysematous from the non-emphysematous portion is irregular but well defined. The anterior inferior edge of the same lobe feels solid and knotty; it is very pale. On section, this solid portion is found riddled with small cavities. The greater number of these cavities contain purulent-looking fluid; their internal wall is smooth and pale; the thin layer of tissue separating them from each other, pale, tough, non-aërated. The largest of the cavities would contain a swan-shot, the smallest a small pin-head. The posterior part of the lobe is dull red, tough, crepitant, and infiltrated with bloody serosity.

The *inferior lobe* is pale and crepitant for one-third of its extent, reckoning from the anterior margin; posterior to that it is dull red, contains but little air, and that only at places. Its surface has a mottled aspect; the darker and lighter portions at some places being separated by distinct lines, at others passing gradually the one into the other. The paler portions are of a dull yellowish hue, friable, readily break down on pressure, and are non-crepitant, sinking in water. A few points only can be cut from the darker portions, which sink in water; the remainder, however, contain less air than natural. At the extreme base of the inferior lobe is a considerable portion of the pale tough tissue riddled with cavities, as in the anterior inferior angle of the superior lobe. A small bronchial tube is traceable into one of these cavities, but the majority have no outlet.

Right Lung.—Weight, 11¼ ozs. The pulmonary pleura is thickened, and of a dull red colour. Recent lymph unites the superior, middle, and inferior lobes to each other.

The *superior lobe* is riddled with small cavities, and closely resembles the anterior inferior portion of the left superior lobe. The inferior lobe feels solid; its section is dusky red, speckled with pale yellowish solid spots, varying in size from a pin-head to a ¼ of an inch in diameter; these spots are irregular in shape, and here and there two or more run into each other. The dull yellowish hue of these pale spots varies in intensity. When the red portion between them is examined with a lens, it is found to be finely speckled with minute yellow points—sanded as it were.

Tongue moist, rather brown.

Pharynx and œsophagus pale and normal in all particulars.

Stomach moderately contracted; rugose; the mucous membrane somewhat thickened, pale, and of natural consistence.

Small intestines.—About fourteen inches above the ileo-cæcal valve, on one of Peyer's patches, is an ulcer 3 lines in diameter, its floor formed of longitudinal muscular fibres, its edges somewhat elevated, and of a deep grey colour; that portion of the patch unoccupied by the ulcer is slightly thickened, its mucous membrane retains its normal consistence. Several ulcers resembling the last described, excepting that their floors are formed of transverse muscular fibres, are situated on the patches between the above and the ileo-cæcal valve. The mucous membrane around the ulcers is in every case of a grey colour, and that covering the patches generally softer than natural, and somewhat thickened. The mucous membrane between the patches is dusky red from minute capillary injection; it is also softer than the mucous membrane a little higher up. The remainder of the small intestines is healthy in colour and consistence. There is no enlargement of the solitary glands.

Large intestines healthy in all particulars.

Mesenteric glands slightly enlarged.

Liver.—Weight 21 ozs.; healthy.

Gall bladder moderately distended with pale orange-coloured bile; its lining membrane healthy.

Spleen.—Weight 4 ozs.; dark and firm.

Pancreas healthy in appearance.

Kidneys healthy.

The urinary bladder was not examined.

This case illustrates the fact, that typhoid fever may prove fatal to a child. I have already adverted to the frequency with which that disease cuts off the young who are attacked by it.

The mode of access of the fever was that very common, *i.e.* it was gradual: so that no day could absolutely be fixed as that on which the illness commenced. No source of contagion was traced. Some doubt might have been entertained on the child's admission as to the nature of the disease under which she was labouring. There was general headache, want of sleep, delirium, confined bowels, strabismus, and impediment of speech, but then the history showed the two latter to be natural to the child, and the presence of the rose spots, conjoined with the full and resonant abdomen, and the presence of the bronchitis and pneumonic rales, removed all doubt as to the nature of the primary affection. Still the question remained, had meningitis been set up as a complication? Headache conjoined with delirium rendered it highly probable that there was morbid vascular action going on within the cranium. Still, remembering the extreme infrequency of meningitis as a local complication in fever, and the constancy with which headache occurs, I felt inclined to believe that the vascular cerebral mischief was not very grave in character. The disappearance of the headache shortly after the child's admission, and the absence of any sign of cerebral disease after death, proved the truth of the opinion first formed.

A large pale tongue is not very common in typhoid fever. The characters present in Cases XXIII., XXX., XXXI., XXXV. are those ordinarily, but not, as some have maintained, invariably, observed in this affection. But the point to which I desire especially to call attention in this case is the condition of the lungs and pleura. The frequency with which local inflammations occur in typhoid fever is most remarkable. *Pleuritis and pneumonia are both of very common occurrence.* The pneumonia is usually double, set up in numerous points of the organs at the same time, commencing from so many separate centres. In such cases, the blastema effused is capable of evolution only into a fluid, and granular corpuscles,—that first formed is the first to soften. The diffusion of the granular corpuscles in the fluid portion gives rise to the purulent-looking matter (pseudo-pus); the still solid blastema to the yellowish friable masses; the hyperæmia which precedes the effusion of the blastema to the deep red patches. In fact, these little cavities are merely minute disseminated abscesses—the consequence of *l'état purulent* of Tessier—that condition being one frequent in, and subsequent to, typhoid and other continued fevers.

I may point out that in this case the mesenteric glands were less seriously affected than usual, and that the ulceration of the mucous membranes was limited to that covering Peyer's patches, the mucous membrane of the large intestines, the pharynx, œsophagus, stomach, and larynx, having entirely escaped. I have before pointed out the frequency with which the mucous membranes of these viscera are affected in conjunction with that of the small intestine.

Duration.

When treating of the duration of typhus fever, I stated that, with reference to acute specific diseases attended by an eruption on the skin, 'so long as the eruption continues, the disease of which it is the diagnostic character exists.' This is as true of typhoid fever as of the other diseases of the class; but then the eruption in typhoid fever may be absent, and when present it is often fugitive. In determining the duration of this affection, then, I have considered it essential to answer the following questions :—

1st. .What is the latest period of the disease at which fresh rose spots make their appearance ?

2nd. What is the latest period of the disease at which a patient may die, and yet no local lesion of sufficient importance to account for death be found ?

3rd. What is the earliest period at which commencing reparation of that lesion, which is the anatomical character of the disease, has been observed ?

In answer to the first question, I may observe, that I have never seen (excepting in case of a relapse) fresh spots make their appearance after the 30th day of disease. Louis states (vol. ii. p. 97, of his great work on typhoid fever), that in *one* case he observed rose spots for the first time on the 35th day of disease; but, on turning to the case to which this statement applies, *i.e.* the fourteenth, it would appear that some error has crept into his calculations, for the subject of that case was admitted into the hospital on the 14th of April. On admission, he stated that he had been ill one week, but on inquiry he was proved to have suffered, more or less, for a fortnight; so that his illness commenced really on the 1st of April. Louis observed rose spots on the 1st of May, *i.e.* at the latest, on the 31st day of disease.

In answer to the second question, my own researches have not made me acquainted with a case fatal after the 30th day in which a lesion of sufficient magnitude to account for death was not detected. Louis details nine cases fatal after the 30th day of the disease. The following is a summary of the structural changes in those nine cases.

In the 1st case.—Suppuration of the mesenteric glands;

evidence of extensive inflammation of the general mucous membrane of the small and larger intestines.   Extensive ulceration of Peyer's patches.

In the 2nd case.—Disseminated abscesses in the lungs. Collections of purulent-looking fluid in the pelves of the kidneys; parotid abscess.

In the 3rd case.—Extensive destruction of the tissues of the left lower extremity from erysipelas.   Evidence of recent pleuro-pneumonia.

In the 4th case.—Extensive cervical abscess.   Multiple abscesses in the liver.   Lymph on and beneath the arachnoid.

In the 5th case.—Extensive solidification of the lungs.

In the 6th case.—Erysipelas of the left leg.   Jaundice; and non-granular consolidation of the lung.

In the 7th case.—Diphtheritic inflammation of the fauces. Lobar granular consolidation of the inferior lobe of the right lung.

In the 8th case.—Perforation of the ileum, and evidence of recent peritonitis.

In the 9th case.—Perforation of the ileum, and evidence of recent peritonitis.

With reference to the third question, I have never seen marked attempts at reparation of the ulcers in the ileum before the 30th day.   Chomel in his *Leçons Clinique Médicale* refers to nineteen cases fatal before the 30th day in which Peyer's patches were ulcerated.   In one only of those nineteen cases was there any attempt at reparation of the loss of substance caused by the ulceration.   He refers to two cases fatal on the 30th day; in one of the two there was commencing cicatrisation; and to fifteen cases fatal *after* the 30th day, in twelve of which the ulcers in the intestine had commenced to cicatrise.

These facts, viz., 1st, that unless in case of relapse, fresh rose spots do not appear after the 30th day; 2nd, that if death occurs after that date, organic lesion sufficient to account for death always exists; and 3rd, that any attempt at reparation of the intestinal ulcerations is, to say the least,[1]

[1] 'To say the least,' for it must be borne in mind that it is often very difficult to fix the exact date of illness in typhoid fever.

of very infrequent occurrence before the 30th day, while, in a large proportion of the cases cut off by intercurrent local disease after the 30th day, the intestinal ulcers are found partially or completely cicatrised ;—these three facts, I say, tend to fix the duration of typhoid fever at about 30 days. That in many mild cases it terminates much earlier little doubt can be entertained, but at the same time,the patient ought never to be considered convalescent till after the termination of the fourth week of disease. Let the reader just reflect that if it were not for the presence of the characteristic pustule many persons labouring under small-pox might consider themselves well after the primary febrile disturbance had run its course. A scanty eruption of small-pox pustules appears, and then, but for its presence, the patients would consider themselves in health. The following case illustrates the fact that all the general symptoms may disappear, and yet typhoid fever be far from its termination.

CASE XXXVIII.—In a man aged 40 years—headache—pains in limbs—rigors—nausea—diarrhœa—violent delirium—loss of sleep—followed by somnolence—eruption of rose spots—absence of delirium—moist, slightly-furred tongue—enlarged spleen—watery stools—reduplicate pulse, varying in frequency from 72 to 96—marked emaciation—restoration to health during the fourth week.

Thomas T., aged 40, a labourer of temperate habits, ten years resident in London, was admitted into the London Fever Hospital, under the care of Dr. Tweedie, Tuesday, November 28th, 1848. He was a tall, thin man, with a dark skin. He appeared to have been taken ill about a week before he came under observation. During that week he had suffered from headache, pains in the limbs, rigors, nausea, and diarrhœa, the latter preceding the use of medicine. On Sunday, November 26th, he became delirious, and the whole of the day before his entrance into the hospital was very violent. On first entering the ward he was with difficulty undressed and put to bed.

He was seen by me on the 29th of November. The nurse then stated that he had slept from 7 A.M. till 8 A.M., but with the exception of that one hour had not closed his eyes since his admission. During the night he was very delirious, getting out of bed every few minutes. At the time of my visit, 2 P.M., his mind was wandering, and he was unable to answer a single question rationally.

He said he had no headache; his head was cool, his face pale; there was no heaviness of expression; no abnormal injection of the conjunctivæ; his pupils were rather small and equal. He was able to leave his bed unassisted with facility; muscular movements were performed without tremor.

The tongue was rather dry, but nearly clean; he had passed two watery stools during the preceding twenty-four hours; there was no abnormal fulness nor resonance of the abdomen, no tenderness nor gurgling, no vomiting; his pulse was only 72, but rather weak; no cough; the heart's sounds and impulse, as well as the breath sound, were natural; the skin was cool and dry; three imperfectly marked rose spots were observed on the back, chest, and abdomen, i.e. one on each.

Soon after I left the ward he fell asleep, and continued dozing, with little intermission, till the following morning. When I then saw him the delirium had entirely disappeared; his mind seemed in all respects normal; he had passed no stool; about twelve rose spots had appeared on the abdomen. On the 1st of December about twenty fresh rose spots showed themselves on the abdomen and thorax, and as many as forty on the back; he had passed two watery stools. There was no delirium, but he thought that he had been in the hospital a fortnight, and that three days had elapsed since he saw me last, instead of, as was really the case, twenty-four hours. His pulse, which on November 30th was 84 and reduplicate—a character it retained so long as he was under observation—rose on December 1st to 96. On the 2nd the rose spots noted on the 30th were much paler, and from thirty to forty fresh ones had made their appearance; his tongue was moist and rather white; he had passed three watery stools; his appetite was returning; the splenic dulness was extensive; he had slept well, and was perfectly rational; he remembered having seen me on the previous day. On the 4th I noted that some of the rose spots marked on the 1st had disappeared; that the others were paler. On the 6th he passed four watery stools. On the 7th December I wrote as follows :—

'Pulse 96; he sits up in bed unassisted, with facility; skin warm; cheeks slightly flushed; tongue moist, somewhat tremulous; no stools. Of the rose spots previously marked two or three only remain; many fresh spots have appeared.'

On the 8th his pulse had fallen to 78; but on the 9th December it had risen again to 96; two or three fresh rose spots were observed, and he passed two watery stools; he had four similar stools on the 10th.

No note was made after 11th December, when his pulse was 96; his appetite good; his bowels had acted once only for twenty-four hours. At the same time I observed that he appeared to have emaciated considerably since his admission. In ten days or a fortnight he left the hospital well.

As I have previously remarked, it is by no means uncommon in small-pox for the severe general symptoms—delirium, etc.—to cease suddenly on the eruption appearing. How far the consentaneous cessation of the delirium and appearance of the eruption in Thomas T. was more than a coincidence may be doubted. I am disposed, however, myself to regard it as something more.

The reader will remember that a similar fact, i.e. the consentaneous appearance of rose spots and cessation of violent delirium was observed in a previous case. Had it not been for the daily eruption of fresh rose spots Thomas T. might have been considered convalescent on the 2nd of December. The specific disease did not cease, however, for at least a week after that date. If the reader will refer to the case of James S. (Case XXVIII.) he will observe that that man might have been supposed to be convalescent at the early part of the second week if reference had been had to the condition of the cerebral functions, the tongue, the physical abdominal signs, or the pulse only—the latter was 72 on about the 8th day of disease; but the presence of rose spots made it certain that the disease had not terminated; and very soon the hemorrhage from the bowels proved that although the febrile symptoms, commonly so called, had ceased, yet the intestinal disease, like the skin eruption, continued to make progress. The disease, the fever properly so called, had not then run its course, although the pulse was only 72, and the mind, in all particulars, was in its normal state.

CASE XXXIX.—In a man aged 17 years—gradual attack of illness—headache—pain in the limbs—diarrhœa—epistaxis —disturbed sleep—partial loss of memory—loss of strength —dry red tongue—rose spots—convalescence during the fourth week.

Edward N., aged 17, a footman, a slim lad, with dark brown hair and eyes, was admitted into the London Fever Hospital, July 17th, 1850. After ailing for some time, the duration of which was not clearly ascertained, he was taken suddenly worse, Friday, July 12th, with increase of headache, which had previously existed, pains in the limbs and bowels, diarrhœa, and epistaxis; the latter was repeated before the lad's admission.

The day after his admission I made the following notes:—

July 18th.—Slight headache; slept but little last night; no delirium; memory defective; cannot tell how long he has been in the hospital; expression inanimate; no flushing of face; special senses unaffected; conjunctivæ pale; pupils natural. Although unable to walk alone, he can reach the close-stool unassisted.

Tongue large, moist, and red at the edges, rather dry in centre, clean. Bowels much relaxed; ten stools before 10 A.M. Abdomen resonant, not particularly full; gurgling in right iliac fossa; no tenderness.

Pulse 96, full and of moderate power; no cough; no abnormal physical chest-signs.

Skin hot and dry. From twenty to thirty rose spots scattered over the abdomen and thorax.

The diarrhœa and a dry red tongue continued the prominent symptoms till the 23rd, when his pulse suddenly fell to 72, and he passed only two stools. Rose spots appeared daily. The pulse never after that date exceeded 70. On the 26th his appetite returned, and I noted as follows on the 27th:—'Pulse 70, soft; expression good; no flush; tongue moist and clean; appetite good; one stool partially formed; sleeps well. The man is most anxious to be allowed to get up.' But fresh rose spots continued to appear till the 31st. In about ten days he left the hospital.

Like James S. (Case XXVIII.) and Thomas T., the subject of the preceding case (XXXVIII.), Edward N. might, had no reference been had to the rose spots, have been considered convalescent some days before the fever, the general disease, and probably also before the specific intestinal lesion had run their course. The recumbent position, i.e. absolute repose in bed, was strictly enforced till all trace of the rose spots had disappeared. This is a practical point of essential consequence to the welfare of the patient; let him leave his bed before the rose spots have vanished, and the chance of severe symptoms coming on is considerable. Many such cases are put down as examples of relapse. The patient is supposed to be convalescent, gets up, commits some trifling error in diet, exposes himself to some injurious external influence, or it may be without either, grave symptoms suddenly appear, and he is said to suffer relapse, whereas in reality the disease had not terminated when the patient was allowed to leave his bed. In fever, to regulate the diet, the temperature and ventilation of the room, the time when the patient shall leave his bed, etc., is often of more moment for the sick man's safety than is the prescribing of drugs. For, let us remember, in no other sense—in a large majority of cases at least—than that in which we say a surgeon cures a fracture can we say a physician cures a fever. The latter, like the former, places his patient in favourable circumstances, and trusts nature to conduct the healing process. Meddlesome medicine is as bad as meddlesome surgery. The surgeon who fixes a limb, the subject of compound fracture, immoveably, covers the wound with a pledget of lint dipped in the fluid nature has supplied, removes every source of irritation, whether within or without, and only interferes further nature failing, all will allow is as scientific a practitioner and as valuable to his patient as the surgeon who, for the purpose of promoting concoction, granulation, or corroboration, handles, probes, and dresses, washes, greases, and powders the wound with tender care, morning, noon, and night.

If the surgeon who places his patient in favourable circumstances for nature to effect a cure is termed a scientific surgeon, while he who is ever interfering is denounced, and justly so, as unscientific, why should the physician dream that he is doing nothing, when, by enjoining or enforcing abstinence, mental quiet, bodily repose, fresh air, and cleanliness, he has placed the patient in circumstances in which nature may effect a cure? or he alone be regarded as scientific who, by the thousand drugs that flesh of the present day is heir to, unloads the liver, empties the bowels, promotes expectoration, excites sweating, induces sleep—who lowers the action of the heart by blood-letting, and produces counter-irritation by the application of cantharides—who, if he does not handle, probe, and dress, certainly washes, greases, and powders his patient, and that, unfortunately, inside as well as outside?

A mild case of fever, like a simple fracture, requires neither bloodletting nor wine, neither the internal administration of pill, powder or mixture, nor the external application of lotion, liniment, or ointment.

CASE XL.—In a man aged 21 years—rigors—chilliness—

Y

loss of strength—vertigo—rose spots—anorexia—diarrhœa —extreme tenderness of abdomen—dry brown tongue— delirium—return of appetite—marked emaciation—signs of pleuro-pneumonia—sloughing of skin over sacrum—recovery, with contraction of right side of chest, 84 days after outset of illness.

George T., aged 21, a fair, thin man, a ploughman, was admitted into the London Fever Hospital, January 23rd, 1849, under the care of Dr. Tweedie. He had always enjoyed health before his present illness; had never lived in London; was at Wandsworth when he fell sick, and had resided there a year. While working in the fields on Saturday afternoon, January 13th, a heavy rain fell; his clothes were wet through. About two hours after, i.e. at 4 P.M., he was seized with severe rigors, accompanied by sense of cold. No further trustworthy history could be obtained.

I saw him for the first time on Thursday, Jan. 25th, i.e. the 13th day of illness, and then made the following notes:—

The nurse reports that he slept the greater part of the night, and for some hours to-day. He himself affirms that he has had no sleep. No delirium; memory defective; thinks he has been in the hospital four days; complexion clear; cheeks slightly flushed; expression listless; nose rather red, slightly swollen, shining; vertigo in erect position; no headache; says he has ' terrible nasty smell and taste, the worst he ever had in his life.' Other special senses normal. He feels very weak, and is unable to leave or sit up in bed without considerable assistance. He lies constantly on his back.

Lips dry; tongue large, pale, moist, centre covered with thick brown fur. No stools the last twenty-four hours; two pale watery stools yesterday; abdomen full, tub-shaped, resonant, generally tender; no appetite; no thirst.

Pulse 120, weak; heart's impulse normal; heart sounds natural; no cough; a little sonorous rale heard on deep inspiration.

Skin rather hot and dry; about four rose spots on the abdomen and thorax, and six on the back. No miliary vesicles.

On the 15th day of disease, the 6th of his residence in the hospital, he thought a fortnight had elapsed since his admission. He still slept well, but fancied he had not closed his eyes. His pulse had risen to 132; the respiration was only 18. His tongue was dry, glazed, slightly furred, fissured; red at the tip; it was not particularly small. The stools were watery in consistence. Some of the rose spots noted on the 13th day had disappeared; the others were paler; about a dozen fresh rose spots had appeared.

The cheeks flushed occasionally. Rose spots were observed on the back on the 20th day.

On the 17th day his pulse had fallen to 120; it continued at that rate till the 22nd day, when it fell to 103. Although he slept well all this time, yet he continued to fancy that he never closed his eyes. There was no actual delirium till the 21st day of disease; he then supposed strange people were around his bed. On the 18th day he passed two solid stools; on the 19th the bowels were confined; on the 20th and 21st two relaxed stools; on the 22nd day the bowels were again confined. During the whole of this time his abdomen was decidedly tender, especially the right iliac fossa, and he frequently complained of pain in the belly. He complained of want of food on the 24th day.

On the 25th day the pulse had again risen to 120, and was very weak; the respiration was 30. He had a troublesome cough, and submucous rale was heard at the base of the right lung anteriorly and posteriorly; some friction sound accompanied inspiration and expiration at the base of the right lung posteriorly; he had passed four watery stools; the tongue was moist, white, and slightly tremulous; the abdomen so tender that he shrank before it was touched. It was very resonant, and preserved the tub-shape noticed on his admission.

On the 27th large liquid crepitation was heard at the base of the right lung; subcrepitant rale was heard as high as the level of the third rib; there was want of resonance at the inferior part of the lung. On the 31st day the physical signs of pleuro-pneumonia were much more extensive, there was absolute dulness as high as the fourth rib anteriorly, friction sound for some little distance above the dull portion. At this time his hands were livid, he lay constantly on his back, and never moved, even in bed, without aid. He had passed two or three stools into the bed during the preceding twenty-four hours. On the 14th of February, i.e. the 34th day of disease, his pulse was 152 and very weak; his respiration 20, and somewhat irregular in depth and frequency. He had slept little the preceding night, was delirious when awake during the night, and occasionally during the day; cheek and nose livid; muco-purulent-looking matter collects at the canthi of eyes; abundant large liquid crepitation as high as the third rib anteriorly on right side. On the 36th day his pulse was from 150 to 160, small and weak; respirations 34; his hands and feet cold and livid; he had no idea where he was. A slough formed over the sacrum on the 40th day.

On the 45th day the dulness of the right chest was much less decided; a little mucous rale anteriorly and posteriorly; his expression of countenance was decidedly improved. On the 52nd day his pulse was 120, and he passed his stools and urine in bed.

From this time he continued to improve daily. The man's appetite continued good from the 54th day, at times even was craving. He ate bread in his beef-tea, rice-pudding, toasted bread, and one or more eggs daily, even when he lay on his back unable to turn, and passing his stools and urine in bed. Yet it was noted that emaciation proceeded daily, in spite of the food taken with evident relish.

Just before he left the hospital, on 82nd day of disease, I made the following note :—'There is still a little cough; the lower part of the right side looks much smaller than the corresponding part of the left side; the chest is compressed from before backwards, and not from side to side. Below the nipple the right measures one inch less than the left side, and the left side expands much more during inspiration than the right. The ribs, anteriorly and laterally, are closer to each other on the right than on the left side, from the extreme base of the right lung to just above the right nipple anteriorly, and to just above the inferior angle of the scapula posteriorly, there is no trace of respiratory murmur; a little obscure crackling and some coarse breath sound for a little distance above the nipple and about the centre of the scapula. At the apex of the right lung the breath sound is less full than on the left side. The vocal resonance and fremitus are decidedly less at the inferior part of the right than at corresponding part of left side.'

The illness of Emma F., Case XXXIII., was prolonged by the supervention of disease during convalescence. No one, seeing she was thrice convalescent, could have confounded the length of her illness with the duration of the attack of typhoid fever for which she entered the hospital.

George T., the case last detailed, was ill 83 days. The typhoid fever terminated some time during the fourth week, but before it had run its course pleuro-pneumonia supervened. This local disease, so common a complication and sequela of typhoid fever, was of great extent and severity in the case of George T. On seeing him during the fifth and early part of the sixth week, with a pulse from 150 to 160 in the minute, and from its feebleness scarcely perceptible, hands and feet livid and cold, mind constantly wandering, stools in bed, urine retained, lower jaw incessantly moving tremulously, and then, added to these general symptoms, the lesions within the chest, revealed by their physical signs, no one could have anticipated the happy result. One favourable symptom alone remained throughout the illness—the patient's appetite was good. Even when lying in a state that death was to be expected every instant, he ate food ravenously, and throughout took what was given him with a relish. The large, loud, liquid rale heard within the chest I now believe to have been an example of what Dr. Walshe has described as pleural rhonchus. On one occasion I was enabled to verify, by an examination after death, the fact, as stated briefly in his work on the Physical Diagnosis of Diseases of the Lungs, i.e. that a large, liquid, superficial rhonchus may be heard in the chest, when, after death, the only physical lesions discoverable are a certain quantity of fluid amid loose adhesions between the pulmonary and costal pleuræ.

The cases of Thomas T. (xxxviii.), James S. (xxviii.), and Edward N. (xxxix.), *illustrate the fact* that the typhoid fever may not have terminated, although the patient seems convalescent, and they teach us to separate the apparent couvalescence of the patient from the termination of the fever.

The case of Jane H. (Case xxxii.) *illustrates the fact* that the intestinal disease may continue to progress long after the fever, properly so called, has terminated—simple ulceration succeeds to specific ulceration—and that, in this way, the illness may be prolonged for months after the fever has ceased.

The case of George T. (Case xl.) *illustrates the fact* that a local inflammation, set up during the progress of the fever, may continue after the fever has run its course, and so the illness be prolonged indefinitely.

The case of Emma F. (Case xxxiii.) *illustrates the fact* that a true relapse may occur, and that affections of a nature different from the fever, as erysipelas, may supervene after the primary disease has ceased, for days or weeks, but before the patient has left the hospital or recruited his strength, and so an erroneous idea be formed of the duration of the fever.

All illustrate the importance of keeping the length of the illness and the duration of the fever distinct from each other in estimating the effects of remedies, etc.

§ 9. TYPICAL CASES OF RELAPSING FEVER.

CASE XLI.—In a lad aged 17 years—sudden sense of weariness—drowsiness—frontal headache—vertigo—loss of appetite—hot and dry skin—furred tongue—on the 8th and 9th days of disease profuse sweating, followed by *sudden convalescence—relapse* on the 17th day of disease—quick pulse —hot and dry skin—frontal headache—white tongue—on the 20th day *restoration to health.*

Henry F., aged 17, a moderately stout fair lad, a street beggar, without settled residence, was admitted into the London Fever Hospital, under the care of Dr. Tweedie, May 31st, 1849. His health before his present illness had been good, with the exception of an abscess in the vicinity of the anus, in 1839.

On Sunday, May 25th, about 7 P.M., he was seized with sense of fatigue and drowsiness; he went to bed and slept well. The next morning he suffered from frontal headache, vertigo, and loss of appetite, and felt sleepy all day. His bowels at this time were regular. He took to his bed on entering the workhouse, on Wednesday, May 29th.

On admission into the hospital, on the 7th day of illness, his skin was hot and dry; tongue furred; bowels regular.

On the 8th day I noted as follows :—

Sweated freely last night for the first time since outset of illness.

Slept but little; mind clear; vertigo in erect position; no headache; conjunctivæ pale; pupils normal; expression natural.

Walks with some little difficulty on account of debility.

Tongue moist, white, loaded; one stool; no appetite; much thirst.

Pulse 72, soft; no cough; no abnormal physical chest-signs; skin warm, no spots; no miliary vesicles.

The following night he again sweated freely; and on the 9th day his pulse was still 72 and soft, and his skin moist.

On the 11th day of disease his appetite was noted to have returned, and his tongue was cleaning.

He was considered convalescent, and no report was made till on the 17th day from the outset, I noted :—

Pulse 120; skin dry and rather hot; slept well last night; no rigors; some frontal headache; tongue white; no stool; some appetite.

Hyd. c. cretâ, gr. iv. st. sumend. ; ol. ricini ʒss., horas tres post pulv.

The aperient acted five times, yet on the following, *i.e.* the 18th day, the pulse was still 120, and the skin hot and dry. During the subsequent night he sweated much, and the next morning the skin being yet moist, was cool, and the pulse only 96; on the 20th day it had fallen to 72; the skin was cool, and the appetite was good; in fact, the lad was well, and continued so till he left the hospital.

CASE XLII.—In a boy, aged 14 years, after exposure to the contagion of relapsing fever—sudden frontal headache—pain in the limbs—rigors—loss of appetite—regular bowels—herpetic eruption on upper lip—rapid pulse—hot skin—*sudden convalescence 9th day—relapse on the 19th day*—nausea—vomiting—sweating—quick pulse—hot skin—*convalescence* with pulse of 48 *on 20th day.*

John D., aged 14, black hair, fair skin, rather thin, a paper-stainer, brother to Peter D., Case XLIIL., and to William D., Case LII., was admitted into the London Fever Hospital, November 13th, 1849, under the care of Dr. Tweedie; he had been an inmate of the hospital six months before.

On Monday, November 11th, about 8 A.M. (having felt quite well when he first rose in the morning), while at work, John D. was suddenly seized with frontal headache and pain in the limbs; at noon he had rigors, and alternately sense of chilliness and heat; his bowels were regular. He took to his bed on Monday morning, and from that time till his admission into the hospital ate nothing. He sweated a little on Tuesday morning; there was no vomiting, and no epistaxis.

On the 6th day of disease I noted :—

Little headache; slept several hours last night, talked while asleep; no delirium; memory good; mind natural; complains of a bitter taste in the mouth; other special senses natural; conjunctivæ pale; pupils normal; no flush of face.

Can leave his bed unassisted with facility, and even walk a little without aid.

Upper lip swollen and red over a spot near half an inch in diameter; tongue moist, furred, white at the edges, dry in the centre; one stool, relaxed and dark; much thirst, no appetite; no vomiting; a little gurgling; splenic dulness vertically four fingers breadth, does not extend below the last false rib; liver dulness of natural extent; no abnormal fulness or resonance, and no tenderness of the abdomen.

Pulse 120, full, of good power; heart's sounds healthy; sonorous rale very *trifling* in amount on deep inspiration; no abnormal dulness of thorax; skin hot and dry, not sallow; numerous minute circular purple spots, unaffected by pressure (flea-bites!) scattered over the whole surface (the lad was very dirty on his admission); no trace of rose spots nor of mulberry rash.

7th day.—Pulse 120; respirations 40; no cough; no sonorous rale; skin hot and dry, no sallowness; sleeps much. From red swollen spot on the upper lip a little serous fluid has been discharged.

Sleeps much night and day, occasionally calls out loudly in his sleep; no headache; no delirium; no flushing of face; tongue dry and of a pale yellowish colour in the centre; three watery stools; liver dulness and other abdominal signs as yesterday; retched much this morning while out of bed, but ejected nothing from the stomach.

Two grains of acetate of lead, and five minims of Batley's sedative, were ordered to be administered, with a drachm of dilute acetic acid every six hours.

8th day.—Pulse 124; sleeps almost constantly; dozing again directly after being aroused; moans occasionally in his sleep. Tongue moist, centre covered with dark thick brown fur; two stools; skin dry and hot; unable to leave his bed unassisted.

All medicine to be omitted.

9th day.—Pulse 72, soft; respirations 18; expression much improved; sleeps well, not too much; many vesicles on the red spot on the upper lip; tongue moist, furred posteriorly; a little appetite; three stools, dark, relaxed. No sweating; skin soft and of normal temperature.

No further note was taken till the 12th day of disease, when the pulse had fallen to 60; the skin was normal in all particulars; the tongue was moist and clean; appetite good; bowels regular, i.e. one stool daily. But, about two o'clock on the morning of the 19th day, he awoke disturbed by nausea, and soon vomited. He subsequently slept, and perspired profusely. He had no rigors. His bowels had acted on the 18th day once, and again during the night. When I saw him on the 19th day, the pulse was 84; skin hot and dry, and an abundant crop of sudamina covered the whole surface of the abdomen and thorax. He had still a little desire for food. A little simple saline mixture, with acetate of ammonia, was prescribed.

On the following, the 20th day, the pulse had fallen to 48; he had slept well; the sudamina were drying up; his skin was of normal temperature; he passed two solid stools, and, with the exception of the tongue being thinly furred, he was well.

CASE XLIII.—In a child, aged 8 years, after exposure to the contagion of relapsing fever—sudden headache—pains in the limbs—rigors—vomiting—sweating—noise in the ears—regular bowels—quick pulse—hot and dry skin—*convalescence on the 9th day.*

Relapse on the 21st day—hot skin—quick pulse—*convalescence on the 22nd day.*

Peter D., aged 7, an intelligent, fair, thin child, was admitted into the London Fever Hospital, November 18th, 1849, under Dr. Tweedie. He stated that he had the 'fever' three months before his admission. On Sunday, November 10th, on first rising in the morning, with headache, pains in the limbs, chilliness, and rigors. On Sunday afternoon he vomited repeatedly, and sweated, according to his own account, all the same night. His bowels were confined.

His two brothers were admitted into the hospital at the same time with Peter D.

On the 5th day of disease I noticed :—

No headache; mind normal; expression natural; colour of face good; noise, as the boy describes, of 'bullocks a-bellowing in my ears;' other special senses normal. Conjunctivæ pale; pupils act healthily. Can walk a few steps unassisted. Tongue moist and white; two stools; ate a little bread to-day; no great thirst; no vomiting; no abnormal fulness nor resonance, and no tenderness of the abdomen.'

Pulse 108; heart and lung-sounds natural.

Skin hot and dry; many minute circular purple spots, unaffected by pressure (identical in appearance with one form of flea-bite), scattered over the whole surface (the boy was in a very dirty condition when brought into the hospital); no trace of rose-spots nor of mulberry rash.

6th day.—Pulse 120; skin hot and dry; complains at the present time of much general headache. Slept for about three hours during the night; none to-day; screamed out frequently during the night, 'My head, my head!' Pupils rather large; conjunctivæ pale; tongue red in the centre, furred posteriorly, tip and edges red; no vomiting; one stool; urine transparent, pale yellow. Six leeches to the temples. The head to be shaved, and cold water kept constantly applied. Two grains of mercury and chalk to be given every six hours.

On the 7th day the head symptoms were much less marked; and on the 8th day the pulse had fallen to 84, but he was still restless, and even somewhat weaker than at previous reports.

On the 9th day he was convalescent, the pulse being only 66, and the skin of normal temperature. There had been no sweating.

Peter D. continued well till the 29th of November, i.e. the

20th day from the commencement of the disease, when he complained of feeling ill. His skin was hot, and his pulse had risen to 84.

On the 21st day, pulse 84; skin normal temperature; tongue moist, slightly furred; no stool.

The following day he was again well.

CASE XLIV.—In a man, aged 18 years—rigors—headache—nausea—vomiting—confined bowels—pain in back and limbs—dry tongue—perspiration—delirium — *convalescence on the 10th day—relapse on the 20th day*—vomiting—delirium—dry brown tongue—relaxed bowels—hot skin—quick pulse—*death on the 24th day*.

After death non-granular consolidation of the left lung—fatty liver—large spleen containing numerous fibrinous deposits—abnormal vascularity of the mucous membrane of the bladder—other organs healthy.

William W.,[1] aged 18, an engineer, was admitted July 21st, 1847, into the London Fever Hospital, under the care of Dr. Tweedie. His illness began July the 17th, with rigors, headache, nausea, vomiting, and confined bowels.

6th day of disease.—Slight headache: pain in the back and limbs; pulse 90. No abnormal physical chest signs; no cough. Tongue dry and furred; bowels open. Skin perspiring. No spots. Mist. ammon. acet. The head to be kept wet with cold water.

7th day.—Slight headache; tongue cleaner; three stools; pulse 70.

8th day.—Has been delirious all night, frequently leaving his bed; eyes suffused. Tongue dry, slightly furred. One stool. Pulse 90. Pil. sapon. c. opio, gr. v. h. s.s.

9th day.—Asleep; passed a restless night; two stools.

10th day.—Pulse 80; sleeps well; tongue clean; one stool. He was noted to be convalescent.

On the 20th day he was seized with vomiting; delirium returned during the night, and on the following morning his tongue was dry and brown. He passed three stools, the vomiting continued, and his skin was hot.

On the 23rd day the following note was made:—

Pulse 112; skin hot and dry. Almost constant talking. Sordes about the teeth; tongue dry and fissured; two stools. He died before the visit on the 24th day of disease.

[1] I am indebted to Dr. W. H. O. Sankey for the notes of this case taken during life. The examination after death was made by myself.

The following notes were made on examining the body of Wm. W. :—

Cadaveric rigidity well marked. Purplish discoloration of the posterior part of the trunk and extremities. Muscles brighter red than ordinary.

Head.—Membranes of the brain normal. A little colourless serosity at the base of the brain, and about 1 oz. in the ventricles. Substance of the brain firm.

Thorax.—A small quantity of transparent yellowish serosity in the *pericardium* ; the membrane itself healthy.

Heart.—Weight 8¾ ozs. Substance, valves, and lining membrane normal. A large fibrinous clot in the right auricle. A similar, but smaller clot in the right ventricle, continuous with one in the pulmonary artery. Similar coagula in the left auricle, ventricle and aorta.

No adhesions of, and no fluid in either *pleura.*

Right Lung.—Weight 25 ozs. ; crepitant throughout. The inferior lobe is gorged with bloody serosity. In the substance of the apex of the superior lobe is a putty-like mass, one-eighth inch in diameter, containing gritty particles.

Left Lung.—Weight 34 ozs. The apex of this lung resembled that of the opposite, except that it contained several little cretaceous and putty-like masses.

The inferior third of the upper lobe is of a deep red colour ; its section is smooth and uniform ; it contains much dark red serosity, and breaks down on pressure rather more readily than a healthy lung ; it sinks in water. The lower lobe, with the exception of its extreme apex, resembles the inferior third of the upper lobe in all particulars.

The *bronchial tubes* of both lungs appear healthy.

The *bronchial glands* are large, dark, and firm.

Abdomen.—There is a little transparent serosity in the peritoneal cavity. The *peritoneum* appears healthy. The *mesenteric glands* are larger than natural ; many the size of small beans, flattened, firm, and pale.

Liver.—Weight 65 ozs. Substance flabby and soft ; mottled externally and internally with delicate yellowish patches. Its capsule is thin and transparent ; it separates with facility from the hepatic substance. (The microscope proved its cells to be loaded with fat.)

Gall Bladder.—Greatly distended with pale yellow watery bile. Lining membrane healthy.

Spleen.—Weight 20½ ozs., dark and tolerably firm. Extending some distance into the substance of the organ at the anterior margin is a mass of pale red colour, friable, having a finely granular fracture ; it feels firmer than the adjacent spleen tissue ; the line of demarcation is well marked. Deeper in the substance of the organ are several smaller masses, resembling in all particulars the one just described; there is also one on the surface near to the inferior margin.

The *pancreas* weighs 2¾ ozs.; it is normal in character.

The *stomach*, small and large intestines, healthy in all particulars. Peyer's patches very distinct, and of a somewhat deeper red than the surrounding mucous membrane.

The *kidneys* weigh 6½ ozs. each; they are healthy in all particulars; no fat to be detected in cells by the aid of the microscope.

Pelves of the kidneys pale.

Urinary Bladder.—Mucous membrane studded anteriorly with red puncta, and posteriorly with somewhat larger red spots, almost continuous with each other. There is no abnormal redness near the urethral orifice.

CASE XLV.—In a man, aged 60 years—repeated rigors —headache — furred tongue — confined bowels — epigastric tenderness — quick pulse —*convalescence on 7th day of disease—relapse on the 16th day*—rigors—quick pulse— hot and dry skin—furred tongue—confined bowels—vomiting of green fluid—free perspiration—permanent *convalescence the 18th day of disease.*

George R., aged 60, a harness-maker, was admitted into the London Fever Hospital, under the care of Dr. Tweedie, November 1st, 1847. He returned from Madras in 1840, where he had resided for forty years; while in India, he was seriously hurt by a fall from his horse. He suffered in 1818 from 'severe dysentery;' a few years after he had some 'disease of the liver;' for these affections he was repeatedly and largely leeched,—200 leeches having been, he says, applied at one time. The abdomen is *covered* with leech-bite scars. During the last seven years his health has been very good.

On Thursday, October 28th, having been exposed to cold and wet the four preceding days, he was suddenly seized with rigors; the rigors were repeated several times before his admission. On the following day he suffered from headache.

On the 6th day of disease I noted :—

Frontal headache; mind normal; expression good; special senses unaffected. Strength somewhat impaired, but he can leave his bed without assistance. Tongue moist, furred; no stool; a little tenderness at the epigastrium; liver dulness occupies the epigastric region; no appetite. Pulse 100; slight cough; little expectoration; no abnormal physical chest signs; heart's impulse feeble. Skin cool; no spots.

Ol. ricini, ʒij., st. s.

He passed a restless night, and was asleep at the time I saw him on the following day. The castor oil had acted three times.

7th day.—Pulse 72; tongue moist, slightly furred; two stools; appetite good; skin cool; complains of slight frontal headache.

8th day.—Pulse 72: little sleep; no headache; complains of severe pain in the back and limbs; he states they are so stiff he can hardly turn in bed unassisted; tongue moist, clean; appetite good; one stool; stiffness of the limbs continued till the 16th day, when, early in the morning, he was seized with rigors. At the time of the visit the pulse was 108; skin hot, dry, and free from spots; tongue dry and slightly furred; there was much thirst; his bowels were confined. Two drachms of castor oil were administered directly.

17th day of disease.—Pulse 90; little sleep; no return of rigors; tongue as yesterday; five stools; vomited some green fluid this morning; skin warm, perspiring freely.

18th day.—Pulse 70; no vomiting; two stools. He was quite well on the 20th day.

CASE XLVI.—In a man, aged 30 years—rigors—headache —pains in the limbs—nausea—want of sleep—vertigo—furred tongue—loss of appetite—free perspiration—*convalescence on the 8th day of disease—relapse on the 18th day*—quick pulse—hot and dry skin—furred tongue—pain in the limbs —permanent *convalescence on the 20th day of disease.*

John F., aged 30, a labourer of temperate habits, was admitted into the London Fever Hospital, December 16th, 1847, under the care of Dr. Tweedie. John F. had resided in London three years, and had till the present attack enjoyed health. His illness commenced on Sunday, December 12th, with rigors, succeeded by heat and sweating, headache, pains in the limbs, and nausea; no epistaxis, no vomiting; the bowels, at first confined, were acted on by medicine before he came under observation. He took to his bed on Monday, the 13th of December, i.e. the 2nd day of disease.

6th day of disease.—Slept but little; no dreaming; vertigo on assuming the erect position; no affection of the special senses.

Tongue coated; three stools; no abnormal fulness, resonance, nor tenderness of the abdomen; no appetite; some thirst.

Pulse 96; trifling cough; skin moist; no spots.

7th day.—Pulse 108; headache increased; tongue loaded; three stools; much thirst; skin perspiring freely.

8th day.—Pulse 60; had a rigor last evening, which was succeeded by heat and sweating; slept well; no headache; tongue clean; two stools.

On the 11th day his appetite had returned, and on the 14th day the pulse had fallen to 48. He appeared in health.

On the night of the 29th December, i.e. the 18th day of illness, he had but little sleep, and on the following days I noted :—

19th day of disease.—Pulse 108; much pain in the limbs; skin hot and dry; tongue moist, thickly furred; four stools; no appetite.

20th day.—About 9 o'clock last evening is reported by the nurse to have had severe rigors, which lasted twenty minutes. About 5 A.M., while at stool, he fainted. At the time of the visit, his pulse was 72; skin warm and perspiring freely.

On the 22nd day the pulse had fallen to 48, and he complained again of pains in the limbs; his tongue was clean; his appetite was returning.

No further note was taken.

CASE XLVIL—In a boy, aged 14 years—headache—pain in the limbs—dry, brown tongue—confined bowels—*convalescence on the* 13*th day.*

Relapse on the 18*th day*—rapid pulse—hot skin—flushed cheeks—vomiting—profuse perspiration—permanent *convalescence on the* 20*th day.*

James D., aged 14, a skin-dresser, was admitted into the London Fever Hospital, under Dr. Tweedie, August 9th, 1847. Without known cause, a week before his admission, he was suddenly attacked with headache and pain in the limbs.

10th day of disease.—Mind normal; no headache; sleeps well. Tongue dry, brown; no stool 24 hours. Pulse 80. No cough; no abnormal physical chest signs; skin cool; no spots.

11th day.—Pulse 80; skin cool; two stools; tongue red; sordes about teeth.

12th day.—Pulse 84; cheeks flushed; two stools.

13th day.—Pulse 72; sleeps well; tongue moist, red; no stool. Hst. aperiens, 3j. st. s.

16th day.—Gradually improving.

18th day.—Pulse 120; skin hot; cheeks flushed; tongue moist; red; three stools.

19th day.—Pulse 96; was troubled with vomiting during the night; tongue dry; two stools. Is now sweating profusely.

On the following day he appeared well.

Attention is particularly directed to the following points connected with the seven cases above detailed :—

1st. The ages of the patients were respectively 7, 14, 14, 17, 18, 30, and 60 years. Relapsing fever, then, limits its attacks to no particular age.

2nd. Two of the cases were brought from the same house. The others, sleeping in common lodging-houses, etc., *might* have been exposed to contagion.

3rd. The case which proved fatal offered no lesion after death by which the fatal termination could be explained.

4th. These seven patients, after having suffered from attacks of simple fever appeared convalescent; continued pretty well for 5, 9, 10, 10, 10, and 12 days respectively; and then had a return of all the symptoms present in the first attack, *i.e.* had true relapse.

§ 10. GENERAL DESCRIPTION OF THE SYMPTOMS AND LESIONS OF STRUCTURE IN RELAPSING FEVER.

Relapsing fever affects persons of all ages. The patient, previously in health, is seized, on waking in the morning, or it may be while occupied about his daily avocations, with rigors, sometimes severe, sense of chilliness, and headache, usually frontal. These are followed by heat of skin; and this, again, is frequently succeeded by sweating; the sweating, however, when it occurs, appears to afford no relief. There is soon pain in the back and limbs, frequent pulse, and a dry and hot skin. The tongue is now white, the urine high-coloured, the appetite is lost, and there is considerable thirst. The patient passes sleepless nights. Vomiting of green bile is generally one of the earliest symptoms. The rigors, headache, vomiting, and pain in the back, might lead one to suppose the patient to be labouring under small-pox; but the pain in the back is rarely so severe, nor is the vomiting so incessant as it ordinarily is in the early period of the last-named disease. The headache is seldom so violent as it is in common 'bilious headache,' in which latter, moreover, it is commonly occipital; the heat of skin and the quick pulse serve still further to separate relapsing fever, at its outset,

from that troublesome affection. The suddenness of the
attack, the rigors, hot skin, pain in the limbs, and white
tongue, distinguish relapsing fever from idiopathic head affections. The patient is generally obliged at once to take to his
bed. He feels not exactly too weak, but too ill to keep
about; frequently affirms only that he is too giddy to walk,
i.e. vertigo, and not sense of weakness, drives the patient to
bed. The sudden transition from health to a sense of disease
warns him that some severe illness is setting in.

By the 2nd or 3rd day the heart often beats 100, 120,
or even 130 strokes in the minute; the patient gets no
sleep; and even, as in the case of William D. (Case LII.),
by the fifth or sixth day, may be violently delirious. The
bowels are usually somewhat confined at the commencement.

After a period varying from five or ten days, a profuse
perspiration breaks out, and in the course of a few hours the
patient appears nearly well. The alteration is most remarkable: in the morning the pulse may have been 120 in the
minute, the skin hot and dry, the head throbbing; in the
afternoon the pulse is 60, the skin cool, the head free from
pain.

On the following day the patient is apparently, in every
respect, free from ailment. His appetite returns, his strength
improves, and we suppose him progressing favourably; when
on from the 12th day to the 20th, reckoning from the outset
of the illness, or on *about* the 7th, counting from the crisis,
the patient having committed no hygienic error, the preceding day having been seemingly in health, or simply weak, is
again suddenly seized with rigors, vomiting of green fluid,
and headache, quickly followed by hot skin, quick pulse,
furred tongue, loss of appetite, and confined bowels; delirium,
perhaps, supervenes, and, in fact, he is in the same state as
on the day his illness commenced. The pulse, which falls
remarkably during the period of apparent convalescence,
often beating, the day preceding the relapse, as infrequently
as 48 strokes in the minute, rises suddenly to 120, or even
higher. After the expiration of two, three, four, or five days,
the patient is again bathed in perspiration, and the next day
is convalescent.

Such is the ordinary course of a tolerably severe non-fatal

case of relapsing fever. But in some cases it presents certain deviations from this, which may be regarded as its normal type. Instead of commencing abruptly, it may make its attack insidiously; *epistaxis* may be among the earliest symptoms; the crisis may be accompanied by diarrhœa, or loss of blood from the nose, and it is said, but I have never seen such a case, by discharge of blood from the bowels, instead of, as is far more common, by sweating. In women the catamenial discharge appears, in some cases, to be critical.

The relapse may be very imperfectly marked; a slight, *even now and then only comparative*, increase in the rapidity of the pulse, and a little greater heat of skin than was observed on the previous day, being all that indicates its supervention.

If blood be drawn during the primary attack or the relapse, it is in many cases more or less buffed, and that without the co-existence, so far as can be ascertained, of any local inflammation.

Yellowness of the skin is by no means an uncommon symptom.[1] The jaundice is sometimes intense; it may be present during the first attack, disappear before the relapse, and not recur; or it may occur only in the relapse. When jaundice supervenes, *the stools retain their natural hue, or are darker than common*; at the same time the urine is frequently loaded with bile.

The skin sometimes has a purplish mottled aspect, an exaggerated resemblance to the skin of young children. Petechiæ are now and then present—flea-bites, which often exist in immense numbers on the trunk and extremities of the poor, have frequently been confounded with them; at the same time, the large size in rare cases of the subcuticular effusions of blood, and the fact noticed by some physicians, that they have made their appearance after the patient entered the hospital, prove that they are due in certain cases to a change in the solids and fluids of the body, and not to the bites of insects.

---

[1] Jaundice is a *very* rare symptom in typhus and typhoid fevers, so rare that I cannot call to mind a single case in which I have observed it, while it is more or less marked in nearly a fourth of the cases of relapsing fever.

z

Neither the mulberry rash of typhus fever nor the rose spots of typhoid fever are ever present in relapsing fever.

Sudden sinking marks the progress of some cases; it is indicated by a deep dusky hue of the face, lividity of the hands and feet, a purple marbling of the whole surface. The trunk feels cool, the hands and feet cold—the patient is in a state of collapse, without having suffered from any severe pain or exhausting discharge. In such cases he is unable to be aroused, to exhibit any sign of consciousness, and not unfrequently dies a few hours—generally from twelve to twenty-four—after the physician had supposed him to be free from danger. Death is, however, a rare termination of relapsing fever; when it does occur, the fatal event may take place during the primary fever or the relapse—I think the former has been in my experience more commonly the case.

Pain in the limbs of a very severe character is not unfrequent at the outset of the disease, but it has been noticed by several writers, and my own observations are in accordance with their experience, that severe muscular pains sometimes cause considerable suffering after the termination of the primary attack, and also after the relapse, *i.e.* after the patient is, in all other particulars, in health.

More or less violent delirium is now and then observed, as Dr. Robertson pointed out, after the critical discharge has taken place.

Vomiting, as I have said, is a frequent symptom in both the first and second attack. The fluid ejected is ordinarily bright grass-green, and very large in quantity. Sometimes the vomiting is almost incessant, and continues during the whole course of the disease. Tenderness at the epigastrium is a common symptom in all cases, but it is especially marked in those to which I have just referred.

If pregnant women are attacked by relapsing fever, a very large majority, if not all, abort. Death sometimes, but by no means invariably, happens under such circumstances.

A second relapse occurs in a few cases; the patient, convalescent about the 7th day, relapses about the 14th; is a second time convalescent by from the 17th to the 21st day; and relapses again from the 21st to the 25th days, for convalescence to be finally established from the 25th to the 28th days. However, in some cases, the disease terminates at the end of a week, the patient experiencing no relapse.[1]

The most frequent local complication, next to enlargement of the liver and spleen, is inflammation of the lung. I have never seen in relapsing fever, any more than I have in typhus fever, an example of meningeal or cerebral inflammation.[2]

Death from uncomplicated relapsing fever is rare. No anatomical character of this disease has been pointed out. The most constant lesion by far is enlargement of the spleen. The size attained by that organ is, I think, on the whole, larger than in either typhus or typhoid fevers. I have found it weigh as much in one case as 38 oz., its size being in proportion to its weight. Pale yellowish pink masses of variable size, firm to the touch, but friable, with a slightly granular fracture, are occasionally found in the substance and near the surface of this organ. As a rule, there is but little congestion of the lungs, the weights of which contrast singularly with the weights of the same organs in subjects dead from typhus fever. The brain and its membranes also are remarkably free from appreciable lesion. A slight excess of serosity beneath the arachnoid and in the lateral ventricles is, however, occasionally observed. The blood, in a few cases, has been found fluid throughout the body. The heart offers no appreciable deviation from its normal condition. The liver is generally large, and the gallbladder contains a considerable quantity of thick dark bile; the ductus communis allows bile to pass freely into the duodenum, even in those cases where jaundice was present at the time of death.

The gastro-intestinal, the laryngo-bronchial, and genitourinary mucous membranes, present all the characters of health. The kidneys are normal.

This description applies only to uncomplicated cases; for,

[1] For the relation existing between these cases and febricula, the reader must refer to the examples of that disease related hereafter (see p. 384 et seq.).

[2] The case detailed by Dr. Stevens of Glasgow, in the *Medical Times*, vol. xxi. p. 156, appears to me to have been an example of hemorrhage into the cavity of the arachnoid.

should any local inflammation have been set up during life, the characters of that lesion will, of course, be present after death ; thus consolidation of the lung and the signs of recent pleuritis are sometimes detected.

§ 11. BLOOD IN RELAPSING FEVER SOMETIMES BUFFED —CRITICAL DISCHARGES.

In his book on the relapsing fever epidemic in Edinburgh, 1817-19, Dr. Welsh states that the blood which he took in such plentiful streams from his patients was buffed. He argues that this condition of the blood proves the propriety of the use of the lancet: *à priori* argument, however, is worth but little in therapeutics. Cruveilhier found, in the bodies of women who died of puerperal fever during an epidemic of that disease, which occurred in Paris some years since, unequivocal signs, as he thought, of pre-existing inflammation. He used the lancet, reasoning *à priori* that it must be useful: the mortality under the treatment he adopted was fearful. Experience alone is a sound basis for therapeutics. *'Ars medica tota est in observationibus,'*—hackneyed as is the phrase of Baglivi, its spirit has yet to be thoroughly incorporated into the members of our profession.

The following record illustrates the fact that, in the cases I have seen, when blood was drawn it was, as in the same disease in 1817-19, buffed.

CASE XLVIII.—In a man, aged 35—headache—pain in the limbs—hurried breathing—quick pulse—hot skin—buffed blood—*convalescent on the 9th day of disease.*

Relapse on the 17th day.—Rapid pulse—hot skin—white tongue—vomiting—delirium—want of sleep—profuse perspiration—*convalescence on the 22nd day of disease.*

Robert M., aged 35, a railway labourer, was admitted under the care of Dr. Tweedie, into the London Fever Hospital, July 22nd, 1847.

He was taken ill without known cause, July 19th, with headache, and pain in the limbs, unaccompanied by any derangement of the bowels.

On the day after admission, my friend Mr. Sankey noted :—

He slept but little last night; headache; mind clear; respiration hurried, some cough; pulse 90; tongue coated; skin free from spots, hot. V S. ad. ʒx.

On the 24th July, *i.e. 6th day of disease*, blood thinly buffed, not cupped, clot large and soft; headache nearly gone; tongue coated; no stool; pulse 90.

On the 8th day the pulse had fallen to 84, and there was considerable pain in the limbs.

On the 9th day the appetite returned; the pulse being still 84.

He was considered convalescent, and no report taken till the 17*th day of illness*, on which, and subsequent days, I noted:— Was seized with rigors last night; pulse 120; skin hot and dry; tongue white, moist; three stools; complains of nausea.

18th day.—Pulse 120; skin hot and dry; no sleep last night; tongue white, moist; has vomited this morning.

19th day.—A little delirium; scarcely any sleep; vomiting continues; two stools; pulse 120.

20th day.—In all respects as yesterday.

Afternoon of 21st day.—Has been perspiring profusely since 10 A.M.; skin cool; pulse 80, soft; tongue cleaner; two stools; no return of vomiting.

22nd day of disease.—Pulse 80; skin sweating; tongue clean; no stools; a little epistaxis this morning; complains of pains in the limbs.

No notes were taken after the 22nd day of disease.

This man derived no marked benefit from the blood-letting, practised on the 5th day of disease. It is true that, on the day after, the headache was less severe; but the reader will have perceived that nature, unaided by the loss of blood, in many cases effected a much larger improvement in a much shorter space of time. Pain in the limbs is often complained of by patients, after the febrile symptoms (commonly so called) has disappeared. In this case, the pain followed both the primary attack and the relapse. On the 9th day Robert M. was considered to be convalescent. No critical discharge appears by my notes to have marked the termination of the primary attack. The relapse set in, as it usually does, suddenly. The febrile symptoms were very severe. The copious sweating on the 21st day was evidently critical. It occurred, so far as concerns the whole illness, on a non-critical day; so far as concerns the relapse, on a critical day; but then, 3, 4, 5, 6, and 7 are all critical days, so that, if a disease terminates in less than a week, it must terminate on a critical day.[1]   Although the sweating was very profuse, yet a second critical discharge, epistaxis, occurred on the 22nd day of disease, the 6th of relapse.

The catamenial discharge is sometimes critical.   I have before stated the fact.   The following cases illustrate it.

CASE XLIX.—In a woman aged 19 years.   Rigors—heat of skin — headache — vomiting — furred tongue — loss of appetite—quick pulse—perspiration—catamenial discharge—convalescent on the *7th day of disease.   Relapse on the 13th day of disease.*   Rapid pulse—headache—hot skin—vomiting—profuse sweating—*convalescence on the 16th day*, with pain in the limbs.

Mary H., aged 19, a domestic servant, was admitted into the London Fever Hospital, September 9th, 1847, under the care of Dr. Tweedie.

On Saturday, September 7th, she was seized with rigors, succeeded by heat of skin, headache, and vomiting.

On the 4th day of disease, no headache ; no pain in the limbs; sleeps well. Tongue furred ; one stool ; no tenderness of abdomen; no appetite ; some thirst.

Pulse 92 ; trifling cough.

Skin warm ; perspiring.

5th day.—Pulse 96 ; a little frontal headache ; tongue slightly furred ; three stools ; catamenia have appeared.

No note was made on the 6th. *On the 7th day she appeared well;* her pulse was only 66, and she had some appetite ; but on the 13th day of disease, pulse 120 ; no sleep ; some frontal headache ; tongue moist, furred ; nausea ; vomited to-day much greenish yellow fluid ; no appetite ; two stools ; some tenderness at the epigastrium ; skin warm, dry ; no spots.

14th day of disease.—Pulse 130 ; no sleep ; headache continues; skin hot, dry ; tongue as yesterday ; two stools ; nausea ; vomiting of greenish yellow fluid continued, about 12 oz. has been ejected to-day. No tenderness at the epigastrium. Prescribed arrowroot with brandy ; mustard poultice to the epigastrium.

15th day of disease.—Pulse 96 ; perspired profusely after the arrowroot and brandy ; slept well ; no headache ; tongue cleaner ; no nausea ; no vomiting.

[1] See *British and Foreign Review*, April 1844, for some able remarks on the doctrine of critical days.

16th day.—Pulse 96; skin cool; complains of pain in the limbs. Tongue clean; no stool.

No further report was considered necessary; the woman was convalescent, and left the hospital in a few days.

It may be observed, that in this case the perspiration did not afford any marked relief. It was not until after the menstrual evacuation, on the 5th day of disease, that the patient was convalescent. As is usual, the relapse took place suddenly. The patient was seemingly in health on the 12th day; on the 13th, her pulse was 120; on the 14th, 130. This extreme rapidity of the pulse, as Dr. Henderson pointed out, is never observed so early in typhus fever without indicating extreme danger, while it by no means indicates danger in relapsing fever. Vomiting of green fluid is a very common symptom in relapsing fever: it was present, to a comparatively trifling extent, during relapse in this case. The profuse sweating with which the relapse terminated occurred on a non-critical day, *i.e.* the 15th day of disease. Pain in the limbs troubled the patient after the termination of the severe febrile symptoms which marked the relapse. Whether the pains are rheumatic or neuralgic in their character has been a question. I am inclined to regard them as neuralgic, or analogous to the pain in the back in small-pox. Certainly I see no reason to believe them to be rheumatic.

CASE L.—In a woman aged 45. Pains in the back and limbs—rigors—vomiting—headache—vertigo—white tongue—quick pulse—slight sonorous rale—hot skin—catamenial discharge—*convalescence on the 7th day of disease—relapse on the 19th day of disease*—rigors—rapid pulse—hot skin—frontal headache—white tongue—slight sore throat—*convalescence on the 23rd day of disease.*

Sarah R., aged 45, was admitted into the London Fever Hospital under the care of Dr. Tweedie, December 9th, 1847. She had enjoyed health till the present attack. On Wednesday, December 8th, she was suddenly seized with pains in the back and limbs, rigors, vomiting of bitter yellow fluid, headache, and vertigo. Her bowels were regular. She was suckling at the time her illness began. Three months before her present illness began, she left Sheffield, and 'tramped' to London, sleeping in Union houses. She affirmed she was of sober habits.

3rd day of disease.—Complains much of general headache; great pain in the back and limbs; vertigo in the erect position; intellect unaffected; expression natural; face flushed.

Is unable to walk more than a few steps in consequence of vertigo.

Tongue moist, white; much thirst; no appetite; one stool; some nausea; abdomen full, resonant, not tender.

Pulse 100; a little cough, trifling amount of sonorous rale on deep inspiration; skin warm, dry, free from spots.

Applic. c. c. temp. et detrah. sang. ad ℥ viii.

4th day of disease.—Pulse 120; skin hot and dry; much less headache; less vertigo; no flush; little sleep. Tongue as yesterday; a little nausea; one stool, confined.

Ol. ricini, ℥ ss. st. s.; hyd. c. cretâ, gr. ii. 6ta quaque hora.

6th day of disease.—Had but little sleep last night; is now asleep. Hyd. c. cretâ, gr. ii. nocte maneque sum.

7th day of disease.—Pulse 84, weak; skin cool; no headache; dozed during night, moaning much in her sleep. Complains of feeling extremely weak. Catamenia appeared last night. Tongue moist, furred; two stools, one of which was passed into the bed, apparently unconsciously. Vin alb. ℥ vi.

8th day of disease.—Pulse 76, stronger; skin cool; slept well last night, less moaning in her sleep; expression improved; tongue moist, nearly clean; three stools in close pan. Catamenia continue.

On the 9th day there was a little appetite.

On the 11th day.—Pulse 70. Sits up in bed unassisted. Tongue moist, clean; appetite good; one stool.

On the 13th day I noted that her pulse was still 70, that her tongue continued clean; and that she gained strength daily.

On the morning of the 19th day she was attacked with severe rigors, which continued for an hour. At the time of my visit I noted:—Pulse 120; skin hot. Complains of frontal headache; face flushed. Tongue white, moist; no nausea; no tenderness at epigastrium; one stool last night; no appetite. Hyd. c. cretâ, gr. iv. st. sum. Haust. ap. horas duas post pil. sum.

20th day.—Pulse 120; skin hot; little sleep; no return of rigors; less headache; face flushed; tongue as yesterday; complains of some sore throat; three stools.

21st day.—Pulse 110; tongue the same; three stools.

22nd day.—Pulse 90; tongue white, moist. Complains of sore throat and pain in deglutition; slight redness of tonsils; one stool.

23rd day of disease.—Pulse 72; slept well; tongue cleaner very trifling sore throat; one stool; appetite returning.

The exact date at which the fever left this woman can scarcely be fixed. The pulse was 120 on the 4th day; no note was made on the 5th day; on the 6th day she was asleep at the time of my visit; on the evening of that day the cata-menial discharge occurred; and when I saw her on the 7th day the pulse had fallen to 84, and the skin was cool; yet she complained of great sense of weakness, and passed stools into the bed. It appears probable that the latter was the con-sequence of the woman's sense of weakness making her prefer to lie quiet. Persons in the class of life of Sarah R., a common tramp, are often very dirty in their habits. Had this case been a solitary example of the disease I am considering, the primary attack might have been held to be simple catarrh; the second tonsilitis. The chest and throat symptoms appear to me, however, to have been secondary to the general disease. In the first attack, the headache was so severe that local blood-letting was considered necessary; while the chest symptoms were so trifling that no remedy was administered for their relief; and, with reference to the sore throat, that was evidently greater on the 22nd day, when the pulse was only 90, than it was on the 20th, when the pulse was 120.

§ 12. PREGNANT WOMEN, AS A RULE, ABORT WHEN AFFECTED WITH RELAPSING FEVER.—DIARRHŒA SOMETIMES CRITICAL.

CASE LI.—In a woman, aged 25 years—headache—pain in the limbs—rigors—heat of skin—bowels regular—abortion on the 6th day of disease—frequent pulse—hot and dry skin —dry, brown tongue—marked prostration—*convalescence on the 9th day of disease—relapse on the 16th day*—frequent pulse—hot and dry skin—furred tongue—diarrhœa on the 18th day—*permanent convalescence on the 19th day.*

Ellen D., aged 25, was admitted into the London Fever Hospital July 28th, 1847. She was taken ill, July 24th, with headache, pain in the limbs and loins, rigors, succeeded by heat of skin; her bowels at the time were regular. Persons in the same house had suffered from ' fever.'

On the 6th day of disease, slept badly, and at 8 A.M. was delivered of a male child. About 12 A.M., headache; mind natural;

tongue coated; bowels open; thirst; little cough; no pain in the chest; pulse 120; skin hot and dry; no spots. Simple saline mixture every four hours.

7th day.—Pulse 120; tongue dry and brown; three stools; skin hot.

8th day.—Pulse 120; appears very prostrate; tongue coated; two stools; skin hot.

9th day.—Pulse 72, soft; skin cool, moist; slightly yellow; very little prostration; tongue moist, slightly furred; three stools.

On the following day the woman appeared in all particulars well, and continued so till the 16th day, pulse 130; skin hot and dry; little sleep last night; tongue moist, slightly furred; three stools. Simple saline mixture every four hours.

17th day.—Pulse 120; skin very hot; tongue moist; two stools.

18th day.—Pulse 120; skin hot; tongue dry and furred; seven stools.

19th day.—Pulse 80. Convalescent.

In this case abortion occurred on the 6th day; the crisis on the 9th day the relapse on the 16th day; critical diarrhœa on the 18th day. The sudden fall in the pulse from 120, its rate on the 8th day, to 72 on the 9th day, and then its sudden rise again on the 16th day to 130, and as sudden fall on the 19th day to 80, is well worthy of note. In relapsing fever, as I before remarked, the degree of rapidity of the pulse is no indication of the amount of danger. This case illustrates the fact, that relapsing fever sometimes suddenly terminates with diarrhœa. Jaundice, trifling in amount, was observed for the first time on the day the primary attack ceased. In some cases pregnant women do not miscarry until the relapse. Death now and then occurs when women miscarry in this affection.

§ 13. STAGE OF RELAPSE OCCASIONALLY ABSENT.

Although relapse is the peculiar, it is by no means an invariable symptom of the fever under consideration. The following case is a good illustration of the fact:—

CASE LIL.—In a man aged 24 years—rigors—extreme vertigo—sense of weakness—sleeplessness—violent delirium

—*herpes labialis*—furred and dried tongue—redness of *velum* —quick pulse—jaundice—convalescence on from the 10th to the 12th day—*No relapse.*

William D., aged 24, dark skin and hair, strong-made, moderately stout, a dealer in iron, brother to John D., Case XLII., and to Peter D., Case XLIII., was admitted into the London Fever Hospital, November 8th, 1849. On Tuesday morning, November 5th, just before leaving his bed he was seized with rigors, followed by heat and sweating. He subsequently got up and went to work, but about 11 A.M. he fell ill and the rigors returned; he tried again to work, but at half-past one A.M. he was so cold that he lay down on the boards before a large fire, and after an hour or two he became warm, and there was no return of the rigors. By 3 P.M. he was unable to walk a very short distance without the aid of two men, and then, as he described it, 'he staggered like a drunken man' from extreme giddiness and weakness. He took to his bed the same afternoon, and then had a dose of aperient medicine, which acted powerfully; the purging continued till his entrance into the hospital. He suffered much from frontal headache; 'could scarcely open his eyes,' no epistaxis; no vomiting.

William D. was a man of very intemperate habits. He drank indiscriminately beer, gin, or rum; as he expressed himself 'nothing came amiss.' He ordinarily swallowed a gallon of porter during the day.

The first night he was in the hospital he slept a little, and at that time was free from delirium.

On the 10th of November, *i.e.* the 6th day of disease, I noted:— Has had no sleep since yesterday. Was very noisy last night; left his bed several times, and struggled with his nurse. Is still occasionally delirious; fancies his relatives were in the ward a few minutes since; yet he remembers past events accurately. Expression lively. A little frontal headache; no flush; complexion thick; conjunctivæ slightly injected; pupils natural; special senses normal. Leaves his bed without aid; but staggers when out of bed. Says he feels very weak. Complains much of vertigo.

A little herpetic eruption at the angles of the mouth and on the upper lip. Tongue dry and furred; very red at the tip; yesterday had pain in deglutition, none to-day; velum pend. palat. and uvula are deep dull red and very dry.

Six stools the last twenty-four hours. No tenderness; abnormal fulness, or resonance of abdomen; no vomiting; no appetite; much thirst; pulse 100; no cough; breath and heart sounds normal.

Skin warm, dry; no rose spots; no mulberry rash. It has a somewhat mottled aspect.

Head to be shaved. Chalk mixture 1 oz., with tincture of opium 10 drops, after every liquid stool. Simple saline mixture every six hours.

Soon after the visit he slept for about ten minutes. Towards evening he became very delirious, and during the night was extremely violent. He ran about the ward, and once even escaped into the courtyard. He then broke the window of the room in which he was placed. The hospital porter had to sit by his bed the whole night.

About 6 ozs. of beer and 70 drops of laudanum were given him during the night, and early the next morning 1½ oz. of gin and three-eighths of a grain of acetate of morphia.

At noon on the following day, i.e. the 7th day of disease, he was lying quietly asleep. He had passed no stool; his urine was dark and very turbid. There was a slight but very decided yellow tint of the whole skin. In about half-an-hour he awoke. His pulse was then 108, weak. There was constant delirium; he fancied he had been in the hospital five and a half days. The pupils were rather small; the conjunctivæ slightly injected. There was no trace on the skin of spots of any kind. Gin, 6 oz., calomel and opium of each a grain, every six hours, and a blister to the forehead. He refused the pill, and one-eighth grain acetate of morphia dissolved in gin was substituted for it.

8th day.—He slept last night from 11½ P.M. to 2½ A.M. He was delirious before and after sleeping; at times, however, he appears very sensible; yet he thinks everything offered to him to drink is poison. Is now (1 P.M.) lying quietly on his left side asleep; has passed two dark watery stools; urine very high coloured, loaded with bile; it contains no albumen. Skin deep yellow; has a bronzed hue.[1] No perspiration since admission.

Acetate of morphia, grain ¼, every eight hours; mustard poultice to the region of the liver; a scruple of strong mercurial ointment to be rubbed into the axilla night and morning.

9th day.—Was delirious all yesterday afternoon. About 6 P.M. he began to sweat, and perspired profusely for about 2½ hours; slept well all night, and a good deal to-day. There has been little, if any, delirium since yesterday afternoon.

Pulse 76; expression improved; skin and conjunctivæ very yellow; tongue dry, rough, yellowish, furred, very red tip and edges; two watery stools; herpetic eruption on lip, has formed a dry scab; sits up in bed with tolerable facility; surface of normal temperature. Has had 1 oz. gin and half pint of porter during the last twenty-four hours.

---

[1] Dr. Chomel pointed out this tint as being frequently observed in relapsing fever.

Omit the morphia; continue the mercury; porter, half a pint.

On the 10th day the pulse was only 72; the skin was of a less deep yellow bronze hue. He was not awake for more than an hour the whole day.

From this time he improved daily. On the 12th day the somnolence had disappeared, the yellowness of skin much less marked. On the 15th day he felt quite well. The jaundice had all but gone, his tongue was clean, and his appetite was good. There was no relapse.

The two brothers of William D. had relapsing fever. Both had distinct relapse; their cases (Nos. XLII. and XLIII.) have been detailed above (pp. 343, 344). Wm. D. had been exposed to the same cause as his brothers,—the illness of James D. commenced on the same day. In Wm. D., however, there was no relapse; the first attack was very severe; it was accompanied by jaundice. The suddenness of the onset of the disease, and the effect it at once exercised on the system at large is remarkable. In a few hours he required the aid of two men to assist him to reach his home, and he staggered like a drunken man. The slight herpetic eruption about the lip was not critical in his case. It was the ninth day before he was convalescent. The jaundice setting in, as it did, just before convalescence, is an important feature. If a case of this kind prove fatal, the bile is found after death to pass readily into the intestine. The violence of the delirium was singular. The patient, eluding the vigilance of the nurse, nearly escaped. He made his way, in his shirt only, into the courtyard of the hospital. The profuse sweat with which the disease terminated occurred on the 9th day, i.e. on a critical day.

Perhaps a better name than relapsing fever might have been framed to signify the disease here described, but I preferred adopting one already used by others who have given a faithful account of the disease in question. Moreover, the name expresses the feature, which, although not constant, is yet, *when present*, the most distinctive of the disease, especially as marking the difference between it and typhus fever, typhoid fever, and febricula.

The question has been raised as to the identity of relapsing and yellow fever. Dr. Cormack is the chief advocate of the supposed identity. The data for determining the problem appear to me to be wanting; for what are the symptoms of yellow fever? If we hold, with Sir William Pym, that there are several diseases confounded under the term yellow fever, with which is it that relapsing fever is to be considered identical?

The repetition of the rigors daily for two or three days in succession appears to approximate certain cases to intermittent fever.

§ 14. A SECOND RELAPSE OCCURS IN SOME CASES.

CASE LIII.—In a woman aged 45 years—rigors—headache —vertigo—vomiting—frequent pulse—furred tongue—bowels regular—*convalescence on the 12th day*—*relapse on the 18th day of disease*—rigors—hot and dry skin—frequent pulse— furred tongue—severe pains in the back and limbs—headache —slight jaundice—*convalescence with pain in limbs on the 22nd day. Second relapse on the 30th day*—rigors—frequent pulse—hot skin—increased cough—*permanent convalescence on the 35th day.*

Sarah S., aged 45, hawker, never free from cough, was suddenly seized on Friday, July 8th, 1848, with rigors, chilliness, frontal headache, and vertigo; her bowels at the time were regular. The rigors were repeated at intervals till she came under observation; she vomited on Friday, Saturday, and Sunday; she took to bed on the Saturday; she had no epistaxis.

On the 7th day she had a hot and dry skin; pulse 112; some headache and vertigo; furred tongue; she had passed two stools. The cough from which she suffered constantly when in ordinary health was troublesome; there was mucous rale and frothy expectoration.

On the 12th, she was convalescent.

She slept well during the night of the 17th day, but on the morning of the 18th day was attacked with rigors at the time I saw her.

Pulse 120; skin hot and dry; tongue moist, furred; two stools; complains much of pain in the back.

On the 19th day the pulse was 130; the pain in the back and limbs unabated in severity; the tongue moist and white; she had passed three stools.

She perspired on the night of the 20th day, but on the 21st

day the symptoms were as on the 19th day. She had passed a restless night, and I found her with pulse 120. Skin hot and dry; considerable headache. Tongue white and moist; nausea, and a little tenderness at the epigastrium. The skin was now faintly yellow. She sweated freely during the night, and on the morning of the 22nd day, I found her free from headache; pulse 96; skin cool; a little appetite; tongue moist, furred in the centre only.

23rd day, pulse 84; complains much of pains in the limbs. In two or three days she was again pretty well; but on the 30*th day of disease* she was again seized with rigors, and on the 31st day I noted:—Pulse 120; skin hot. Slept but little last night. Cough troublesome; some sonorous rale; sputa frothy, rather tenacious. Tongue moist and white; two stools.

During the five subsequent days the pulse ranged from 130 to 104. The cough continued very troublesome, and on the 33rd day had, at one point, a slightly rusty aspect. On the 35th day, the sputa were muco-purulent, and on the 38th day she was well; cool skin, quiet pulse, moist and clean tongue, and good appetite. A little cough remained.

The disease in Sarah S. deviated little from its ordinary course; convalescence was rather tardy in being established. Six days subsequent to the date when she was considered to be convalescent she relapsed. The pulse on the second day of the relapse was 130, offering another example of the little value of a rapid pulse as a ground of prognosis in the disease under which Sarah S. laboured. The second relapse, like the first, was accompanied by very frequent pulse. Primary bronchitis, with a pulse of 130 on the third day, would not have terminated as the second relapse did in the case under consideration on the 7th day. In the first relapse this woman was slightly jaundiced—a symptom of considerable diagnostic value.

§ 15. DEATH SUBSEQUENTLY TO THE TERMINATION
OF THE RELAPSE.

CASE LIV.—In a man aged 32 years—rigors—headache —pain in the limbs—vertigo—furred tongue—anorexia— rapid pulse—hot and dry skin—convalescence on the 11th day of disease.

Relapse on the 16*th day of disease*—rigors—rapid pulse—

loss of appetite—hot skin—vomiting—convalescence on the 22nd day—erysipelas of the head and face on the 35th day—death on the 47th day of disease. *After death*, a clot in the cavity of the arachnoid—slight opacity of the arachnoid—serosity beneath mucous membrane of epiglottis and adjacent parts—large firm spleen—mucous membrane of cæcum and colon thickened and grey—liver tough, dark, and coarse in texture—other organs healthy.

Alexander M'D., aged 32, of temperate habits, a ship steward, was admitted into the London Fever Hospital, June 17th, 1848, under the care of Dr. Southwood Smith. He stated that, after having slept out in the rain during the night of Monday, June the 12th, he was seized on the following day with rigors and headache. On Wednesday he suffered from pain in the back and limbs. His bowels at this time were regular. He took to his bed on Thursday, *i.e.* the third day of illness.

About two years before his present attack he had, while at Calcutta and Madras, dysentery, followed by liver complaint and dropsy.

On the 18th June, *i.e.* the 7th day of disease, the following notes were made:—'Slept at intervals during the night; sleep disturbed by dreams. Some headache; vertigo on assuming the erect position; mind and special senses normal; muscular powers little impaired; tongue furred, dry in the centre; much thirst; no appetite; two stools; slight tenderness of abdomen. Pulse 120; occasional cough; expectorates a little greyish frothy mucus. No pain in the chest; skin hot and dry; no spots.

Mist. salin. eff. Hydr. c. cretâ, gr. ij; pulv. ipecac. co., gr. vj., M. h.s.a.

Alexander M'D. continued to improve daily till the 23rd of June, *i.e.* the 11th day of illness, when his pulse was only 78, and appeared convalescent.

No further note was made till the 16th day, when he was attacked with rigors, followed by heat of skin, quick pulse, and loss of appetite.

On the 18th day the skin was hot, the pulse 108, and there was occasional vomiting.

By the 22nd day his pulse had fallen to 84, his appetite had returned, and he was again noted to be convalescent.

On the 35th day he was attacked with erysipelas of the head and face. He died on the 29th of July, *i.e.* the 47th day from the commencement of his illness, and the 25th after convalescence from the relapse.

The body was examined 6½ hours after death, the weather being temperate.

There was no *rigor mortis*. The integuments of the head, neck, and face were pale. A considerable amount of serosity was found in the subcutaneous cellular tissue of the same parts, but no trace of pus.

Head.—A little red serosity escaped from the cavity of the arachnoid. On dividing the *dura mater* a delicate film of coagulated blood lay on the surface of the arachnoid, covering the convex surface of the left hemisphere. Firm, old adhesions united the two layers of the arachnoid in the vicinity of the longitudinal fissure. The arachnoid itself was slightly opaque. There was no abnormal vascularity of the *pia mater*. A little colourless transparent serosity was found in the ventricles. The substance of the encephalon was firm, as in health.

Pharynx.—Its mucous membrane was pale and considerably elevated by a quantity of transparent yellow serosity, which occupied the meshes of the sub-mucous cellular tissue. Much similar fluid was found in the sub-mucous tissue at the base of the *epiglottis.*

Larynx.—The epiglottis itself, the arytæno-epiglottidean folds, and *chordæ vocales* were much thicker than natural; the *rima glottidis* was a mere chink. The mucous membrane between the epiglottis and the *chordæ vocales* was finely injected. A large amount of yellow serosity was found beneath the mucous membrane of the whole larynx.

The *right and left lungs* weighed respectively 15 and 12½ ozs.; they were perfectly healthy in appearance.

Several of the bronchial glands had passed into a state resembling dry mortar.

A few old adhesions united the pulmonary and costal *pleura* on either side.

The *pericardium* contained about ½ ozs. of transparent yellow serosity.

The *heart* weighed 9½ ozs.; its substance and valves were healthy in all particulars. A large firm clot was found in the right auricle and ventricle. A smaller clot on the left side.

The *liver* weighed 2 lb. 5½ ozs. It was dark in hue, abnormally tough. The lobules seemed large and the texture of the organ coarse.

The *gall bladder* contained a moderate amount of dark, thick, orange-coloured bile.

The *spleen* weighed 24½ ozs., and was adherent on all sides. The adhesions were old and firm. The substance of the organ was pale, and broke down with difficulty. The capsule was considerably thickened, especially about the centre of its convex surface.

2 A

The *pancreas* weighed 3½ ozs.; it was pale and firm; apparently healthy.

The *right kidney* weighed 6½ ozs.[1] Its capsule was thin, and separated with facility. On section the substance of the organ was dark in hue, but perfectly healthy in structure. There was no abnormal vascularity of the lining membrane of the pelvis.

The *left kidney* weighed 6¾ ozs. In other particulars it resembled the right.

The *urinary bladder* was distended, its. lining membrane pale, and in every respect normal.

The *œsophagus* was healthy in appearance; its mucous membrane had a purplish-violet hue inferiorly.

The *stomach* was contracted; very rugose. Its mucous membrane was mammillated throughout its whole extent. It was normal in consistence.

The *small intestines* were healthy in all particulars.

The mucous membrane of the *cæcum* was of slate colour; the ascending and transverse *colon* of a palish grey. The solitary glands were visible throughout, whiter than the surrounding membrane, each gland surrounded by a dark margin, and having a dark grey central point.

The mucous membrane of the *large intestines* generally was rather softer, and slightly thicker than natural.

This was a well-marked case of relapsing fever in a man aged 32 years. Vomiting was a prominent symptom in this, as in several of the previous cases. Although vomiting may and does occasionally occur in the course of both typhus and typhoid fevers, yet, compared with its frequency at the outset of the first attack of relapsing fever, and during the relapse, it is rare in the two former diseases. The erysipelas, from which the man died, commenced thirteen days after the termination of the relapse, and was probably in no way dependent for its origin on his previous state. There was no trace of disease of Peyer's patches, that is to say, the anatomical character of *typhoid 'fever* was absent; in fact, the case is here adduced to show that in mild cases of relapsing fever no serious lesion of the viscera is discoverable after death. The only structural change which could be referred to the preceding attack of relapsing fever was the large size of the spleen, and even that I think may with greater probability be

---

[1] On this, as on other occasions, the kidneys were weighed *without* their capsules.

considered to have been partly due to old disease and partly to the erysipelas, as a consequence or accompaniment. *In the acute febrile specific diseases generally, of which erysipelas is one, there is a tendency to enlargement of the spleen.* The importance of this fact pathologically has not, it appears to me, been sufficiently dwelt on by writers. The circumstances which determine this enlargement, and the laws which regulate it, are within the legitimate scope of pathological research. Louis' reasoning on his own observations, in *one* of these diseases, appears to warrant the conclusion, that the softening and increase in size are not the consequence of inflammatory action. As is common, if not constant, in erysipelas of the head and face, the fauces and, by continuity in *this case*, the larynx also became affected with erysipelatous inflammation. The tendency of that variety of inflammation to induce effusion of serosity, an event of no moment in the subcutaneous tissue, is, in this situation, a cause of death.

The grey hue, and thickened state of the mucous membrane of the large intestines, studded with the abnormally visible solitary glands; the tough and coarse-grained condition of the liver, and the old disease of the spleen, *i.e.* its thickened capsule and trabeculæ, and firm, pale adhesions, were doubtless the remains of the ' dysentery and liver complaint' from which Alexander M'D. had suffered at Calcutta two years before his entrance into the hospital.

§ 16. SUDDEN COLLAPSE.

Relapsing fever occasionally terminates in sudden collapse—this may occur during the primary or secondary attack. Death, under these circumstances, takes place with fearful rapidity. Between such cases and some detailed in these papers there is as much apparent difference as there is between English and Asiatic cholera.

§ 17. DEATH DURING THE PRIMARY ATTACK.

CASE LV.—In a female aged 15 years—rigors—headache
—pain in the limbs—nausea—vomiting—furred tongue—
quick pulse—slight cough—sleeplessness—delirium—epistaxis—somnolence—*death* on the 12th day of disease.

Thirty hours after death.—Moderate cadaveric rigidity—
large liver—large spleen—other organs healthy.

Ellen F., aged 15 years, a female servant, was admitted into
the London Fever Hospital, May 11th, 1847, under the care of
Dr. Tweedie.　On Thursday, May 6th, she was seized with rigors,
headache, pain in the back and limbs, nausea, and vomiting; her
bowels were regular at that time.

May 12th, *i.e. 7th day of disease.*[1]—Complains of headache;
slept well last night; mind natural; tongue coated in the centre,
red at the tip and centre; two stools; no appetite; some thirst;
no tenderness of abdomen; pulse 112.　Some cough and mucous
expectoration; a little sibilous rale; no abnormal dulness of
thorax; skin warm, free from spots.

A blister was applied to the chest, and a mixture containing a
small quantity of tartar emetic ordered.

On the 8th day of disease I noticed that she had had no sleep
the preceding night; had been and was still delirious; had
repeatedly attempted to leave her bed, for the purpose of wandering about the ward; the headache was gone; profuse epistaxis
had occurred subsequently to the visit on the 7th day, and again
on the 8th day; in all about 1½ pints of blood had been lost.　She
had passed three stools.　Cold was applied to the head.

On the *9th day of disease* she was asleep when I visited the
ward.　She was reported to have passed a quiet night, and to have
had three stools.

On the 10*th day of disease* I noted, 'Slept but little last night;
complains of sense of prostration; mind wanders occasionally; is
at present perfectly conscious of everything around; pulse 120;
cough and abnormal physical chest signs trifling; tongue covered
with dry fur; three stools in bed.

11th day.—Expression dull; sleeps much and heavily; conscious when aroused; pulse 136; three stools; one of them in
bed; no spots.

A blister was applied to the forehead.　4 ozs. of wine ordered
to be given in divided doses during the succeeding 24 hours, and
a draught, with carbonate of ammonia, every 4 hours.

[1] The note on this day was made by my friend Dr. Sankey.

On the following morning she died.

The body of Ellen F. was examined thirty hours after death, the weather being temperate and dry.

The body was well made; the cadaveric rigidity moderate in amount; there was no appearance of decomposition. A layer of fat about 1 in. in thickness covered the abdominal muscles.

Head.—There was no abnormal injection of the pia mater; no excess of serosity beneath the arachnoid; the red points in the substance of the brain were not more numerous than usual. About 1 drachm only of serosity was found in the ventricles of the brain. The fornix and septum lucidum were of normal consistence; the velum interpositum transparent. In fact, the meninges and substance of the cerebrum and cerebellum were in *all* particulars perfectly healthy.

The *pericardium* contained a little yellow serosity. It was natural in all respects.

The *heart* pale, soft, and flabby, was in other points normal: it weighed 8½ ozs., a fibrinous clot stained purplish was found in the right auricle, ventricle, and pulmonary artery. There were no adhesions of, and no fluid in, either *pleura.*

The *lungs* were crepitant throughout, slightly darker posteriorly than anteriorly; the right weighed 19 ozs., the left 15 ozs. They were quite healthy in appearance.

The *bronchial mucous membrane* was somewhat redder than natural, but of normal consistence.

The *bronchial glands* healthy in aspect.

The *peritoneum* was healthy in all respects.

The *liver* weighed 4 lbs. 2 ozs., *i.e.* 66 ozs.; generally pale; the congestion of the separate lobules was hepatic. The liver cells, examined by the aid of the microscope, appeared healthy.

The *gall bladder* contained a considerable quantity of thin, golden-yellow bile. Its lining membrane was healthy.

The *spleen* was large; it weighed 12 ozs., and was somewhat firmer than ordinary.

The *pancreas* was flabby; it weighed 2¾ ozs.

The *kidneys* were pale and flabby, but in other respects normal.

The *uterus* was healthy; the ovaries contained several small cysts filled with transparent serosity.

In the *stomach* was a little gruelly-looking fluid. The consistence of the mucous membrane of the organ was natural; it was mammillated in the vicinity of the pylorus. The large vessels in the cardiac three-fourths were particularly large and distinct.

The mucous membrane of the *duodenum* was somewhat greyish in hue.

The *jejunum* and *ileum* were normal in colour, consistence, and thickness. There was no thickening nor trace of disease of any kind of Peyer's patches. The solitary glands at the lower part of ileum were distinct, but not morbidly so.

In the large intestine the solitary glands were somewhat more distinct than ordinary; the mucous membrane generally seemed healthy in all particulars.

At the time Ellen F. entered the hospital, relapsing fever was epidemic; she presented all the symptoms of the primary attack of that disease. Vomiting occurred at the outset; epistaxis on the 7th and 8th days, *i.e.* at a time when it often appears critical. The bronchitis present on the girl's entrance into the hospital was trifling in amount. There was no trace of the mulberry rash of typhus, nor of the rose spots of typhoid fever.

The large spleen and liver, the absence of cerebral and pulmonary congestion, and the generally healthy condition of the other organs, *i.e.* taken in conjunction with the symptoms, rendered the nature of the disease of which Ellen F. died unquestionable.

The frequency with which nasal hemorrhage occurs in several of the acute specific blood diseases, and the large size of the spleen in a large number of cases of the same affections, are facts of considerable interest—whether they are in any way related, and, if so, the relation that they bear to each other, is worthy of investigation.

§ 18. DELIRIUM OCCASIONALLY THE MOST PROMINENT SYMPTOM IN THE RELAPSE.

Case LVI.—James S., aged 30, was admitted into the London Fever Hospital, November 6th, 1846, under the care of Dr. Southwood Smith; he had been ill four days.

His pulse on admission was 104; the skin hot and dry; diarrhœa, which seemed critical, occurred on the 7th day; and on the 8th his pulse was only 60, his skin was cool, and he appeared convalescent.

James S. continued well till the 16th day, when he was suddenly attacked with vomiting, and in the night became delirious, ran about the ward, endeavoured to turn other patients out of their beds, announced in loud terms that he was a member of the swell-mob, and, in proof, attempted to abstract the watch of one of his medical attendants. On the following day, although his manner was still agitated, his pulse was only 74. He was not permanently convalescent till about the 21st day from the outset of the illness.

§ 19. RELAPSING FEVER IN 1850.

The larger number of the cases of relapsing fever narrated in these papers were collected in 1847, when that disease was epidemic. However, I have already given the histories of three cases, which occurred in 1846, 1848, and 1849 respectively. I shall now subjoin the cases of two boys and their father, admitted into the hospital in 1850, to show that, although this affection was more common in 1847 than at present,[1] it retains to-day all its characteristic features unchanged.

CASE LVII.—In a boy aged 8 years—sudden illness— headache—frequent pulse—furred tongue—*convalescence on the 7th or 8th day.*

Relapse on the 14th day of disease—headache—frequent pulse—hot skin—vomiting—confined bowels—permanent convalescence on the 17th day of disease—accompanied for some days by an irregular pulse.

Robert N., aged 8, a pale, thin child, was admitted into the London Fever Hospital, September 25th, 1850, under the care of Dr. Tweedie. Two years since he had ' the fever;' all the family had it at the same time.

On the Saturday preceding his admission, September 21st, after going to his bed, he was seized with headache, and did not leave his bed after; he took some senna tea, which acted freely the next day.

On September 25th, *i.e.* 5th day of disease, I noted as follows:— 'Expression natural; mind normal; conjunctivæ pale; pupils natural; is unable to walk without aid; tongue moist, furred; no stool to-day; no abnormal fulness, resonance, nor gurgling of abdomen; no tenderness of the same; pulse 120; no cough; no abnormal physical chest signs; skin cool; no mulberry rash; no rose spots; numerous small crimson spots on thorax and abdomen, unaffected by pressure (flea-bites ?).

[1] This was written in November 1850; and it was further pointed out, that during the month of October, several cases of relapsing fever were admitted into the hospital.

Ol. ricini. ʒij.

6th day.—Pulse 90 ; skin cool ; sleeps well ; tongue moist, clean ; two stools.

7th day.—Pulse 80 ; feels well ; no appetite ; three stools.

9th day.—Pulse 72 ; appetite good ; one stool.

On the 14th day of disease I noted, 'Early this morning he awoke one of the patients, crying with headache. He was quite well when he went to bed. The nurse saw him at 11 P.M. ; she paid especial attention to him, because relapse was anticipated.'

At the time of the visit: Pulse 124 ; skin hot ; face flushed ; tongue moist, very slightly furred ; three stools the last twenty-four hours ; no vomiting ; has had no rigors and no chilliness.

15th day.—Pulse 120 ; skin hot, dry ; sleeps much ; tongue moist, white ; no stool since yesterday ; no abnormal fulness, resonance, nor tenderness of abdomen.

Ol. ricini, ʒij. st. sum.

16th day.—Pulse 112 ; skin warm and dry ; sleeps well ; no headache ; no delirium ; vomited twice last evening ; tongue moist, white ; no stool.

17th day.—Pulse 64 ; skin cool ; no sweating ; tongue moist, white ; vomited once yesterday after the visit.

Hyd. chlorid. gr. ij. ; pulv. scammon. gr. vi., M. st. sum.

18th day.—Pulse 56 ; skin cool ; two solid stools ; appetite good.

19th day.—Pulse 60, irregular in frequency ; no stool ; tongue moist, white.

20th day.—Pulse 54 ; tongue moist, clean ; one stool ; good appetite.

22nd day.—Pulse 54, irregular in frequency ; no stool ; appetite good ; well.

The sudden rise in the pulse, at the outset of the relapse, to 124, and its sudden fall from 112 on the 16th day to 64 on 17th day, is worthy of note. No critical discharge appears to have marked either the termination of the primary attack or of the relapse. Irregularity in the frequency of the pulse at the termination of the relapse is occasionally observed ; I do not remember, however, another case in which it occurred in a very young subject.

CASE LVIII.—In a lad aged 17 years, sudden illness—slight headache—sense of weakness—frequent pulse—nausea—tenderness of epigastrium —vomiting of green fluid—slight jaundice—*convalescence 8th day.*

Relapse on the 16th day—hot and dry skin—frequent pulse—slightly furred tongue—vomiting of yellow fluid—*permanent convalescence on the 19th day.*

James N., aged 17, a hawker, thin and fair, the brother of Robert N., had 'the fever' at the same time with the other members of his family, *i.e.* two years since. Admitted into the London Fever Hospital September 25th, 1850, under the care of Dr. Tweedie. On the Saturday preceding his admission, bowels confined at the time of attack.

On September 25th, *i.e.* the 5th day of disease, I noted:—' Expression natural, conjunctivæ pale, pupils normal; no mental aberration; slight headache (*at vertex*); feels very weak, but is able to walk with a little aid; tongue moist, furred, white; no stool for twenty-four hours; no appetite; some thirst; pulse 96; no cough; no abnormal physical chest signs; skin cool; no mulberry rash, no rose spots; no crimson spots (*flea-bites*) *i.e.* such as seen on his brother Robert N.,' Case LVII. Ol. ricini, ʒij. st. s.

6th day.—Pulse 100; skin rather hot; slept well; frontal headache; tongue the same; nausea; some tenderness at epigastrium; three stools.

7th day.—Pulse 72; skin cool; no spots; no sweating; conjunctivæ rather yellow; complexion sallow; vomited some green fluid several times during the night; slight tenderness of the epigastrium; two watery stools; appetite returning.

8th day.—Pulse 66; no vomiting; appetite trifling; no stool; tongue cleaning.

9th day.—Pulse 56; skin cool; no sweating; faint sallowness of conjunctivæ; tongue moist; still slightly furred; two stools; no appetite.

10th day.—Pulse 70; skin natural; no sweating; tongue moist, clean; no stool for twenty-four hours. Ol. ricini, ʒij. mane sum.

11th day.—Pulse 96; four stools; appetite returning.

12th day.—Pulse 60; skin natural; tongue clean; appetite good; no stool.

13th day.—Pulse 60; two stools.

15th day.—Pulse 52; tongue clean, and otherwise as before.

16th day.—Pulse 96; skin hot and dry; slept well; tongue moist, slightly furred; appetite good; no spots of any kind on the skin. Ol. ricini, ʒij., st. sum.

17th day.—Pulse 84; skin rather hot; tongue same; one stool; appetite good.

18th day.—Pulse 108; skin hot and dry; tongue the same; no stool. Ol. ricini, ʒiij., st. sum.

19th day.—Pulse 64 ; skin natural ; slept but little ; vomited three times yesterday much yellow fluid, before the oil was administered ; tongue moist, white, thickly furred ; four stools.

20th day.—Pulse 54 ; slept well ; tongue cleaner ; no vomiting ; two stools.

22nd day.—Pulse 54 ; skin natural ; no stool ; tongue clean ; appetite good ; no vomiting.

The pulse fell between the 6th and 7th days twenty-eight beats ; between the 15th and 16th days it rose forty-four beats. Had this case not been watched carefully the relapse might not have been observed till the 18th day ; at that time, a pulse of 108, hot and dry skin, and repeated vomiting of yellow fluid, would have fixed the attention of the most inattentive. On the following day the pulse had fallen to 64, i.e. forty-four beats ; and on the 20th day, the frequency of the heart's action was only half that it presented on the 18th day.

Trifling jaundice, i.e. sallowness of the skin, and a more decidedly yellow hue of the conjunctivæ, were observed on the 7th day of disease.

This boy presented no trace of those little crimson spots, the exact nature of which is yet matter for inquiry.

Who can doubt that if this lad had been bled, or that if any favourite specific had been administered to him on either the 7th or 18th days of disease, that the marked diminution in the frequency of the pulse, and the general improvement on the 8th and 19th days, would have been attributed to the remedies employed. Oh, the pitfalls that everywhere lie hidden for the therapeutist ! Surely *he* need keep fast hold on the thread of rigid induction.

Case LIX.—In a man, aged 41—nausea—loss of appetite —rigors—chilliness—vomiting of yellow fluid—headache— skin sallow—conjunctivæ yellow—furred tongue—enlarged spleen—*convalescence by the 8th day.*

Relapse on the 16th day of disease—pain in the limbs— hot skin—white tongue—nausea—retching—profuse sweating—miliary vesicles—frequent pulse—permanent *convalescence on the 20th day of disease.*

James N., aged 41, a fair, thin man, of tolerably temperate

habits (two pints of porter daily), by trade a carman, was admitted into the London Fever Hospital, October 12th, 1850, under the care of Dr. Tweedie. He had been residing at 2 Smith's Court. In 1847, he had, at the same time, with other members of his family, an attack of 'the fever;' since then he had enjoyed the best of health.

On Sunday, October 6th, while in the act of sitting down to take tea, he felt nausea; lost his appetite. Slept well on Sunday night. On Monday, on first rising, he felt a cold chill around his loins, and general sense of illness. At this time his bowels were rather confined. He went to work, and while so engaged was attacked with cold chills and rigors. In the evening he had some medicine, after which he vomited much yellow fluid. On Monday night he took to his bed. From that time till admission he suffered from frontal headache, hot skin, alternating with chills.

The following notes were taken.—

October 13th, i.e. the 8th day of disease.—States that he was much worse the day before, than on that of his admission into the hospital, and the nurse says he was then much worse than at the present time.

Slept from 12 last night till 4 A.M.; mind clear; complexion sallow; conjunctivæ yellow, cheeks slightly flushed; can walk unaided, but feels rather weak; tongue moist, large pale, loaded posteriorly; no tenderness of epigastrium; no appetite; no nausea; no stool for three days; splenic dulness seven fingers' breadths vertically; no abnormal fulness, resonance, or tenderness of abdomen.

Pulse 72, soft; no cough; no abnormal physical chest signs.

Skin cool, damp; no mulberry rash nor rose spots; numerous hemorrhagic points, purple, unaffected by pressure, with well-defined edges (flea-bites?).

Ol. ricini, ʒiij. st. s. Mist. acid. sulph.

14th October, i.e. the 9th day.—Pulse 72; skin natural temperature; tongue clean; three stools; less sallowness; no miliary vesicles.

On the 17th October, i.e. the 12th day, his appetite was good, and on the 18th a note was made that his pulse was 72, and his bowels regular. He was now very anxious to be allowed to get up, as he felt quite well.

On the 19th October, i.e. the 14th day, his bowels acted, and he seemed on the following day as well as ever; he was not, however, allowed to leave his bed. His diet consisted only of beef-tea, bread, and rice-pudding.

At 3 A.M. on the morning of the 21st October, i.e. the 16th day of disease, he awoke with pain in the legs and back, and did not sleep after; he had neither rigors nor headache; there was some nausea; he felt very hot; and in the morning the skin was hot, the tongue white, and he complained of great sense of weakness. There was now loss of appetite, and he kept his bed all day; he retched much in the afternoon, ejecting, however, only a little white frothy fluid.

At 10½ A.M. a dose of castor oil was administered; it acted once half an hour after it was taken, and again in the evening. About 5 P.M. he broke out into profuse sweat; the clothes and sheets were quite wet through. He then slept from 10 P.M. till near 1 A.M., and after 1 A.M. felt quite comfortable and well; the pains, he said, all left him.

22nd October, i.e. 17th day of disease, 8½ A.M.—Pulse 96; skin warm, dry; a few miliary vesicles on groins; no stool since last evening; no nausea; tongue white and moist, thickly furred; no pain in limbs; spleen 5 inches vertically; no yellowness of skin.

On the 23rd October, i.c. the 18th day of disease.—Slept none; no delirium; no local pain; feels very low; expression dull and rather anxious; sweated a little last night; no miliary vesicles; vomits everything he takes; no green fluid; constant nausea; belly soft, not tender; skin hot and dry; no stool; leaves bed unaided with difficulty. A saline aperient draught, some saline effervescing draught; a simple enema, and a mustard poultice to the pit of the stomach were prescribed.

On the 19th day.—Pulse 96; passed a restless night; slept about one hour; says he sweated about the head last night, not elsewhere; tongue moist, loaded; seven stools, watery (after draught). Vomited occasionally until this morning; no vomiting to-day. The mustard poultice has left a deep stain, studded with dark crimson points, unaffected by pressure.

25th October, i.e. the 20th day of disease.—Pulse 84; no local pain; slept well; feels nearly well; no vomiting; tongue clean; one stool; sweated last evening for an hour about head and face; spleen 2½ fingers' breadth.

On the 21st day he was regarded as convalescent.

This man, James N., was father to the two boys, Robert and James N., i.e. the two immediately preceding cases. Like his two sons, James N. had relapsing fever; all three had probably been exposed to the same cause, and all three had the same disease,—the father subsequently to the sons. Moreover, a man, who removed the children to the workhouse before they were sent to the hospital was, at a later period, admitted into the latter, labouring under the same disease as James N. and his sons. This man did not reside in the house of the N.'s; but he lived in the same court—one of the London Fever Preserves.

With reference to James N., father, he was evidently just convalescent from the primary attack when I saw him on the 8th day of the disease. He was exceedingly ill for two days during the relapse, certainly worse than the notes appear to represent him. James N., sen., was kept in bed after the 9th day of disease, simply because I was anxious that no cause, such as exposure, error in diet, etc., should interfere with the natural course of the disease. In spite, however, of every precaution, he relapsed. The disease ran precisely the same course in the father and the elder son; they were both convalescent from the first attack on the 8th day of disease; both relapsed on the 16th day; and in both permanent convalescence was established on the 19th or 20th days. Both, also, it is worthy of note, were slightly jaundiced towards the termination of the primary attack. In the younger child primary convalescence was noted on the 7th or 8th day; relapse occurred a little earlier than in the father and elder brother, i.e. on the 14th day instead of the 16th day; and permanent convalescence was established by the 17th day, instead, as in their cases, by the 19th or 20th day.

Cases such as these (and I have seen very many similar during the last two months)[1] must, I think, satisfy the sceptical of the existence of relapsing fever as a disease distinct from typhoid or typhus fever.

James N., and his two sons, had fever two years before their present illness. The species of fever from which they suffered at that time could not, of course, be ascertained. It is clear, from the evidence of others, that relapsing fever not unfrequently affects the same individual a second time, and that sometimes even within a few months after the termina-

---

[1] Note of November 1850. I may here state, that I have not seen, during the past year, a single exception to the law that when more than one person suffers from typhus, typhoid, or relapsing fever, in consequence of exposure to a common cause, they all suffer from the same fever. Several families have lately been admitted into the hospital, every member suffering with relapsing fever. For analysis of cases occurring anterior to November 1849, see *Trans. Med. Chir. Society*, vol. xxxiii. (*supra*, p. 149).

tion of the first attack. Dr. Christison—then Mr. Robert
Christison—when clinical clerk to Dr. Welsh, is stated by
that physician, in his work on the epidemic of 1817 and
1818, to have suffered twice from the disease under consideration. In this particular, relapsing differs from typhus
and typhoid fever.[1] Moreover, it is to be borne in mind,
that an attack of either of the three fevers has no effect in
protecting a person from an attack of the others. Dr. Bartlett
details cases in which typhoid and typhus fevers affected the
same individuals in succession. Several examples of typhus
fever following relapsing fever, and *vice versa*, are mentioned
by the various historians of the Scotch epidemic of relapsing
fever of 1843.[2]

The subjoined case will illustrate the facts, that an attack
of typhus fever does not protect an individual from relapsing
fever, and that an attack of relapsing fever is no protection
against typhus fever.

CASE LX.—In a man, aged 25 years—vertigo—pains in
limbs — headache — confined bowels — vomiting — *convalescence on the 8th day—relapse on the 16th day of disease*
—rigors—frequent pulse—hot skin—furred tongue—headache—vomiting—severe pain in the limbs—permanent *convalescence on 18th day of disease.*

Edward B., aged 25, a labourer, was admitted into the London
Fever Hospital, December 1st, 1847, under the care of Dr.
Tweedie. On Friday, November 26th, he was attacked with
vertigo, pains in the limbs, slight rigors, and headache. His
bowels had been confined the two preceding days; he vomited for
the first time the day before his admission. He took to his bed
on the fourth day of illness, because he felt too weak to keep
about.

On the 7th day of disease.—A little headache; vertigo; unpleasant taste (fishy) and sense of disagreeable odour; other

---

[1] I have before referred to and illustrated the fact, that typhoid fever
may relapse; but such cases, as far as my experience reaches, are rare. [I
saw a case since these papers were published which relapsed three times,
and finally recovered.—*Note* 1893.]

[2] See Dr. Henderson's paper in the *Edinburgh Medical and Surgical
Journal* for 1843. On the Epidemic of 1843, by R. Cormack, M.D. On the
Scotch Epidemic Fever of 1843, by R. Wardell, M.D.

special senses normal; intellect unaffected; expression natural; strength slightly impaired, but he can walk unaided; complains of some pain in the shoulders and hips; tongue moist and covered with thin white fur; two stools; appetite good; no abnormal fulness, resonance, nor tenderness of abdomen; pulse 70; a little cough; trifling muco-purulent expectoration, some sonorous rale heard on deep inspiration; skin cool; no spots of any kind.

On the following day his pulse had fallen to 60, his tongue was clean, and there was no headache and no vertigo.

On the 16th day I found that he had shortly before I saw him been seized with rigors; his pulse was 120, skin hot, tongue furred, bowels confined, and there was a little nausea. He was complaining of severe headache. Half an ounce of castor oil was ordered to be given directly.

17th day of disease.—Pulse 120; headache rather less severe; rigors were repeated yesterday evening, and he had little sleep last night, tongue moist, furred; one stool; has vomited once; nausea; pain and tenderness at the epigastrium; *complains of much pain in the limbs*; head to be shaved; a mustard poultice applied to the epigastric region, and some simple saline effervescing mixture given every four hours.

18th day.—Pulse 60; skin cool and moist; little headache; slept but little last night; tongue as yesterday; no stool; less nausea; no vomiting; no tenderness at the epigastrium.

19th day.—Pulse 60; no headache; two stools; tongue clean. The man was now convalescent, and in a few days he left the hospital well.

On the 19th of January 1848, he was re-admitted with typhus fever, and had mulberry rash; from this, also, he eventually recovered.

Edward B., on his admission, was evidently recovering from some slight ailment. The pains in the shoulders and hips, seeing that his pulse was only 70, and that he evidently had been suffering much from general disturbance of the system, and that his illness commenced with vomiting, might perhaps have raised a suspicion as to the nature of his disease; all doubt was removed by the relapse. The pain in the limbs, although considerable, was not so long continued as it is in many cases, and was perhaps less severe; not unfrequently it is a most distressing symptom.

Two boys, aged respectively 13 and 19 years, brothers, were admitted into the hospital in 1849 with well-marked typhus fever. The elder died of erysipelas which supervened during early convalescence; the younger recovered. Both had been inmates of the hospital in 1847. At that time both had equally well-marked relapsing fever.

FEBRICULA.

§ 20. TYPICAL CASES OF FEBRICULA.

CASE LXI.—In a lad aged 15 years—severe headache—loss of appetite—vomiting—slight epistaxis—vertigo—furred tongue—pain in abdomen—frequent pulse—*convalescence on the 7th day of disease.*

John K., aged 15, a plasterer, had enjoyed health till he was attacked, without known cause, on first waking, May 7th, with severe headache and loss of appetite; in the course of the day he had some pain in the abdomen, his bowels were at this time confined; he vomited several times. On May 9th, while in the act of vomiting, he lost a little blood from the nose. Two pills taken on this day acted on the bowels. There had been no rigors, and no pain in the back. He had attended at a dispensary till his admission into the hospital, May 11th, 1848, under the care of Dr. Tweedie, on which day he walked from Whitecross Street to the hospital, a distance of about a mile and a half.

The following notes were made :—

May 12th, *i.e. the 6th day of disease.*—Some headache; vertigo in the erect position; mind and special senses normal; slight heaviness of expression; feels weak, but is able to leave his bed unaided.

Tongue moist, covered with thick white fur; no appetite; no thirst; complains of occasional pain in the abdomen; has passed one scanty, hard stool; pulse 96; physical chest signs normal; skin hot, no rash.

7th day of disease.—Pulse 84; a little appetite; two stools; otherwise as yesterday.

8th day of disease.—Pulse 60; tongue clean; appetite good; three stools.

CASE LXII.—In a man aged 18 years—frontal headache—pain in the limbs—rigors—slightly relaxed bowels—sleeplessness—vertigo—frequent pulse—hot skin—*convalescence on the 6th or 7th days.*

Thomas M., aged 18, a healthy man, a labourer, was admitted

into the London Fever Hospital, May 19th, 1848, under the care of Dr. Tweedie.

On Wednesday, May 17th, after sleeping in the streets for four nights, in want of food, etc., he was attacked with severe frontal headache, pain in the limbs, rigors, and slight relaxation of the bowels. He did not take to bed till his entrance into the hospital.

The following notes were made :—

May 20th, *i.e., the 4th day of disease.*—Severe frontal throbbing headache, sometimes so severe that it appears to take his sight away; little sleep; bitter taste in the mouth; mind normal; vertigo in the erect position, so that he is unable now to leave his bed without assistance; cheeks flushed; tongue moist, white; much thirst; little appetite; no stool; no pain nor tenderness of the abdomen; pulse 120; physical chest-signs normal; skin hot and moist; no trace of mulberry rash or rose spots.

5th day of disease.—Pulse 84; skin warm, perspiring freely. Slept well; little headache. Tongue as yesterday; three stools.

6th day no note.

7th day of disease.—Pulse 60; sleeps well; no headache; tongue moist, clean; appetite good; two stools.

CASE LXIII.—In a female aged 34 years—vertigo—head-ache—rigors—chilliness—heat of skin—pain in the limbs—loss of appetite—thirst—sleeplessness—frontal headache—frequent pulse—furred tongue—*convalescence on the 6th or 7th day of disease.*

Mary W., aged 34, a hawker, the mother of four children, but unmarried, was admitted into the London Fever Hospital, August 14th, 1847, under the care of Dr. Southwood Smith. She affirmed that her habits were temperate; that she had never been drunk in her life.

She had been 'tramping' lately, sleeping in common lodging-houses. She reached London for the first time the day her illness commenced. She entered the hospital on the first day of illness. I did not see her till the fourth day. Between the time of her admission and the date at which I saw her the following symptoms were present. Vertigo; headache; rigors; sense of chilliness frequently repeated; heat of skin; pain in the limbs; confined bowels; loss of appetite; extreme thirst; little sleep. She had taken shortly before admission half an ounce of sulphate of magnesia, which acted three times; on the next day an aperient powder and a senna draught were administered.

Aug. 17th, *i.e. 4th day of disease.*—Great frontal headache;

2 B

vertigo in erect position ; no *tinnitus aurium* ; no injection of conjunctivæ; no pain in the limbs ; mind natural ; slept but little last
night; tongue white and moist ; no stool to-day, several yesterday ; slight fulness of abdomen, said to be natural.

Pulse 120 ; no cough ; no abnormal physical chest-signs ; skin
warm ; no mulberry rash, no rose spots.

5th day of disease.—Little sleep, and that disturbed by dreams;
intense headache ; vertigo in erect position. Complains of a 'cold
shivering' sensation running through her every minute or two.
Tongue moist, covered with thick white fur ; much thirst.

6th day.—No note was made.

7th day of disease.—Slept well last night; no delirium; no
headache ; tongue cleaner; less thirst ; no appetite; pulse 72;
skin cool and moist. She reports that she perspired profusely
last night, since which she has felt much better. Complains, for
the first time since admission, of great pain in her joints when
they are moved. No swelling nor redness; the next day she
was well.

CASE LXIV.—In a woman, aged 20—headache—sense
of languor—vertigo—sleeplessness—delirium—headache—
pains in the limbs—tongue dry, furred, yellow—frequent
pulse—hot skin—trace of albumen in urine on the 8th day
—*convalescence on the 9th day of disease.*

Mary C., aged 20, a large-made, stout, fair woman, a domestic
servant, was admitted into the London Fever Hospital, August
13th, 1847, under the care of Dr. Southwood Smith. She was
a native of Roscommon, and had resided in London only four
months.

On August 9th, while engaged at the wash-tub, she was
suddenly seized with headache, and general sense of languor. On
the 10th she was unable to quit her bed on account of great
giddiness on assuming the erect position. So far as could be
ascertained, there had been, before she came under observation,
no epistaxis, no rigors, no abnormal affection of the special
senses.

From the outset she had slept but little ; the bowels, at first
confined, were subsequently relieved by medicine.

The following notes were made :—

August 15th, *i.e. the 7th day of disease.*—Has been very delirious
the last two nights, not sleeping at all ; slept a little this morning;
mind rambles on first waking; answers questions rationally;
memory appears good ; mind now quite natural ; severe headache;
vertigo ; no abnormal affection of the special senses ; pupils

natural; conjunctivæ injected; face slightly flushed; raises herself in bed without any aid; complains of severe pain in the hands and arms. Tongue dry and smooth, with yellow fur down the centre, edges moist; great thirst; no appetite; two relaxed stools; no tenderness of the abdomen; slight fulness; pulse quick; no cough; no abnormal physical chest-signs; skin hot and damp; no mulberry rash; no sudamina.

8th day of disease.—No sleep during the night; much noisy delirium; her head was shaved this morning; since then she has slept a little; pulse 84; skin cool; urine deep orange—specific gravity 1·016; it contains a very small quantity of albumen; no trace of lithates.

9th day of disease.—Some sleep last night; no delirium; no headache; gets in and out of bed unassisted; skin cool, moist; no spots of any kind; tongue moist, cleaning anteriorly, thickly furred posteriorly; pulse 72.

10th day of disease.—Slept well; no delirium; expression good; moves freely unaided; tongue moist, almost clean; no appetite; three stools; pulse 72; skin natural.

§ 21. GENERAL DESCRIPTION OF FEBRICULA.

Febricula is not contagious; it has no specific cause, but attacks an individual, sometimes after having exerted himself more than ordinarily, sometimes after slight excess, and frequently without known cause. It commences with rigors, generally slight, often imperfectly marked, yet occasionally severe. Chilliness, headache, pains in the limbs, and sense of fatigue follow, and these are soon succeeded by a hot and dry skin, frequent pulse, generally from 96 to 120, thirst, want of appetite, white tongue, slightly confined bowels, and drowsiness; in some cases, however, the patient sleeps but little; rarely in adults, more commonly in children, trifling delirium is observed on first waking from their restless slumbers. There is no cough, no abnormal physical breath or heart sounds; the abdomen is indolent, and preserves its natural degree of fulness and resonance.[1]

---

[1] An eruption is referred to by Duvasse, viz., that of the *taches bleuâtres* as present in some cases of febricula. This same eruption had been previously described as occasionally to be seen in cases of typhoid fever. Forget, of Montpellier, among others, had especially mentioned its occurrence in the latter disease. My own observations enable me to confirm the statements of these writers. I have seen the *taches bleuâtres* in both febricula and typhoid

These symptoms increase in severity for the space of three or four days; the rapidity of the pulse increases till it reaches from 100 to 120; at the same time it is full, hard, and perhaps bounding; the tongue is covered with a thick white fur; anorexia is complete; the bowels rarely act without medicine; the urine is scanty and high coloured; the face retains its normal expression, or it is slightly anxious and oppressed; there is rarely any prostration.

After the expiration of five, six, or seven days, the feverish symptoms disappear as suddenly as they began,—a critical discharge, a deposit of lithates, or a copious sweat, in many cases marks the moment when the patient regains his health.

The chief variations observed in the disease are, 1st, in the mode of attack,—thus, now and then it commences insidiously; and, 2ndly, in the duration, which in some cases is only two or three, but in rare cases is eight or ten days; in some cases the headache, in others the restlessness, and in others, again, pain in the limbs, as though the patients had been bruised, are the predominant symptoms, and give a complexion to the case. Epistaxis, the catamenial flow, and diarrhœa are now and then the evacuations which occur at the crisis. In some cases the disease terminates at once without any critical discharge; and in others it ceases so gradually, that the exact day on which the patient regains health cannot be fixed.

A herpetic eruption on the lips not unfrequently occurs at the time the general symptoms are about to abate.

---

fever. It is important to be acquainted with the characters of these spots, as the inexperienced may, in some cases, confound them with the mulberry rash, though ordinarily they are readily to be distinguished.

The *taches bleuâtres* do not pass through the same stages as the mulberry rash; they never present the characters of its first stage; they are from the moment of their appearance on a level with surface of the skin; they are irregular in outline, and are larger than the separate spots constituting the mulberry rash; they are unaffected by pressure, have a delicate bluish aspect, are of a uniform hue over their whole extent, and, in the few cases I have seen, were much less abundant than the spots of the mulberry rash. In one case, in which some doubt as to their nature was entertained, and which case I saw in consequence, they were nearly confluent about the groins and lower part of the abdomen, and might readily have been confounded with the true mulberry rash; the abdomen and back I believe to be their most frequent seat.

Febricula, uncomplicated, *is never 'fatal.* Local inflammations are occasionally set up in its course, and then either the local disease terminates with the general affection, or the critical evacuation terminates the fever, while the local lesion, excited and kept up by that condition of the system, terminates at the same time.

In such cases the order of events is as follows:—Rigors, chilliness, hot skin, frequent pulse, in a day or two inflammation—say of the substance of the lung—in a week from the outset a profuse sweat, followed by a sudden fall in the temperature of the skin, and in the rapidity of the pulse, and, consentaneously, by a marked improvement in the chest symptoms; the breathing is less oppressed, the cough less troublesome, perhaps almost disappears, the physical signs cease to make progress, the patient believes himself well, and is, in fact, very quickly restored to health. These are the cases which have misled many in estimating the value of remedies on the progress of inflammation of the lungs, etc., and have also led to the idea that a copious sweat, an attack of epistaxis, or a diarrhœa, has been the means of relieving a pneumonia, and, as a consequence, to the employment of remedies to procure sweating, etc., in pneumonia.

It is by no means an uncommon event for a patient to be sent into the hospital with a pulse of 72, a cool skin, and slightly furred tongue, and yet bringing with him a certificate to testify that he is labouring under severe fever, such certificate having been granted when the severity of the general symptoms warranted the expectation that the patient would be long ill.

The close relation, if not identity, of the symptoms present in the primary attack of relapsing fever, and those which occurred in the cases above described, as illustrative of febricula, must strike every reader, and the question naturally arises, How are cases of febricula to be distinguished from cases of relapsing fever in its first stage? and how are they, even eventually, to be separated from those cases of relapsing fever which do not suffer relapse? My answer is, that I know no absolutely distinctive feature; that my own observations do not enable me to afford an answer to this question. Doubtless, however, an analysis of a more careful collection of cases than that I have, might afford answer. The relative condition of the spleen ought to be made a subject of special research, and much light might also be thrown on the subject by investigations into the causes of the two groups of cases here described respectively under the terms ' relapsing fever ' and ' febricula.'

A fever lasting only about twenty-four hours has been described by medical writers under various names.[1] By some it has been regarded as a primary general affection; by others, the constitutional disturbance has been considered as simply indicative of local inflammation, or of local irritation, as it has been called. I propose to express, by the term febricula, that condition of the system which is manifested by a hot skin, a quick pulse, and white tongue, continuing from two to eight days, and, so far as our powers of observation go, unable to be referred to local disease as its cause.

If we take cases from the two extremes of the two groups, the distinction I have made between relapsing fever and febricula will be found a natural one, and if, symptomatologically or nosologically, they are unable in some cases to be separated, yet pathologically, using that word in its wide sense, the difference is evident. Thus, let us take the two following cases :—

CASE LXV.—A man, aged 24, moderately stout and strong-made, by trade a brickmaker, walked from the neighbourhood of Highgate to the hospital, with the aid of his wife. He had been working in the open field, exposed to an autumn sun; and six days before he came under observation had been attacked with headaches, chilliness, and pain in the limbs, his bowels being at the time regular. When he came to the hospital his skin was hot and dry; he was suffering from severe frontal headache; his conjunctivæ were slightly injected, so that his eyes had a somewhat ' ferrety look ; ' he could ; walk, but his gait was feeble and unsteady; he felt ill, and looked oppressed and somewhat anxious ; he could give a collected account of his past and present sensations. When put to bed he was restless, tossing about. His urine was scanty, clear, and high-coloured; his bowels had acted in the

---

[1] I would direct the reader's attention to a very excellent description of febricula by M. Duvasse, in an inaugural thesis, published in Paris in 1847. M. Duvasse considers what I have regarded as one affection to be divisible into two, viz., ephemera and synoque, but they appear to pass by insensible gradations into each other, to differ only in intensity.

morning; there was no desire for food, but considerable craving for fluids; no nausea, no vomiting, no abnormal fulness, resonance, nor tenderness of the abdomen; his tongue was covered with white fur, and was somewhat tremulous; his pulse was 100, full and of good power; there was no cough, no pain in the chest, no sonorous nor sibilous rale, no friction sound.

On the following day he felt almost well; the skin was of nearly normal temperature; the expression natural, the general strength improved; all pain in the head and limbs gone; the tongue was yet white, but the appetite had returned; the pulse was 80 only; the urine loaded with lithates. On the following day he was allowed to get up, and he continued well.

CASE LXVI.—A man, aged 24, strong-made, by trade a brick-layer, came under observation in August 1847. Admitted from a house whence two others had been removed with the same symptoms. Three days before he came under observation, he had been attacked with rigors, headache, pain in the back and limbs, nausea, and vomiting. On the 4th day of disease, hot and dry skin; jaundice; frontal headache; disturbed sleep; pulse 120; tongue white, moist; frequent vomiting of green fluid; bowels open; tenderness at epigastrium. On the 6th day, epistaxis; and on the 7th, profuse sweating; apparent convalescence, with cool skin and pulse of 60, on the 8th day. On the 15th day, rigors; severe pains in the back and limbs; headache; nausea; vomiting; loss of appetite; thirst; hot and dry skin; pulse 120; bowels open.

On the 19th day, profuse sweating; and on the 20th, permanent convalescence, with a pulse of 50 and a cool skin.

These two cases differ in cause; in the one the disease was attributable to over exertion under a hot sun: in the other to contagion; they differ also in symptoms, and they differ finally in their course.

Influenced, then, by cases such as these, I have been led to describe as different two affections, the non-identity of which, I confess, I am not absolutely prepared to *prove*.

GENERAL CONCLUSION.

Let me now briefly recapitulate the object of this essay, and the conclusions I have desired the reader to form.

The object was to illustrate, by cases collected at the bedside, the fevers commonly confounded under the term 'con-

tinued fever.' I say, commonly, for, although some writers
in this country have distinguished typhus fever from typhoid
fever; and others have distinguished relapsing fever from
typhus fever; and others, again, have separated febricula
from typhus fever, yet neither of these distinctions has yet
been drawn in any of the systematic works on medicine;
and no one, so far as I am aware, has formally stated his
belief that these four affections are as many distinct diseases;
as distinct from each other, that is to say, as are measles,
scarlet fever, and small-pox; the poison of the one being
by no combination of circumstances capable of producing,
inducing, or exciting the others.

The four diseases thus attempted to be separated from
each other may be briefly thus defined:—

Febricula.—A disease attended by chilliness, alternating
with sense of heat, headache, white tongue, confined bowels,
high coloured scanty urine, hot and dry skin, and frequent
pulse, terminating in from two to seven days, and having for
its cause excess, exposure, over fatigue, etc., *i.e.* the cause of
febricula is not specific.

Relapsing Fever.—A disease arising from a specific cause,
attended by rigors and chilliness, headache, vomiting, white
tongue, epigastric tenderness, confined bowels, enlarged liver
and spleen,[1] high-coloured urine, frequent pulse, hot skin,
and occasionally by jaundice, and terminating in apparent
convalescence in from five to eight days—in a week a relapse,
i.e. a repetition of the symptom present during the primary
attack.

After death spleen and liver are found considerably enlarged, absence of marked congestion of internal organs.

Typhoid Fever.—A disease arising from a specific cause,
attended by rigors, chilliness, headache, successive crops of
rose spots, frequent pulse, sonorous rale, diarrhœa, fulness,

[1] In my paper in the 33rd volume of the *Medico-Chirurgical Transactions*,
it is stated there are 'no abnormal abdominal signs' present in relapsing
fever (r. p. 142, *supra*). The error arose from my having been in the habit,
when taking notes of cases at the bedside, to use the above expression, to
signify for the sake of brevity,—no abnormal fulness, nor gurgling in the
abdomen. The rules of the Society did not permit writers to correct their
own papers for the press. Had I seen the paper, in proof I should not, I
think, have allowed the error to pass uncorrected.

resonance and tenderness of the abdomen, gurgling in the right iliac fossa, increased splenic dulness, delirium, dry and brown tongue, and prostration, and terminating by the 30th day. After death,—Enlargement of the mesenteric glands, disease of Peyer's patches, enlargement of the spleen, —disseminated ulcerations, disseminated inflammations.

Typhus Fever.—A disease arising from a specific cause, attended by rigors, chilliness, headache, mulberry rash, frequent pulse, delirium, dry brown tongue, and prostration, and terminating by the 21st day. After death.—Disseminated and extreme congestions; in young persons, enlargement of the spleen.

I do not mean to say that in every case of either of these diseases all the symptoms here enumerated will be present, or that, in many cases, other symptoms will not be super-added; but I give the above as the ordinary diagnostic characters of the diseases,—symptoms which, if present, leave no doubt on the mind of the observer of the name of the disease. Just as, if chilliness, succeeded by heat of skin and running from the eyes and nose, and harsh cough, should be followed, on the 4th day, by an eruption of port-wine red spots, arranging themselves more or less crescentically, and then the whole, of these symptoms should disappear on from the 7th to the 9th day of disease, no one would entertain a doubt that the patient was labouring under measles; and that, although measles may affect a person, and yet some of the above symptoms be absent; or although, in particular cases, additional symptoms may be present. I intend, then, the foregoing brief descriptions of febricula, relapsing fever, typhoid fever, and typhus fever, to apply to those diseases as much as, but no more than, the above description applies to measles.

As my object was simply to illustrate the different continued fevers of the country, it is only with reference to here and there a point; *e.g.* the frequency with which the mulberry rash is absent from individuals of different ages affected with typhus fever, that I have attempted to prove any of the statements I have made with reference to the frequency with which particular symptoms or lesions are present or absent, the invariable connection between certain symptoms and certain changes of structure, etc., etc.   At the same time, in some instances, the cases adduced prove the fact they illustrate; the case is at once the illustration and the proof; e.g. the two cases of simulated perforation of the intestine (pp. 303, 311).

At the outset I stated that I should touch but slightly on the question of treatment.   This was not from my undervaluing the usefulness of therapeutical agents in some of the diseases here illustrated, but rather because I felt that so much had been written on the treatment of fever,—so often had it been argued *post hoc propter hoc*,[1]—so greatly had some erred, it appeared to me, in substituting general impressions of the efficacy of drugs for rigid logical induction, that I determined to make few therapeutical assertions unsupported by that weight of argument in the shape of facts I knew I had it in my power to adduce in evidence; to arrange and to analyse those facts is a work of time, and the pages of a weekly journal are unsuited for their publication.   Such are the arguments that have influenced me in postponing the consideration of treatment—a subject so easy to write on, so difficult to discuss philosophically.   But this much I hope . the reader will have gathered from these papers, that henceforth, whether the therapeutics speak dogmatically in the loose and easy phraseology of general terms, or, having worked out his results by rigid induction, he lay before his reader the process by which he arrived at his conclusion, as well as the conclusion itself,—I say, whether he intends to load the literature of fever with another *ipse dixit*, or to add a truth to those which have been dug out by constant toil,—

---

[1] Let the reader refer to Dr. Welsh's book *On the Efficacy of Blood-letting in Fever*, and compare the cases contained in the appendix to that work—the larger majority of which are examples of relapsing fever—with the cases of relapsing fever narrated in this paper.   In the former, the pulse often fell after the blood-letting, and the patient rapidly regained his health ; in the cases I have given, as marked and as sudden improvement ensued within a week when no blood-letting was employed.   The pulse in my cases often fell in a few hours from 120 to 60.   Whenever in his cases the fall occurred after the loss of blood, Dr. Welsh attributed it to the loss of blood.   Relapse frequently occurred after blood-letting in the epidemic described by Dr. Welsh ; and it was forthwith argued that the relapse was the *consequence* of the blood-letting ; in the cases I have detailed relapses were frequent, and yet no blood-letting had been employed.

whichever be his purpose, he must distinguish from each other diseases having a different origin, a different course, different symptoms, and leading to or accompanied by different lesions, and not confound all under one common name because they possess in certain cases, as common symptoms, a brown tongue, frequent pulse, and loss of general power.

I cannot conclude without briefly adverting to the labours of others on the subjects embraced by them. As I said at their commencement, I lay no claim to originality. At the same time, *every statement I have made rests on my own observations.*

It would not be consistent with my object to enter into a lengthened account of the share taken by different observers in bringing our knowledge on the subject of fever to what appears to me to be its present comparatively advanced condition, but I will refer those who are desirous of learning the various steps by which we have gained our position, to Dr. Bartlett's work on *The Fevers of the United States*, and to Dr. Paterson's *Essay on the Epidemic Fevers of* 1847-8; to the former for a literary history of typhoid and typhus fevers, to the latter for a brief history of the relapsing fever; and finally, to M. Jules Duvasse's Thesis, Paris, 1847, for a history of febricula, termed by him *Fièvres Ephémère et Synoque.* These writers show pretty clearly that neither of the above four affections can be regarded as a new disease; that all have been frequently described, *now* as varieties of prevailing epidemics, and *now* as new diseases; and from my own researches into the histories of past epidemics of fever, I have no hesitation in averring my confident belief, that an explanation of the great difference observed by different historians in the progress, mortality, and lesions of fever,—the difference of opinion entertained as to its communicability by observers of unquestionable honesty of purpose and soundness of judgment,—that the difference of opinion expressed as to the admissibility of particular modes of treatment,—that an explanation, I say, of these differences is not to be sought in variations in a hypothetical epidemic constitution, but in the differences which exist in the essential nature of the four diseases commonly confounded under the term 'continued fever.'

ON THE ACUTE SPECIFIC DISEASES,

BEING THE GULSTONIAN LECTURES

DELIVERED AT THE ·

ROYAL COLLEGE OF PHYSICIANS OF LONDON

IN MARCH 1853

GULSTONIAN LECTURES

ON THE ACUTE SPECIFIC DISEASES.[1]

LECTURE I.

Necessity for analysis of observed facts—Sydenham on Acute Diseases—His classification of fevers—Epidemic constitution—Comparison of small-pox with measles— Analogies with plant life—The two main divisions of acute diseases having definite duration and attended by disseminated lesions—General symptoms—Rigors— Temperature of skin—Pain in back—Headache— Mental condition—Malaise—Pulse-rate—Influence of perspiration on pulse-rate—Local lesions—Cutaneous eruptions—Lesions of internal organs—Duration— Mode of determination—Its definite limit—Specific cause—Contagion—Pathological affinities.

SIR,—Among the *idola specûs*, the father of the inductive sciences ranked the tendency of some minds to fasten on the differences of things to the neglect of their agreements, and of others to perceive the agreements and pass by unheeded the differences—to divide where nature has drawn no line, and to generalise where nature has bestowed no unity.

Physicians, like other philosophers, have sometimes paid homage to these idols of the den; and, from their inability to resolve into their simple elements, the very complex phenomena they study, are peculiarly tempted by these—to use Bacon's figurative language—'seducing familiar spirits.'

To avoid the errors thus indicated, a review of the principles and facts that guide us in determining that a series of individual cases are really identical, and ought to be called by one name, or that a series of diseases ought to be grouped

---

[1] From the *Medical Times*, March and April, 1853.

into one class from a supposed relationship existing between
them, is from time to time, as our pathological knowledge
advances, essential.

And such a review is well suited to an occasion like this.
To prove the frequency of particular symptoms and lesions
of structure in any given disease, the duration and mortality of the same,—the influence on its course and termination, of age, sex, season, etc.,—the curative effects of various
remedial agents,—to prove any one of these, or any similar
points, an analysis of recorded observations is essential.
Mere enumeration can give a correct answer to the most
simple questions only; in reference to all others, a comparison of various enumerations, and an analysis of the items
used in the enumerations, are essential for the formation of a
correct conclusion.   But neither numerical analyses nor a
close examination of the facts used in the analyses can be
efficiently made in a verbal discourse; and it is for this
reason, therefore, that lectures are suited especially for the
dogmatic teaching of established doctrines, and for general
surveys of admitted facts and their relations.

Just as no two animals are absolutely alike, and no two
plants the same in all particulars, so no two cases of disease
are in all points identical.   Nature knows only individuals.
And yet, to use the words of the Preface, so replete with
wisdom, affixed by Sydenham to the third edition of his
Observations on Acute Diseases, 'it is necessary that all
diseases be reduced to definite and certain species, and
that with the same care which we see exhibited by botanists
in their phytologies; since it happens, at present, that many
diseases, although included in the same genus, mentioned
with a common nomenclature, and resembling one another
in several symptoms, are, notwithstanding, different in their
natures,and require a different medical treatment.' For the purpose of effecting this desirable division of diseases, Sydenham
laid down certain rules, which may be briefly stated thus :—

1st. Every physiological hypothesis must be laid aside.
'No man,' he remarks, 'can state the errors that have been
occasioned by these physiological hypotheses.'

2ndly. The clear and natural phenomena of the disease
should be noted. 'They should be noted,' he says, 'accu-

rately, in all their minuteness; in imitation of the exquisite industry of those painters who represent in their portraits the smallest moles and the faintest spots.'

3rdly. The peculiar and constant phenomena must be enumerated apart from the accidental and adventitious.

4thly. The season of the year in which the disease occurs ought to be observed; that is to say, the external conditions which may possibly cause the disease, modifications in the symptoms, local complications, etc., are to be considered.

Thus, Sydenham thought all diseases might be divided into definite species, and time has tended to confirm his opinion; for, by a close adherence to these rules, the existence of several species of the same class, and as well defined as the two he so sagaciously divided, and of which he gave such truthful descriptions, have been established. And the especial objects I propose to myself in the lectures I have had the honour of being appointed to deliver, are to point out what appears to me to be the real differences which separate these particular species from each other, and to indicate the true affinities of these same species to each other,—the grounds of their union into class, and the foundation of their division into species. And I choose this subject, in the *first place*, because I feel that it becomes a junior Fellow of the College to select for these lectures the subject of which his personal experience has been most extensive;—that he ought here to treat only of matters concerning which he may hope that his own knowledge is inferior to that of his hearers in a less degree than on any other; and, *secondly*, because it affords an opportunity, not only of pointing out the agreements as well as the differences of these species, but also of indicating the diseases which, in practice, have been often confounded with certain of them, and the diseases, on the other hand, for which some varieties of these species have been themselves mistaken—a confusion which has fostered the opinion, that the limits of these species are ill-defined, and their symptoms most variable.

It is from Sydenham that many of the leading ideas now current concerning the acute specific diseases are derived. He divided acute diseases into two great classes, viz., stationary and intercurrent fevers. The latter, he held, occurred at

2 c

particular seasons, and owed their origin to appreciable atmospheric changes,—e.g. temperature and moisture.

Pleurisy and quinsy were adduced by him as examples of this class. In the present day, the majority of the diseases arranged by Sydenham under the head of intercurrent fevers are believed to be essentially local affections, the constitutional disturbance or fever which accompanies them being regarded as symptomatic.

Of stationary fevers, Sydenham distinguished two kinds, viz., the typical or proper fevers, and the twin sisters of the typical or the variable fevers. The typical or proper stationary fevers preserved their essential characters through a series of years, only from time to time they varied in some particulars a little; and yet, ever amid the prevailing variety, cases in all points identical with the model or type of the disease occurred. Of these typical or proper stationary fevers, small-pox and measles were the best-defined species. In the epidemics of these diseases which Sydenham witnessed, both presented, for a while, deviations from what he considered to be their most perfect form; but still, notwithstanding these deviations, they preserved their *essential* characters. Sydenham never doubted the essential identity of the measles of the dysenteric constitution of 1669, 'the most perfect of their genus,' with those of 1674, which 'adhered less to their proper type.'

What I have termed Sydenham's second class of stationary fevers, was constituted by those diseases which, in the present day, have been termed continued fever. The diseases of this class he held to be most variable in all their characters, —varying in symptoms and in the treatment they required with each change in the constitution of the atmosphere, and, consequently, with each change in the prevailing epidemic.

By epidemic constitution, Sydenham signified some state of the atmosphere arising from ' certain hidden and inexplicable changes within the bowels of the earth,'—a condition originating, that is to say, neither in heat, cold, wet, nor drought,—a condition known to exist only by its effects in determining the origin, or spread, or peculiarity in symptoms, of any one of the stationary fevers, and of their ' twin sisters,' the variable fevers, which accompanied them. Now, the tendency of more recent investigations has been to remove the whole of the diseases included in the group of variable fevers into that of 'typical or proper' fevers,—to erect from the individuals of this class a series of distinct species.

Taking small-pox and measles as the type of the proper stationary fevers, I propose to examine what are the peculiarities of these two diseases which render them thus fitted to be the type of a class, and why they are separated from each other as distinct species; what general characters they have in common, and what are the special characters which divide them; what it is which constitutes their bond of union, and what are the grounds of their separation.

In both general constitutional disturbance precedes the occurrence of any local lesion; both are attended in their progress by local affections; both have a limited and definite course; and, from those suffering from either, a something capable of inducing a disease identical with itself in all essential points is evolved. The general constitutional disturbance is manifested by increase of temperature, rapidity of pulse, loss of muscular power, and sense of malaise. The great peculiarity of the local affection is its disseminated character.[1] Thus, inflammation of the skin commences in innumerable points unconnected with each other. Many parts of the mucous membranes suffer at the same time, not of one tract only, but of several; and that not by extension, but by the establishment of separate centres of diseased action. Organs at a distance from each other, and not known to be especially related, suffer simultaneously; the spleen increases in volume, the lymphatic glands enlarge, and the lungs are frequently inflamed at several points of their substance.

In both there is a more or less sudden commencement, and in both, after the lapse of a certain number of days, if the case be not fatal, restoration to health. The disease terminates usually on, and invariably before, a given day; while certain lesions appear at a fixed time after the outset of the constitutional disturbance.

[1] Quelques médecins ont comparé l'état de l'intestin (i.e. in typhoid fever) à celui de la peau dans les affections exanthématique, mais je ne sache pas qu'aucun ait rapproché les unes des autres toutes les phlegmasies qui se montrent ainsi disséminées, et deduit de ce rapprochement les conséquences qui ressortent généralement de la comparaison de faits analogues.'—Chomel *Leçons de Clinique Médicale Fièvre, Typhoïde*, p. 442.

Both have their origin in the action of a specific cause. Just as a plant produces a seed from which another plant essentially identical with the parent may spring, so from every case of these two diseases is evolved a something,— a seed which can develop a disease essentially identical with the parent disease.

But by neither the seed of the plant, nor the seed of the disease, can this power of development be exercised, unless the conditions of development be given. An acorn could never develop into an oak if it lay on a dry stone, exposed to the light of the sun; nor the seed of small-pox develop small-pox if deposited in the blood of a man who had recently suffered that disease. The power of development would be there in both cases; the conditions of development would be wanting.

In the power of propagating themselves, and themselves only, lies the test of the specific difference of plants. In the power of reproducing themselves, and themselves only, also lies the test of the specific difference of these two diseases. Could it be shown that from the same seed, under different conditions of development, might spring the oak and the lily, then would naturalists admit, no matter how dissimilar in external characters, that these plants were specifically identical. So, in regard of these diseases, could it be shown that the something, the seed evolved from a person labouring under either, could, the conditions of development being different, develop the symptoms of the other, then must small-pox and measles be held to be specifically identical. But the power of reproducing themselves, and themselves only, *is* possessed by small-pox and measles, as it is by the oak and the lily, and therefore the diseases, like the plants, are held to be distinct species.

But the conditions of development being different, from the same acorn may spring an oak the most perfect of its kind, and one the most diminutive in size and ungainly in form, and the seeds, again, from either of these, may develop, under different external conditions, into the perfect or the anomalous tree; and for this reason it is that the perfect oak and the anomalously formed oak are held to be mere varieties of oue and the same species; and so in reference to small-pox and measles. As a person exposed to the effluvia of the most perfect of either kind may be affected with the most anomalous form of the same kind, while another, exposed to the emanations arising from a third person affected with the anomalous form, may have the perfect disease, the anomalous and typical diseases themselves are held to be merely varieties of one and the same species.

Typical small-pox and anomalous pox spring up indifferently from the same seed, the conditions of development only being unlike.

Typical measles and anomalous measles spring up indifferently from the same seed, the conditions of development only being unlike. Hence the typical and anomalous diseases are mere varieties of the same species. But the seed of measles cannot develop small-pox, nor that of small-pox measles, however the conditions of development be varied, and therefore it is that they are held to be true species.

Having thus eliminated in respect of these types of the proper or typical stationary fevers of Sydenham, their common invariable characters, it will be seen that an enumeration of these points of conformity constitutes a definition of a perfectly natural order of diseases, viz.:

Acute diseases of definite duration capable of reproducing themselves and attended in their course by disseminated lesions of structure.

The distinct species of disease referable to this order are far more numerous than those included in it by Sydenham; to it unquestionably belongs one disease he ranked only as a moderate effervescence of the blood, viz., scarlet fever; and I think it may now be proved, that to it also belong all those fevers which Sydenham described as the twin sisters of measles, of small-pox, of dysentery, etc., those which may be termed the variable fevers. In fact, that we have now reached that stage of pathological knowledge, where we are able to include almost all the epidemic diseases that affect in our day the inhabitants of Great Britain in Sydenham's order of typical or proper stationary fevers, and to group them into species, and to show that each of these has preserved through series of years, and, consequently, during many changes in the

epidemic constitution of the atmosphere, and many changes
in the conditions of its development, its essential symptoms,
run its definite course, been attended by the same lesions of
structure, and continued capable throughout of reproducing
itself in all its integrity.

In this order or class or genus are to be included the
following well-defined species :—Small-pox, erysipelas, measles,
typhus fever, scarlet fever, typhoid fever, and relapsing fever.
It is not to be supposed that there are no other species belonging to this group.   Cholera, to which it may be that autumnal
diarrhœa bears the same relation that febricula does to typhus,
glanders, yellow fever, and plague, may possibly, nay, probably, belong here; but at the present moment we are
scarcely in a position to assign to them so definite a place.
There is another, it appears to me, equally natural group of
diseases, to which I shall have occasion hereafter to refer
more particularly, from the fact of cases of the species which
I would include in it being often confounded with some of
those of the acute specific diseases.   This order, however, for
the sake of comparison with that just described, I shall now
define, and thus :

*Acute diseases of definite duration attended in their
course by disseminated lesions of structure, but incapable of
reproducing themselves.*

As examples of this order I may mention :—
Acute tuberculosis.
Acute purulent diathesis, or pyogenic fever.
Acute cancer.

I have spoken of the diseases of the order I first defined
simply as acute specific diseases, yet our present knowledge
almost justifies the term of acute specific blood diseases; for,
although actual observation has failed to demonstrate any
constant change in the composition of that fluid in any one
of these diseases, yet there is no question that the blood is at
the outset either the medium for the circulation of the seed,
poison, materies morbi, ferment, or whatever be the particular
principle on which the development of the phenomena which
indicate the existence of these diseases depends; or, that
from the very first the infectious principle produces such a
change in the blood itself, that that fluid is so altered in

quality as to produce the phenomena of the disease. But that, whatever be the condition of the blood at the outset of these affections, it does, in the progress of severe cases, undergo some change, is a matter of direct observation, for chemically and microscopically it then differs from healthy blood.

There are several indirect evidences also of an abnormal condition of the blood in the diseases of which I am speaking; *e.g.* the alteration of the animal temperature and the departure from health of the various secretions from the very first; the deviation from its natural size and consistence of the spleen in so large a proportion of cases, and the disseminated character of the structural changes,—the simultaneous occurrence of so many functional derangements, and subsequently of so many organic lesions.

Leaving, however, this point as beyond the purpose I have in view, I propose now to consider the peculiarities manifested by each of the species which I have enumerated as belonging to the group of proper stationary fevers, with reference to the several points which constitute, considered generally, the grounds for their combination into one class or genus, taking typical cases of each for the terms of comparison, and

1st. Of the general symptoms which precede the local lesions of structure, and, during the whole course of the disease, are out of proportion to them in severity—Rigors, abnormally high temperature; pain in the back and limbs; headache; mental disturbance; increased frequency of pulse; loss of muscular power, and general sense of illness; these, it may be said, are common to all, but still they present marked differences and peculiarities with regard to each of the species in question.

A severe *rigor* often ushers in an attack of small-pox, of erysipelas, and of relapsing fever. Rigors are very common, but rarely severe at the outset of typhus fever; they are of infrequent occurrence in measles and scarlet fever.

In typhoid fever rigors are replaced by a frequently repeated sense of chilliness. A rigor occurring so long after the outset of the disease as that which ushers in the relapse in relapsing fever, would, in typhoid fever, as has been proved by Louis, indicate the establishment of some serious local complication.

The *temperature* of the skin, which from the very first is much higher than in health in scarlet and relapsing fevers, is in typhus fever peculiar in kind—pungent, biting, but not particularly high. In small-pox it often, and in typhoid fever occasionally, falls considerably after the appearance of the eruption.[1]

The severity of the *pain in the back* in small-pox is, as is well known, singularly great; in erysipelas it is often complained of a good deal. In typhus fever the pain is usually more severe in the limbs than in the back, while in relapsing fever it is commonly present and often severe in both situations. In typhoid fever, scarlet fever, and measles, the pains in these parts are generally from first to last trifling.

Present in all these diseases, *headache* varies in severity and duration in each. Thus in small-pox it is severe at the moment of invasion, but quickly disappears; in relapsing fever, it continues through the whole of the primary attack and of the relapse; in typhus and typhoid fevers it is one of the more constant symptoms at the outset, and in both disappears spontaneously, but some days earlier in typhus fever than in typhoid fever. Headache is by no means a prominent symptom in typical cases of scarlet fever or measles.

The *mind* in scarlet fever, measles, and relapsing fever is unaffected, or active delirium, mild in character, occurs at night.

In typhoid and typhus fevers the power of collecting, directing, and fixing thought first fails, then the power to appreciate the duration of time,—periods of time that elapse between given events are to the patient's imagination lengthened, minutes seem hours, hours days, and days weeks, and rarely, *if ever*, the reverse. In typhus fever this mental incapacity gradually merges into the lower form of delirium.

---

[1] I speak only of the temperature as determined roughly by the hand. The results obtained by Traube and Zimmerman by the daily use of the thermometer, lead one to anticipate large advances in our knowledge from the more extensive employment of that instrument.—(Note of 1853.)

The same happens in some cases of typhoid fever. Occasionally, however, as in small-pox, active delirium is one of the earliest symptoms in typhoid fever, and then, as in small-pox, it ceases when the 'eruption appears. This probably never occurs in typhus fever.

In small-pox and scarlet fever, measles and relapsing fever, the *general sense of illness* may be extreme; at the same time the patient loses the power of exerting to any considerable extent his muscular powers; he feels and is really weak. In typhoid fever, the loss of muscular power is yet greater; but it is in typhus fever that this is from the first the most marked. In small-pox, measles, scarlet fever, erysipelas, and relapsing fever, the patient ordinarily assigns as the cause for keeping his bed a sense of general illness. In typhoid fever, this is often the case; but, in typhus fever the all but constant reply to the question, Why did you take to bed ? is, ' Because I was too weak to keep about.'

A *frequent pulse* is a symptom common to all the acute specific diseases,—one of their bonds of union; but it is also one of the grounds of their distinction.

On the next page is a table representing the pulse typical of some of these diseases :—

TABLE I.—TYPICAL PULSE IN

Day of Disease	Scarlet Fever					Typhoid Fever					Typhus Fever					Relapsing Fever					Day of Disease
1																					1
2																					2
3		120	120	120	130														120	120	3
4	120	120	120	96	120														120	90	4
5	120	120		84	108										84				124	90	5
6		90	96												96	70			72	72	6
7	84	84			96		120				100	114	120	120	102	60	84				7
8	84	96				100	100	100	106	76	100	120	120	120	108		80			72	8
9	80	80				100	96	100	120	98	108	130	120	120	120				60		9
10		70				124	90	100	110	78	120	138	120	120	120	120	120	120		84	10
11						100	96	96	110	90	120	134	120	108	120	60	120	84	194	48	11
12						100	96	84			120	108	120	88	120	60	60	60	120		12
13						124	100	96	110	96	120	100	96	90	120				112		13
14						100	96	96	96	98	120		96		108				64		14
15						108	96	96	80	98	120	72	84	76	108			120	56		15
16						108	96		116	96	96			78	84			84	60		16
17						108	96		100	108	100				70			60	54		17
18							96		108	96	96							60			18
19						108			100	108	96	92									19
20						108	96		100	108	Conv.	92									20
21						108			100	108											21
22							76		100	150											22
23									98												23
24						140			108		120*										24
25						96	84		110		130										25
26						130					130										26
27						90	96	96	96		130							120			27
28											90							100			28
29											72							104			29
30																		60			30
31																		60			31
32																					32
33																					33
34																					34
35																					35
36																					36
37																					37
38																					38

* Erysipelas of Nose.

In *scarlet fever*, the pulse at the very outset of the disease attains its maximum rate of frequency, continues at the same rate for a certain number of days, and then gradually falls.

In *relapsing fever*, the pulse also attains its maximum rate of frequency from the first, beats at the same rate for a certain number of days, and then suddenly falls to its rate in health, or below that. Again, after a limited number of days have elapsed, it suddenly doubles the frequency of its beats, and then a second time, after a limited number of days, falls below the standard of health.

I may remark here, with reference to the very slow pulse observed after the first and second stages of relapsing fever, that the extremely infrequent pulse is due not to any slowness of contraction of the muscular substance of the heart, for the first sound is not lengthened, but to the duration of the pause,—that each beat of the heart appears to be normal, but the time that elapses between the beats is prolonged, *i.e.* the pulse is really infrequent, not slow.

The reverse of this is true in reference to the length of the first sound of the heart, and the duration of the pause in some cases of slow pulse in cerebral disease.

Again, as to the ratio between the pulse and the respiration in these cases, the pulse being extremely infrequent, the respirations may preserve their ordinary frequency, fall very slightly, or be a little more frequent than in health. So that, instead of bearing to each other the ratio of 1 to 4, the pulse is often little more than twice as frequent as the respirations, and the two may be almost equal in frequency; thus, I have seen the pulse during the stage of convalescence from relapsing fever 36 only, when the respirations were 30 in the minute, no heart, lung, or cerebral disease being present.

The influence of change of position, of muscular exertion, on the frequency of the pulse in these cases is illustrated by the following facts: the pulse being 48, the patient lying on his back, rose, on his assuming the erect position to 116, the respiratory movements at the same time being scarcely more frequent than they were while the patient was in bed.

In *typhus fever* the pulse slowly rises in frequency to a

certain point, preserves that rate of frequency for a variable period, and then as slowly falls.   It is well here to remark, that whenever an increase more than may be accounted for by error in observation, *e.g.* four or six beats in the minute in the frequency of the heart's beats occurs after the first fall in frequency in typhus fever, that increase is the precursor or accompanies the development of some complication. Thus, in the sixth case tabulated, erysipelas commenced with the rise in the pulse.   A sudden fall in the rapidity of the heart's beats in typhus fever is occasionally the consequence of intracranial disease, *e.g.* hemorrhage into the cavity of the arachnoid.

In *typhoid fever* the pulse rises and falls in frequency in a most irregular manner,—to-day 120, to-morrow 90, the next day 120,—and this apparently without any relation to the increase or decrease of the general or local affections without appreciable cause.

The different influence of free perspiration in diminishing the frequency of the pulse in relapsing fever and in typhus fever, is illustrated by a comparison of this table, which is copied from a Report on Continued Fever, by Dr. Flint, Professor of Medicine in Buffalo University, United States, and the above table, compiled from my own observations in regard of the pulse in relapsing fever; for, in the cases there tabulated, the sudden fall in the pulse was preceded by profuse sweating :—

Influence of Perspiration on the rate of Frequency of the Pulse in Typhus Fevers.

No. of Cases.	Day before Perspiration.	Day of Perspiration.	Subsequent Day.
1	120	120 A.M. 116 P.M.	100
2	108	104	104
3	132	124	118
4	108	100	88
5	128	128	120
6	156	134	128
7	110	120	104
8	106	126	135
9	90	100	108
10	111	108	96

It is, then, manifest that those general symptoms which the diseases of this class have in common, and the possession of which serves, in some measure, to prove their affinity when closely examined, indicate their want of identity.

2nd. The same affinity and yet want of identity is observed in regard of the local affections.

In six of the seven—viz. small-pox, measles, erysipelas, scarlet fever, typhoid fever, and typhus fever—the skin is the seat of disseminated vascular engorgement. In reference to relapsing fever, some difference of opinion on this point exists. Cases of relapsing fever, as of other diseases, rarely come under observation till after the period at which the German observers of this disease state the rash they saw in it had disappeared.

In a large proportion of the cases of relapsing fever I have seen there have been minute hemorrhagic points, i.e. petechial spots, scattered over the surface; but whether these were the result of disease or of the bites of insects I am unable to determine. The patients that fell under my observation were of the very lowest class; but a similar state of skin was observed in Edinburgh, and, in a few of the cases I have recorded, there were on the skin purple spots so large as to preclude the idea of their having had an external origin.

But although all these diseases—at least save one—agree in having an eruption on the skin, the nature of the eruption varies in each. In small-pox it is a specific suppurative inflammation; in scarlet fever it is diffused vascular engorgement, commencing in the most minute points; in measles it is also vascular engorgement, but commencing in spots of some size; in typhus fever there is a similar distension of the capillaries of the skin at detached spots at the outset, but terminating, before the conclusion of the disease, in a large proportion of cases, in rupture of one or more minute vessels in each spot. In typhoid fever the eruption is due apparently to an increased flow of blood only to detached points; and rupture of the vessels at those points never occurs. The spots I have seen in relapsing fever have been evidently caused by cuticular hemorrhage. In erysipelas the skin affection appears to be inflammatory in nature, and it is accompanied by one of the effects of inflammation, viz. effusion of serosity.

Peculiarities in respect of the parts of the skin affected.— The eruption in each of these diseases appears first on particular parts of the body, or limits itself throughout to particular parts. In small-pox and measles the eruption shows itself first on the chin, nose, or forehead, and thence invades the whole face. In small-pox the skin of the wrists next suffers, while in measles the rash gradually passes from the face to the neck, thence to the trunk, and subsequently to the extremities. In scarlet fever the eruption breaks out first on the root of the neck, upper part of the chest, loins, and outer aspect of the arms. In typhus fever the back of the hands are the seat of the earliest spots; subsequently, the trunk and extremities, and it appears on these parts almost simultaneously. In typhoid fever spots scarcely ever appear on the face, and rarely on the extremities. They are, perhaps, more numerous on the posterior surface of the trunk, but their characteristic appearance is best seen on the anterior.

In erysipelas the inflammation commences about the centre of the face—*e.g.* over the lower part of the nasal bones—the point of the nose, or the centre of the upper lip, or a little to one side of these parts.

As to the period after the outset of the disease at which the skin affection appears, its course and duration.—In relapsing fever, if there be a specific skin affection, it appears on the first day of illness; the rashes of scarlet fever and of erysipelas show themselves on the second; that of small-pox on the third; of measles on the fourth; of typhus fever on the fifth; of typhoid fever on the eighth. While in relapsing fever the duration of the rash is less than twenty-four hours; in measles, three or four days; in scarlet fever, six or seven days; in erysipelas, seven or eight days; in small-pox, ten or twelve days; in typhus fever, ten or twelve days; and, in typhoid fever, twelve to twenty days.

In their course these skin affections present certain peculiarities. Thus, in scarlet fever, measles, and small-pox the eruption disappears first from the parts first affected; so that in scarlet fever, for example, the legs are brilliant scarlet when the face and trunk have resumed their normal tint.

The eruption seated on the back of hands in typhus fever often disappears in twenty-four hours, while that which studs the remainder of the surface continues of one uniform shade over the whole extent to the last. In erysipelas the inflammation of the skin spreads from one spot gradually in all directions, ceasing to extend only with the cessation of the disease. Typhoid fever offers this peculiarity, that successive crops of spots follow each other at short intervals, the fresh spots being intermingled irregularly with the old, and the spots which appeared first never continuing till the close of the affection.

The scarlet tint of the rash in scarlet fever; its dusky red hue in erysipelas; its lake-like shade in measles; its mulberry aspect in typhus fever, and the rose colour of the spots in typhoid fever; the broad patches of eruption in scarlet fever and erysipelas; the circular, irregularly distributed spots in typhoid fever; the crescentic arrangement of the spots in measles and small-pox, and their orderless coalescence in typhus fever; the limited extent of the eruption in erysipelas and typhoid fever contrasted with its wide diffusion in the other disease—these are characteristics of form, colour, and extent which need only, from our familiarity with them, to be mentioned.

In regard, then, to the skin affection in the diseases under consideration, we observe in each certain peculiarities in respect of nature, situation, date of appearance, colour, form, extent, and duration. With reference to the internal disseminated affections, the *mucous membranes* suffer the most markedly in scarlet fever, typhoid fever, erysipelas, and small-pox. In measles, however, it is the conjunctival, nasal, buccal, and bronchial; in scarlet fever and erysipelas, the faucial; in small-pox, the nasal, buccal, laryngeal, and tracheal; and in typhoid fever, the bronchial and intestinal. Again, the nature of the affection of the mucous membranes varies in each; in measles, it is active congestion, with abundant secretion from the membrane; in erysipelas, inflammation of a peculiar type, with dryness of the surface of membrane, and serous effusion beneath it; while in small-pox the tendency is to suppuration; and in scarlet fever and typhoid fevers, to ulceration. In typhus fever, the mucous membranes suffer congestion only in common with other structures, if seated in depending parts of the body. Disseminated inflammations of the *serous membranes* are remarkably common in typhoid and scarlet fevers; comparatively rare in measles and typhus fever. Enlargement of the spleen is common in and to all; while in typhoid and scarlet fevers and erysipelas it is especially that the lymphatic glands suffer.

3rd. The *duration* of all these acute specific diseases is limited, neither lasts longer than a month, and many have completed their course long before that time. Neither one continues more than a given number of days.

As to the mode in which this is determined, from the sudden commencement and abrupt termination of relapsing fever, and the fact that it is usually uncomplicated, there is no difficulty in fixing its duration.

The data for determining the duration of all the other diseases of this class are derived, *first*, from a consideration of the time that elapses between the first symptom of illness and the disappearance of the eruption; and, *secondly*, from a consideration of the appearances found after death. The eruption is one of the specific effects of the action of the exciting cause, *i.e.* of the poison, seed, or other principle of infection, or of the condition of blood directly produced by that exciting cause (and its continuance is ordinarily equal in duration, after its first appearance, with that of the specific disease). The length of the disease is then at least the period during which the specific eruption is present, plus the period occupied by the general symptoms anterior to the outbreak of the skin affection.

The second class of data for determining the duration is derived from the examination of the bodies of those who die of these diseases.

Thus, all of these acute specific diseases are general diseases, and all may prove fatal without any lesion of structure of sufficient moment to account for death being found. Death results, that is to say, in a certain number of cases of each of these diseases, from the direct action of the poison which induces them, *i.e.* from the changes directly induced on all the tissues and organs of the body by that poison, or by the blood altered by that poison. Now, it is evident that death from this, or these causes, can occur only during the period that the disease itself lasts; therefore, if there be a period in each of these affections, *after which*, if death occur, changes of structure of sufficient moment or extent to account for death are always found, then the specific disease must be held to continue at least up to that time, whatever be the duration of the eruption. Now, experience proves, that in several of these diseases there is such a time, and has shown, moreover, that it is never later in each of the diseases than the time when the eruption fades in typical cases. Thus, the eruption of scarlet fever has disappeared in typical cases, by the ninth or tenth day of disease. If death occur in scarlet fever before the latter date, then experience shows that in a certain proportion of cases, no appearances are found of sufficient importance to account for death; while, if death occur after that date, then death may invariably be explained by the lesions discovered. If, in typhus fever, death ensue within twenty-one days after the first symptoms of illness, then may no deviation from healthy structure, such as experience proves to be capable of producing death, be discovered; while, after twenty-one days, extensive alterations of structure are constantly found.

If a case of typhoid fever prove fatal before the twenty-eighth day of disease, then may slight ulceration of the mucous membrane covering Peyer's patches, some enlargement of the mesenteric glands and spleen, be the only aberrations from the normal condition exposed by the most careful examination of the body; while, after the thirtieth day of disease, aberrations from healthy structure of the gravest character may always be demonstrated after death.

On the table are parts of the small intestines from two females, who died respectively on the fifth and fourteenth day of typhoid fever. In neither preparation is the intestinal disease very grave in character, yet scarcely any other change of structure was detected. For the one preparation I am indebted to my friend Dr. Sankey, and for the other to my friend and colleague Dr. Parkes.

It is, then, by a consideration of the period that elapses between the outset of the disease, when the invasion has been sudden, and the cessation of the eruption; and the period after the first symptoms, when also the invasion has been sudden, at which, if death occur, no lesions of structure to account for death are to be found, that we determine the duration of the acute specific diseases.

By the aid of the latter of these two points, it is, especially, that we are enabled to separate the duration of the illness from the duration of the specific disease. Practically, with regard to some of these diseases, this separation is generally, because readily, effected; the duration of the specific disease being determined by the duration of the symptoms of invasion, and of the eruption, the physician seeks for the complication by which the symptoms of illness are kept up. No one would say scarlet fever had lasted for seven weeks, because a person suffering from that affection had pleurisy established in its course, which pleurisy, passing into a chronic state, ran a course of six weeks. If such a case proved fatal, it would be at once admitted that the patient had died of a disease which had commenced during the progress of the scarlet fever, and continued after the latter had ceased. The same admission would be equally correct, even though the disease of which the patient died was one of those which, in a mild or severe form, invariably accompanies scarlet fever, e.g. the throat affection; thus, in a case I saw lately, sloughing and ulceration of the fauces—established by the action of the specific disease—continued to progress after the latter had itself ceased, and ultimately caused the patient's death two or three weeks after the scarlet fever had terminated. I say with regard to scarlatina and some other of these diseases, this separation of the duration of the specific disease from the duration of the illness is made, and consequently the former can have assigned to it as definite a duration in complicated as in uncomplicated cases,—in those unattended by an eruption as in those attended by an eruption. But with regard to typhus and typhoid fevers, the line in question has not been drawn, and we find, consequently, the duration of the latter said to be sometimes as much as sixty days, and that when no relapse has occurred. This confounding the duration of the illness with the length of the specific disease is an error into which I think some of the most able writers on these diseases have fallen. In typhoid fever, as in scarlet fever, there are two classes of lesions of structure discovered after death—1st, those which are invariably present; and, 2ndly, those which are more or less frequently the result of the disease. An instance of the former is ulceration of Peyer's patches; of the latter, pleurisy and pneumonia. Now, having been established in the course of the specific disease, either one of these may continue to progress after that has termiuated, and all the general effects of ulceration of the small intestines, or of thoracic inflammation, be the result. The pulse may continue frequent, the skin hot, and the patient be delirious, and yet the fever may have ceased, the specific disease have terminated.

Determined by the data to which I have referred, each of the acute specific diseases has a definite duration, *i.e.* with regard to each there is a date capable of being fixed absolutely, by which time the patient either dies, or, so far as concerns the specific disease, recovers.

The duration is different for each species; thus, for measles it is seven or eight days; for scarlet fever, eight or nine days; for erysipelas, about fourteen days; for small-pox the same, supposing in all four the eruption to have made its appearance on the typical day; while, without regard to the date of the appearance of the eruption, it is in typhus fever twenty-one days, and in typhoid fever thirty days.

If, therefore, health be not restored soon after these dates, we may be certain that some other than the primary affection is the cause of the continuance of the symptoms. And, again, if for either of these diseases a specific exist, or a special treatment be proper, it is manifest that that specific or that treatment can be expected to exert a favourable influence only during so many days from the onset of the first symptoms as the specific disease has been proved to exist.

The conclusion as to the duration of typhoid fever at which I arrived from a consideration of the points just referred to, has recently been fully confirmed by a consideration of a different class of facts.

Dr. Zimmerman lately published two papers in the *Deutsche Klinik*,[1] on typhoid fever. He determined the

[1] November 1852.

duration of the disease thus: He noted the temperature of the patient daily, and found that the thermometer indicated that the fever ceased some time between the 21st and 28th days; that is to say, then, for the first time after the commencement of the illness, the thermometer being introduced into the mouth, the mercury stood at the point at which it stands when placed in the mouth of a healthy person. Up to the same date of the disease, the patient was proved by the balance to lose weight daily, while from that date he was proved to gain weight rapidly: thus a patient who weighed before his illness 170 lbs., on the 22nd day of disease weighed only 119 lbs., and on the 26th day only 117 lbs. On the 30th day he was found to have gained 3lbs., i.e. he weighed 120 lbs., and on the 39th day his weight was 124 lbs.; no alteration in his diet of sufficient consequence to account for the increase having been made.

4th. The last point common to all these diseases is, that they have a *specific cause*. But although all are capable of reproducing themselves, there is not one which does not sometimes arise under circumstances in which it is impossible to trace the existence of any source of contagion,—that is to say, there is not one which does not sometimes appear to arise spontaneously. But the frequency with which this happens differs considerably. It rarely happens that cases of small-pox, the disease not being epidemic, are unable to be traced to their origin. The inability to refer the disease to contagion is more common in respect of cases of scarlet fever, measles, and typhus fever, while the contagious nature, even of erysipelas and of typhoid fever, has been called in question. Nay, it was long held that typhoid fever differed from typhus fever for this reason among others, that while the latter was contagious, the former possessed no power of reproducing itself. The memoir of M. Piedvache, 'Recherches sur la Contagion de la Fièvre Typhoïde, et principalement sur les Circonstances dans lesquelles elle a lieu, par Joseph Piedvache, Paris, 1850,' has for ever laid this doubt. That observer has shown, that if the conditions of development be given, typhoid fever has the power of reproducing itself, and has adduced several instances in which persons in attendance on cases of typhoid fever not only contracted the same disease, but, having been removed while ill to houses situated miles distant from the primary case, and where no fever existed, communicated the disease to their relatives and friends. As a rule, those only had the disease who, in imperfectly ventilated rooms, were in close and continued communication with the sick man.

But let the cases of that disease collected together be numerous, and the attendant fully exposed to the effluvia, and it will spread among them in the best ventilated places as freely as typhus fever. For example, the number of nurses who suffered from typhoid fever during the time I visited the London Fever Hospital was as great as the number of those who had typhus fever, while, during the same time, one of the medical attendants had typhus fever, and just before one had died of typhoid fever.

It would appear that the seeds of these specific diseases differ from each other, like the seeds of plants, not only in requiring more or less different conditions for their development, but also in the facility with which their germinating powers are destroyed.

I cannot call to mind a single instance of a case of smallpox being received into the wards of a general hospital without the disease spreading to one or more of those in relation or proximity to it; while I can remember only two instances of the extension of typhoid fever when cases of that disease were scattered through the wards of a *general* hospital; and in these cases it was the friends of the patient —the mother, in one instance, who had watched by her son night and day—who suffered.

The following facts, given by Dr. Flint of Buffalo, are of interest, as bearing on this point and some others connected with the means of the propagation of the contagious diseases. At North Boston, Erie county, United States, in 1843, resided nine families. Taking a tavern for the centre, seven of the nine lived within an area of 100 rods in diameter.

All the inhabitants, with the exception of the members of one family, were in the habit of frequenting the tavern. A feud existed between the master of that one and the tavern-keeper. A man labouring under typhoid fever (a disease previously unknown in North Boston) took up his residence at the tavern September 21st, and died October 29th

Between October 19th and December 7th, twenty-eight persons in this little community had typhoid fever. Three families only escaped the disease, viz. the two residing the farthest from the tavern, and that of the man who had a quarrel with the tavern-keeper, and who, consequently, never visited at his house. Now, a fact of interest in this case is, that all the families in which the disease appeared drew their supply of water from the well of the tavern, while two out of the three that escaped had their water from other sources.

The man at feud with the tavern-keeper was accused of having poisoned the well of the tavern. He resided nearer than any of the others to the tavern. None who visited the village simply for the purpose of rendering assistance to the inhabitants contracted the disease.

In concluding this review of the typical causes of the acute specific diseases, I would observe, that, as the pathological tendency

of small-pox is to produce inflammation and suppuration;
of measles   „   active congestion;
of scarlet fever   „   inflammation and ulceration;
of typhoid fever   „   inflammation and ulceration;
of typhus fever   „   congestion and extravasation of blood;
of erysipelas   „   inflammation and effusion of serosity;

it is probable that the pathological affinity of typhoid fever [1] is with scarlet fever rather than with typhus fever or relapsing

---

[1] I have been repeatedly asked, Why give names so nearly alike to things so distinct as typhoid and typhus fevers? The former name, moreover, it has been said, is very inappropriate.

Two circumstances have prevented me from proposing another name for typhoid fever; 1st, the fact of the disease having been described by that name in the classical works of Louis, Chomel, Jackson, Bartlett, and others; and, 2nd, my inability to find a name for it so appropriate as to justify the attempt to displace the old one.

Dr. Babington proposed to me the name 'febris tympanica;' Dr. Hare that of 'sepomia,' to express the disease in question. Nervous fever was the old English name.

Many of the German and some English writers have adopted the term 'typhus abdominalis;' to this term I object strongly, because, especially, it involves a theory concerning the nature of the disease maintained by no sound authority.

fever; and that the pathological affinity of typhus fever is with measles rather than with typhoid fever or relapsing fever; while the symptomatological affinity of relapsing fever is with the class of diseases in which intermittent fever ranks, rather than with typhus fever or typhoid fever, although etiologically its place is among the acute specific diseases.

In my next lecture, I propose to consider the essential and determining causes of the deviations from their types of particular cases of the acute specific diseases; and to give a brief sketch of some of the varieties thus produced.

LECTURE II

Varieties of acute specific diseases — A. Their essential causes—Differences in severity—Influence of specific local processes—As to skin affection—As to laryngeal and intestinal lesions—Occurrence of local complications. B. Determining causes of variations—Vital conditions of patient—External condition—Atmospheric changes—Epidemic constitution—Endemic influences. C. Phenomena of variations—In Small-pox—Typhoid fever—Scarlatina—Measles—Typhus fever—Relapsing Fever—Erysipelas.

In practice, deviation from the types of the acute specific diseases that I compared in my last lecture, continually present themselves; and I propose now to consider, in regard of these varieties—

A. Their essential causes.

B. Their determining causes.

And C. their phenomena.

A. The essential causes of the differences in the symptoms and lesions of structure of the acute specific diseases may be referred to three heads, viz.:—

(a) To differences in the severity of the general specific disease.

(b) To variations in date of origin, extent, severity, course, and duration of the specific local processes, and to their immediate effects.

(c) To the presence and varying degree of severity of functional or organic complications.

(a) Of the deviations from their type produced by differences in the severity of the general specific disease, scarlet fever and typhus fever afford the most frequent and striking illustrations; and for these two reasons, viz.—1st, that, in both, death is not unfrequently caused by the general disease, independently, that is to say, of any change of structure; and, 2nd, that, in both, the general disease is often of the most trivial character, and runs its course unattended by any grave or prominent local affection.

To this head are probably to be referred those differences in the suddenness of the access of these diseases sometimes observed. The more severe the general disease, the more suddenly do the patient's powers succumb to the impression produced on them; and when, towards' the termination of the disease, grave constitutional symptoms occur for the first time, they are usually due—in a great measure, at least—to the severity of the specific local processes, or to the establishment of complications.

(b) As to the influence of the specific local processes. The skin affection is occasionally wanting in all. Arranged in the order of the frequency with which it is present in the adult, these diseases stand thus:—

Small-pox—measles—typhus fever — erysipelas — scarlet fever—typhoid fever.

Being present, the eruption in the same diseases varies infinitely in amount, and, to some extent, even in appearance. Thus, only two or three rose-spots may be present in typhoid fever, and not more than half-a-dozen pustules in small-pox; while in the same diseases, nearly the whole surface may be covered with their characteristic eruptions. In typhoid fever, a minute vesicle may in very rare cases be seen on the apex of what appear, from their colour, size, seat, and course, to be rose-spots; and the pustules of small-pox are occasionally represented by papulæ or by watery blebs. And, again; who has not hesitated now and then to say, judging from the eruption alone, whether a given case was one of measles or of scarlet fever?

This table, from Rilliet's paper,[1] exhibits the great variations that occur in reference to the date of the appearance of the eruption after the first symptoms of measles.

[1] *Gazette Médicale*, 1848.

Day of Disease on which the Eruption appeared in Three hundred and ninety-five Cases of Measles.

On the 1st day	in	11 cases.	On the		7th day in 34 cases.
,, 2nd ,,	,,	29 ,,	,,	8th ,,	12 ,,
,, 3rd ,,	,,	57 ,,	,,	9th ,,	35 ,,
,, 4th ,,	,,	77 ,,	,,	10th ,,	4 ,,
,, 5th ,,	,,	76 ,,	,, 10th to 13th	,,	12 ,,
,, 6th ,,	,,	42 ,,	,, 13th to 16th	,,	6 ,,

The duration of the eruption is equally variable. Sometimes it vanishes in twenty-four hours; in other cases its duration is singularly prolonged. Thus, in one of Rilliet's cases, it attained its height as late as five days after its appearance; and, in one detailed by Reveillé-Parise, fifteen days after its commencement. Sometimes it almost disappears, and then returns more intensely than at first.

In scarlet fever the date, after the first symptoms of illness, of the appearance of the rash varies much. Often present on the 1st day, it is not unfrequently delayed till the 3rd day, and, in one of the cases referred to in the table, it appeared for the first time on the 7th day. Rilliet and Barthez say that, in the cases they watched, the eruption now and then disappeared on the 5th day, and that it sometimes continued out even to the 10th day. This table shows the period of the disease at which I noted the appearance of the rash in twenty-four cases—

Day of Disease on which the Rash appeared in Twenty-four Cases of Scarlet Fever.

On the 1st day	in	7 cases.	On the 5th day	in	1 case.
,, 2nd ,,	,,	10 ,,	,, 6th ,,	,,	1 ,,
,, 3rd ,,	,,	2 ,,	,, 7th ,,	,,	1 ,,
,, 4th ,,	,,	2 ,,			

And the following table the day of the disappearance of the rash in fifty-four unselected cases, including all those that have come under my care in the Hospital for Sick Children :—

Day of Disease by which the Rash had Disappeared in Fifty-four Cases of Scarlet Fever.

On the 5th day	in	1 case.	On the 10th day	in	8 cases.
,, 6th ,,	,,	3 ,,	,, 11th ,,	,,	4 ,,
,, 7th ,,	,,	5 ,,	,, 13th ,,	,,	2 ,,
,, 8th ,,	,,	13 ,,	,, 14th ,,	,,	2 ,,
,, 9th ,,	,,	12 ,,	,, 16th ,,	,,	2 ,,

In typhus fever the eruption may appear as early as the
3rd day; sometimes, however, it is delayed till so late as
the 9th day. This table shows the date of its disappearance
in sixty-eight unselected cases—

*Day of Disease by which the Mulberry Rash had Disappeared
in Sixty-eight Cases of Typhus Fever.*

On the	7th day	in	1 case.	On the 16th day	in	8 cases.
,,	8th ,,	,,	1 ,,	,, 17th ,,	,,	8 ,,
,,	9th ,,	,,	2 ,,	,, 18th ,,	,,	5 ,,
,,	10th ,,	,,	1 ,,	,, 19th ,,	,,	5 ,,
,,	11th ,,	,,	3 ,,	,, 20th ,,	,,	5 ,,
,,	12th ,,	,,	3 ,,	,, 21st ,,	,,	4 ,,
,,	13th ,,	,,	2 ,,	,, 23rd ,,	,,	1 ,,
,,	14th ,,	,,	9 ,,	,, 25th ,,	,,	2 ,,
,,	15th ,,	,,	8 ,,			

In typhoid fever the eruption may be seen as early as the
5th day of disease, while spots sometimes appear for the
first time as late as the 20th day, and fresh spots as late as
the 32nd day.

The day of appearance, and the duration of the skin
affection, in small-pox, are comparatively constant, but the
modifications in the other symptoms produced by its extent
and severity are very great.

'Very many patients,' says Dr. Gregory, 'die between the
8th and 12th days of the eruption, from the combined effects
of cutaneous and cellular inflammation.'

The specific local process of the skin modifies the symptoms
of small-pox; 1st, by interfering with the due performance of
the functions of that structure; and, 2nd, by exciting
symptomatic constitutional disturbance.

Erysipelas is another of these acute specific diseases in
which the external local process is in some instances so severe
as to modify greatly the phenomena of the disease. Sometimes the inflammation, instead of causing œdema only of the
subcutaneous tissue, leads to the exudation of pus blastema;
the constitutional disturbance is in such cases fearfully
increased by the severity of the local process, and the duration of the general illness greatly prolonged.

As to the symptoms due to the internal specific local
processes, they also may be altogether absent. We see measles

without catarrhal symptoms; scarlet fever without sore throat; small-pox without any affection of the nasal, buccal, or laryngeal mucous membranes; typhoid fever without diarrhœa; erysipelas without pain in deglutition,—and in all we see the symptoms of the internal affections most intense. The influence of the internal specific processes in modifying the symptoms is well seen in some cases of small-pox and typhoid fever.

In small-pox, about the seventh day of the eruption, severe symptoms, arising from the specific process established in the larynx and trachea, are not uncommon. The patient up to that time has perhaps suffered severely, but yet from no symptoms calculated to awaken alarm in the inexperienced. A little hoarseness, some hard cough, first dry, and subsequently accompanied by tenacious mucous expectoration, are all that indicate the presence of the specific lesion, which in two or three days more proves fatal.

The laryngeal, like the skin affection, modifies the symptoms of small-pox in two ways—

1st, By exciting symptomatic constitutional disturbance, and so adding in appearance to the severity of the specific constitutional disturbance; and,

2nd, By interfering with the due performance of the respiratory function.

The specific intestinal and mesenteric diseases often give a complexion, as it were, to cases of typhoid fever; and they do so—

Sometimes by inducing direct abdominal symptoms of a more severe character than occur in typical cases; e.g. great pain, distention of the abdomen, or extreme sensibility to pressure.

Sometimes, by leading to diarrhœa, or to hemorrhage from the bowels, and so depressing the powers of the patient that he is unable to bear up against the specific general disease.

In some cases the hemorrhage itself proves directly fatal; thus, I have seen a man suffering from typhoid fever at a time when his general powers were little impaired, when he was able to sit up and converse freely with those around him, suddenly lose so much blood from the bowels as to be reduced in half-an-hour to a state of extreme exhaustion, and then, in the course of a few hours, be carried off by a return of the hemorrhage.

And sometimes by causing perforation of the peritoneum. When this occurs, the patient may sink rapidly from acute general peritonitis, or more gradually from a more chronic form of the same disease.

The primary breach of surface of the intestinal mucous membrane seems to be effected in three modes—

1st, By thickening and softening of the mucous membrane, and then the detachment of the softened membrane, in the form of molecules of inappreciable magnitude. 2nd, By the effusion of lymph on and into the mucous membrane, and the separation of the former with minute portions of the latter,—still portions of some size. 3rd, By the detachment of large sloughs. In these latter cases there is always, at an early stage of the disease, a deposit of protein matter—using that word in its largest sense—in the submucous cellular tissue. This substance is friable, of a pale yellowish colour, and now and then marked with vascular striæ, apparently the vessels of the tissue in which it is placed. It has been called typhus matter, and is susceptible only of the lowest form of cell-development. It is probably rarely, if ever, absorbed from the submucous tissue, and never enters into permanent relation with the structures amid which it is placed. Before the thirtieth day of disease, the whole of this matter is ejected; and in this wise, by its accumulation in the submucous tissue, the nutrition of the mucous membrane is so seriously impaired that it dies, and then both it and the foreign matter are thrown off in the form of a slough of considerable size. Sometimes the whole of the newly-deposited protein matter is separated at the same instant, at others it comes away in several pieces. But however this may be, when the whole of it has been thrown off, the mucous membrane is found to have been detached from the submucous tissue to a greater extent than it has been destroyed; so that, if a portion of intestine, on which is an ulcer in this stage, is placed in water, the edges of the ulcer float upwards, as in this preparation put up by my friend Dr. Sankey, and this from University College Museum.

Destruction of the other coats of the intestine is effected thus—by ulceration, or, as ulceration is pathologically termed, by molecular death, the inferior layer of the submucous cellular tissue is destroyed, and then the floor of the ulcer is formed of the muscular fibres of the intestine. These fibres swell, grow intensely red, soften and then die molecularly, and so the peritoneal coat is exposed.

The actual perforation of this membrane may be the result of the continuance of the process by which the muscular coat was destroyed, viz. molecular death, and then one or more minute rounded apertures are formed in the floor of the ulcer; more commonly a portion of the peritoneum of some magnitude dies, and then a slough dyed with the intestinal fluids may be found in some cases attached to one point of the aperture; and lastly, but so rarely that it has been denied by some, rupture of the delicate layer of peritoneum that constitutes the floor may take place. Of this perforation of the intestine by rupture I do not myself remember ever to have seen an example in typhoid fever; but I have seen an unequivocal case of the kind in a child the subject of tubercular ulceration of the large intestine; and, from the tenuity of the floor of the ulcer in some cases of typhoid fever that have fallen under my observation, I cannot doubt the possibility of its occurrence in that disease. The fact of such an accident being possible should teach us to be careful in manipulating the abdomen of patients in an advanced stage of typhoid fever.

As the destruction of the walls of the intestines progresses lymph is sometimes deposited on the external surface of the peritoneal coat corresponding to the ulcers, without adhesions to surrounding parts being effected. But in some cases adhesions are formed, and then perforation of the intestinal walls may take place without any escape of the intestinal contents into the peritoneal cavity. Sometimes, again, adhesions unite adjacent folds of the intestine, and the borders of these folds adhering to the parietal peritoneum, a circumscribed cavity is formed. Opening into such a cavity an aperture is sometimes found communicating with the interior of the intestinal canal. In such cases a considerable period may elapse between the perforation and the escape of the contents of the intestines, and the death of the patient, and then most extensive organic changes may be discovered after death. In such a case I have seen large tracts of the parietal peritoneum destroyed by ulceration and sloughing.

But, however perforation of the intestine is effected in typhoid fever, and whatever adhesions take place, it may be laid down as a law, to which nothing on record affords an exception, that ultimate recovery is never accomplished, and that, sooner or later, death is the consequence of intestinal perforation. The adhesions, as Rokitansky says, are never permanent.

To describe the general appearance and the structure of the glandulæ agminatæ, or Peyer's patches, is here needless; every one is familiar with them. But there are one or two points in connection with these structures to which I must advert, because errors respecting them have found their way into very able works; for example, Dr. Flint's reports. I allude especially to their anatomical characters, and the signification of their degree of visibility.

(1) In young children Peyer's patches are always readily seen, and about the period of the first dentition, are often very distinct. Their extreme visibility in the intestines of these subjects, as well as in those of some adults, is ordinarily due to the prominence of the ridges of mucous membrane between the pits in which the sacculi lie. This is well seen in this preparation of the intestines of a young child who died of bronchitis; in this preparation, from the College Museum; and in this preparation from the Museum of University College, of the intestine of an adult killed (while in health) by an accident.

(2) In aged persons, and in some adults less advanced in years, Peyer's patches readily catch the eye, in consequence of their being smooth, and of an opaque dull white hue. In such cases they are sometimes less prominent than the adjacent membrane.

When the patches have lost the projections between the pits, and have not experienced that conversion of structure which is indicated by the appearances just mentioned, they may readily be passed by unnoticed; nay, may require to be sought for carefully before they can be discovered. Under these circumstances they have been sometimes said to be absent.

(3) A third cause of the facility with which Peyer's patches are seen is, that they sometimes remain pale when the vessels of the mucous membrane around them are injected with blood.

(4) While a fourth reason of their distinctness is the presence on them, in some cases, of small blackish grey, or black points, giving to them an aspect which has been compared to the recently shaven beard. This appearance is produced by the action of the intestinal gases on the blood contained in the capillaries which lie in the folds of mucous membrane surrounding the pits containing the sacculi.

No one of these four conditions of the glandulæ agminatæ, or Peyer's patches, is connected with any particular disease, though the last mentioned occurs whenever the circulation through the vessels of these parts has been delayed for any length of time. This much is certain, that they have no connection with the lesions proper to any form or species of fever.

In the mesenteric glands exudation matter is sometimes found identical in appearance with that in the submucous tissue of the intestine. Like that it is susceptible only of the lowest cell-development, and therefore incapable of forming a permanent part of the organism. From its situation it cannot, like that in the submucous tissue, be ejected. It appears to undergo two changes, viz. softening and fatty degeneration.

By its softening it forms a purulent-looking fluid, and constitutes a variety of pseudo-abscess. The fluid thus found may be absorbed, or the peritoneum over it may give way, and peritonitis, general or partial, be the result.

Masses of typhoid matter in the mesenteric glands soften first at the circumference, so that a lump of unsoftened matter is often found bathed in a purulent-looking fluid.

By fatty degeneration I mean a metamorphosis, or conversion into fat, of the exuded protein matter by a re-arrangement of its elements,—a change which protein matter of low organisation, or without the power of developing into tissue, constantly experiences. This conversion into fat may be effected either before or after softening has taken place, and the fatty matter thus formed may subsequently be absorbed. In fact, fatty degeneration is one mode in which solid fibro-albuminous substances are brought into a state suitable for absorption. The process by which the healing of the typhoid ulcers is accomplished is of interest, practically and pathologically. It seems to be this: The floor of the ulcer, after every part of the substance deposited during the progress of the specific disease has separated becomes smooth, and of a pale bluish-white colour—it is covered with a delicate layer of healthy organisable lymph—to this layer, which extends under the detached mucous membrane at the edges of the ulcer, the latter adheres (gradually from without inwards, *i.e.* from the circumference towards the centre). If the intestine be now placed in water the edges of the ulcer no longer float upwards. After a time, all that remains is a flat, smooth, shining, and somewhat depressed surface, to which the transition from the mucous membrane around is imperceptible. At first this smooth surface is, unlike the natural mucous membrane, fixed to the subjacent coat, so that it cannot be moved on the latter. Ultimately, however, it can be so moved, and is then scarcely to be distinguished by the unaided eye at least from normal mucous membrane. It is important to remember that constriction of the intestine has never been known to result from the healing of a typhoid ulcer.

Occasionally, in the progress of typhoid fever, a deposit similar to that which is seated in the intestinal wall and in the mesenteric glands is found in other parts; the spleen, walls of the gall bladder, lungs, and kidneys are the organs in which I have seen such deposits. By their consequences, these deposits may lead to modifications in the primary disease.

Thus, in the spleen it may soften, form a pseudo-abscess, and ultimately induce general inflammation of the peritoneum, either by bursting into the abdominal cavity, or by exciting inflammation of the serous membrane covering itself, and then that inflammation spreading over the whole extent of the membrane. A case of the latter kind lately proved fatal under my care in University College Hospital.

(c) The third cause of the modifications in the symptoms

of the acute specific diseases is the occurrence of local complications.

By the term complications are signified those affections which may exist as substantive diseases; e.g. pleurisy, pneumonia, hemorrhage into the cavity of the arachnoid, and also those extreme functional derangements of particular organs, which are out of proportion to the severity of the general disease.

Of the influence of these local complications, in causing deviations from their type, measles, typhoid fever, and scarlet fever afford frequent examples. The symptoms and course of measles are singularly modified by the occurrence of pneumonia; thus, if severe pneumonia be established during the stage of invasion, the eruption in many cases never appears, and when it does appear it is pale and of short duration. If the pneumonia be set up after the eruption has appeared, then the course of the latter is considerably shortened: it quickly disappears. Neither bronchitis nor enteritis, according to Rilliet's observations, have any such effect on the course of the eruption.

In cases of typhoid and scarlet fevers, it is by no means uncommon to see aberration in the functions of the brain manifested by violent delirium or extreme depression, when from an examination of that organ we are satisfied that it was the seat of no more vascular engorgement than the brains of those who die without having exhibited any such symptoms. This extreme cerebral excitement is often witnessed when the other symptoms do not warrant the opinion that the case is one of great gravity.

In a diagnostic point of view it is well to know, that after the patient becomes delirious in the acute specific diseases, he never complains of headache, and rarely admits its existence, even when questioned concerning it, while in cases of intracranial inflammation headache is constantly, and often loudly, complained of after delirium has commenced.

B. These, then, being the essential causes of the chief deviations from their typical form of the acute specific diseases, it remains to consider the circumstances which determine the severity of the general specific disease, the extent and severity of the local specific processes, and the supervention of complications.

These are—

(a) The vital conditions of the patient. (b) The external circumstances by which he is surrounded.

(a) The influence of the vital conditions incident to age in modifying the severity of the general disease, and the specific local process, is well seen in typhus fever.

The mortality from typhus fever in persons between the ages of six years and fifteen years is very trifling, not more than two or three per cent. The mulberry rash in the same class of persons is either absent, or pale in hue and scanty in quantity, except in rare cases. While the mortality in persons more than fifty years of age is about fifty-six per cent., and in them the mulberry rash is always present, and ordinarily dark and abundant. Typhus fever, too, very often proves fatal to those past the middle period of life without any local complication having been established in its course, while this never happens in the young. Nay, an abundant rash, a brown tongue, and marked prostration, are uncommon symptoms in typhus fever when it affects children.

Other instances of the modifying power of the vital condition of the patient over the phenomena which follow the introduction of the specific element into the system are offered by the fact, that strumous children, when the subjects of scarlet fever, suffer much more frequently than others from acrid discharges from the eyes, ears, and nose; from swelling of the parotid and the parts in its vicinity; and that women who contract scarlet fever in the puerperal state, comparatively speaking, rarely recover. It cannot in any of these cases be supposed, that the difference in the severity of the general disease, or the specific local processes, depends on a difference in the poison, or in the quantity of the poison. It can depend solely on the different conditions of the recipients.

In some persons, again, from constitutional idiosyncrasy, great general disturbance is produced by comparatively slight local disease. Now, if in these persons any local complication be set up in the progress of a specific disease, or if the specific local processes be severe in nature, then the sympathetic constitutional disturbance, superadded to the specific disease, materially modifies its symptoms. This same constitutional idiosyncrasy is manifested in the excitement which particular organs suffer in some individuals from a cause which has no influence in producing the same symptoms in others. In some the brain is peculiarly prone to sympathise, as it is called—a term which probably signifies, in these cases, that the presence in the blood of an element which produces no aberration from the functions of the brain in one individual, is, in another, from a difference in the susceptibility of that organ to that stimulus, sufficiently potent to produce delirium, etc.

These differences may be illustrated by a reference to the differences observed in the effects of alcoholic drinks on the cerebral functions in different individuals.

(b) The external conditions on which deviations of the acute specific diseases from their types depend, are—

1st. Readily appreciable atmospheric changes. These changes modify the symptoms and the course of the acute specific diseases, by inducing intercurrent affections as complications, e.g. pneumonia in measles.

2nd. The epidemic constitution. This, it is said, manifests its influence, not only by determining the prevalence of particular diseases, but also by impressing on them peculiar modifications. *Now*, almost every case requires the administration of powerful stimulants; *then* the lancet is the chief agent in diminishing the mortality. Our ideas, however, on the meaning of the term 'epidemic constitution,' are undergoing considerable change. But, granting the epidemic constitution to be something totally distinct from directly appreciable atmospheric changes, there is every reason to believe that its influence in determining differences in the type of these diseases has been greatly overrated.

First, because under one name several diseases have been, in times past, confounded, and what was due to difference of disease was referred to difference of type. The fever for which the lancet was used so freely in 1818, without injury to the patient, was relapsing fever; and the estimation in which blood-letting was held rested on the fact, that nature terminated the apparently severe attack, aided or unaided by the treatment, in less than a week. Stimulants have been held in high repute in late times, because the disease we have had to treat has been typhus fever. The constitution of the air has favoured the prevalence now of one and now of the other; but the sporadic cases of either which occurred during the prevalence of the other, required the same treatment that they did when they themselves were epidemic. Cases of relapsing fever that occur when typhus prevails need no wine, and cases of typhus fever that occur when relapsing fever is epidemic, need stimulating as much as they do when typhus is itself epidemic; just as sporadic cases of scarlet fever that occur during an epidemic of measles require the treatment fitted for scarlet fever, and the reverse.

A second reason why such great powers in modifying the acute specific diseases were assigned to the epidemic constitution by the old observers, was, that variations in the symptoms resulting from intercurrent affections, induced by appreciable atmospheric changes, were not, from imperfections in the art of diagnosis, separated from the variations dependent on differences in the severity of the specific diseases themselves.

3rd. The third class of external circumstances which modify the acute specific diseases, are endemic influences, under which head I would include imperfect ventilation, overcrowding, and want of drainage. The effect of these is to increase the severity of the general disease, to impress on it a typhoid type. A striking proof of this is afforded by the sudden change in the type of the symptoms often seen on removing the poor from their close-crowded rooms to the well-ventilated wards of an hospital.

C. Such, then, being the essential and determining causes of the modifications of the acute specific diseases, I have now to pass briefly in review some of the varieties of these diseases which result from the influence of these causes.

SMALL-POX.—I have already remarked that the deviation from the type of small-pox in the confluent variety is due to the extent and severity of the specific local process.

Symptomatologically considered there are three, and pathologically considered two, distinct varieties of small-pox included under the term 'malignant small-pox.'

In the first symptomatological variety, the severity of the general specific disease is evidenced by the patient dying before any local disease whatever is established.

In the second, the severity of the general specific disease is manifested by the softened state of the solids, and the ready solubility of the organised elements of the blood; the effects of which are hemorrhage from innumerable small vessels in various parts of the body, the effusion of serosity dyed red by dissolved hæmatosin, and diminution of muscular power, cardiac as well as voluntary. The cerebral functions in these cases are often unimpaired.

The third variety is characterised by so-called typhoid symptoms, *i.e.* by frequent pulse, dry and brown tongue, low delirium, and great prostration—characters which it owes either to the severity of the general affection—for they are sometimes present when the pustules are few in number and distinct—or to the presence of severe local complications. Thus, in a case I witnessed of this kind, when the patient was progressing favourably, the evidence of pneumonia being established, was quickly followed by typhoid symptoms. On examination after death the interlobular septa of the lung were found infiltrated over a considerable space with purulent-looking fluid.

TYPHOID FEVER.—The cases of typhoid fever met with in practice may be grouped under the following heads:— The typical, the mild, the grave, and the insidious, simulative or latent.

Time permits me only to sketch the last; and this I shall do at some length, because I believe the cases included in it are often misunderstood.

The insidious, simulative, or latent variety of typhoid fever usually commences most gradually, the patient being altogether unable to say on what day he first felt unwell; nay, sometimes he cannot fix within a week or ten days the outset of his illness; rarely is he able to say what the first symptoms from which he suffered were. He seeks aid from the physician because he feels ' poorly;' he deferred seeking aid before, because ' he hoped to shake it off.' His bowels have been, he says, somewhat 'out of order,' his head has ached a little, and perhaps he has had trifling cough. He thinks he must have caught cold. Now and then one or other of the symptoms mentioned are especially complained of. Less commonly pain in the limbs and back are trouble-

some. The patient has not given up his ordinary employment, but he feels, as he describes it, 'not up to it.' He lies
in bed as late in the morning as his occupations permit him;
when he rises, feels weary and fatigued, and at night scarcely
able to undress himself. His appetite is lost; more or less
diarrhœa is usually present; sometimes, however, the bowels
are constipated. The tongue is often large, pale, and but
slightly furred. It is generally somewhat tremulous. If the
case be not understood, the patient gradually growing less
able to exert himself, ceases to leave the house, or, if he still
goes out, it is for a short time only. The greater part of the
day he spends in bed or on a couch. At night he is restless,
and disturbed by thirst and a sense of heat—'eaten up by
fever,' as he calls it.

In this state, if the case go on favourably, the patient
continues one day better and another worse, but always losing
flesh for about a month, and then he begins to mend, and
after another week or two feels pretty well.

For many years some of these cases puzzled me much.
A pulse somewhat quickened only, a tongue not greatly
differing from that of health, and no marked heat of skin,
trifling frontal headache, a little sonorous rale, and slight
irregularity of the bowels, seemed local ailments altogether
insignificant, and yet the patient continued ill, and often
appeared worse to his friends than to me, for they saw him
at all times, I only when he was aroused to exertion. I have
supposed the case to go on well; but in some instances it
terminates fatally by hemorrhage from the bowels, or perforation of the intestine, and then the patient dies in a few
days, to the surprise of those who have watched the progress
of the case.

In these latent cases the physician has often but to be
aware of the possible nature of the illness to detect it. The
confirmation follows immediately on the suspicion; for, if
the surface of the abdomen and thorax be carefully examined,
in a large number of cases the rose spots, which, when well
marked, are as characteristic of typhoid fever as are the
small-pox pustules of small-pox, may be detected.

But in a certain proportion of cases, on the most careful
search, not the trace of a spot can be seen.

Still the diagnosis may usually be made with certainty. The conjunction of frontal headache with diarrhœa is rarely observed except in cases of typhoid fever; and, if to these symptoms be added a sense of weakness disproportioned to that which might be occasioned by the diarrhœa, trifling sonorous rale, with a want of steadiness in directing or keeping up, even for a short time, trifling muscular effort, *e.g.* a little unsteadiness of the tongue when fully protruded, a little wavering of the hand when the arm is extended—the diagnosis of typhoid fever may be considered absolute, even though the heart's beats be scarcely quickened, the tongue be moist and almost clean, and the patient able to leave his room for the greater part of the day. Ordinarily, in the cases of which I am speaking, the abdomen is somewhat more resonant than natural, a little ' blown,' as it is called, and gurgling, on careful manipulation, may be detected in the right iliac fossa; the splenic dulness, too, is extensive.

In some cases which commence, as the one I have just sketched, after sixteen or seventeen days have elapsed, the febrile symptoms become more marked, and in a few days the tongue is brown, sordes collect about the teeth, and prostration is considerable; then the disease is said to run into typhus fever.

In other cases cough and sonorous rale are the most prominent symptoms, and then the patient may be supposed to be labouring under a mild but protracted form of bronchitis. A fourth set of cases, from the presence of redness of the tip and edges of the tongue, and the marked character of the intestinal disorder, are called by some 'mild gastric fever,' or ' muco-enteritis.'

While, in a fifth set, the symptoms are so trifling that the patient and his friends resort for an explanation of his illness to those English disorders, a bad cold or an attack of the bile, while the medical attendant sees protracted influenza, irritative dyspepsia, or error in diet.

SCARLATINA.—Passing by those forms of scarlatina which are never fatal, I will enumerate the apparent causes of death in the fatal cases I have examined.

For this purpose I may divide the cases into two groups, viz. those which proved fatal during the first week, and those which proved fatal after the first week. Of the first group some died before the appearance of the rash.

The following are the particulars of a case of this kind which came under my observation in 1851 :—

A man about fifty years of age, his wife and three children, resided in two small rooms opening into each other, in an imperfectly drained house.

Between May 15th and 29th the woman and the three children were attacked with scarlatina. The man slept during the whole time in the same bed with his wife and sick children. On June 1st, about noon, *i.e.* after eating, drinking, and sleeping in an atmosphere highly charged with the emanations from those suffering from scarlatina for seventeen days, this man complained of sore throat.

On the 2nd, about noon, he became suddenly insensible, and near midnight was admitted into University College Hospital. At that time there were a few dusky red patches on the skin, the surface was cold, the pupils large, and the pulse scarcely to be felt. The man continued very restless to the last, and at no time after he came under observation could he give any account of himself. An hour or so before death petechiæ appeared on the skin.

He died at 3 A.M. on the 3rd, *i.e.* less than forty hours after first suffering sore throat.

When the body was examined on the 4th, the whole surface had a purplish mottled aspect. Small spots of extravasated blood were found in the cutaneous tissue under the pleuræ, pericardium, endocardium, peritoneum, and gastro-intestinal mucous membrane.

The tonsils were enlarged, and, in common with the mucous membrane of the *velum pendulum palati* and pharynx, highly vascular. The spleen was large, and there was some engorgement of the vessels of the pia mater.

In some of the cases I have examined which proved fatal during the first week, the rash being fully developed, careful examination after death has not enabled me to detect any great change of structure. In some of these cases the general symptoms have inclined to an inflammatory, and in others to a typhoid type. In neither set of cases were the symptoms referable to the specific throat affection very

prominent during life. The structural changes of extent
or severity that I have found in other cases fatal during the
the first week have been—

(a) Sloughing of the tonsils.

(b) Ulceration of the pharynx and larynx.

(c) Intense redness of, and granular lymph—the croupose
lymph of Rokitansky—on, the mucous membrane of the
pharynx, larynx, and stomach.

(d) Abnormal vascularity of the cellular tissue, and lymphatic glands in the vicinity of the parotid gland, and of
the cellular tissue uniting the lobules of the gland itself,
with excess of serosity in the same tissues.

(e) Blood on the free surface of the arachnoid, without
evidence of the rupture of any vessel appreciable by the
unaided eye.

The grave structural changes I have found in those cases
which have proved fatal after the first week—i.e. after the
rash had disappeared, have been—

Sloughing and ulceration of the fauces and pharynx;

Post-pharyngeal abscess;

And the condition which is often termed 'parotid bubo.'

Under this latter term are comprised the following pathologico-anatomical conditions—viz. inflammation and suppuration of the cellular tissue around the gland, and also

Inflammation and suppuration, chiefly of lymphatic glands
over or near to the parotid gland. In either of these cases
the purulent fluid may be diffused among the structures;
infiltrate them, that is to say, or it may be circumscribed or
collected into an abscess.

Lastly, inflammation and suppuration of the parotid gland
itself. In these cases the pus is diffused through the cellular
tissue, dissecting the lobules of the gland from each other.

The remaining serious lesions I have found, after the disappearance of the rash, have been the effects of local inflammation, especially pleurisy and pneumonia, and collections of
pus in several parts of head, trunk, and extremities.

The death, then, in all these cases, can readily be referred
to the extreme severity of the general specific disease, to
excess of the local specific process, or to the occurrence of
complications.

In *scarlatina simplex* and *scarlatina sine eruptione* the specific general disease is moderate in degree, and the specific throat or skin affection trifling in amount or absent. The complete absence of any affection of the fauces must, I think, be very rare, for no instance of it has fallen under my observation. In a tolerably large number of cases, the patient has complained of sore throat: but inspection of the part in all such cases, has proved the presence of abnormal redness. In scarlatina anginosa the severe and inflammatory character of the throat affection gives a peculiar aspect to the case. The skin affection may, at the same time, be highly or imperfectly developed.

Under the head of *scarlatina maligna* are included several symptomatologically and pathologically distinct varieties of scarlatina.

1st. That variety in which death takes place a day or two after the first symptoms of disease.

2nd. That in which the specific local processes of the skin and throat are fully, but not excessively developed, and the patient dies comatose, or sinks suddenly, while the rash is well out, or immediately it has faded.

3rd. That, in which the eruption is dusky; petechiæ stud the skin; the tongue is dry and brown, the pulse rapid and feeble, and the prostration extreme, and at the same time a tendency is manifested to gangrene of the throat and also of all parts exposed to pressure.

4th. That in which, at a very early stage of the disease, acrid discharges escape from the nose, eyes, and ears; the tonsils are greatly increased in size, and, in common with the uvula, *velum pendulum palati*, and pharynx, are red; the parts behind the rami and angles of the lower jaw are considerably swollen; the pulse rapid and feeble; and the rash more or less imperfectly marked.

In this variety, which is so common in strumous children, all the mucous membranes referred to are the seat of ulceration. I have seen, under these circumstances, a patient recover after losing the sight of both eyes from destruction of the cornea, and having the sense of hearing greatly impaired by ulceration of the membranæ tympanorum.

MEASLES.—A case of measles, in which the disease has assumed a typhoid type, or a case of measles in which death has been caused by the specific disease, or a fatal case of measles, in which no local complication existed, has not fallen under my observation.

As in scarlet fever, either of the specific local processes, viz. the skin eruption or the catarrhal symptoms, may be absent, or, being present, may vary in severity. But it is chiefly from the presence of complications that marked deviations in particular cases of measles from their type arise, and to cases with such complications, chiefly, that the term 'malignant' has been applied.

TYPHUS FEVER.—Cases of typhus fever deviate from the type of the disease chiefly in the greater mildness or severity of the general symptoms, and in the extent and intensity of the specific skin affection. As a rule, the milder the case, the less marked the rash. The danger of the disease is in proportion to the gravity of the general affection, local complications rarely occurring in mild cases to modify the features of the disease. The general symptoms are sometimes so trifling, that the patient hardly needs to keep his bed; while, on the other hand, they are sometimes so severe, that the patient dies within a few hours, constituting the 'typhus siderans' of some authors. The only complication which I have seen causing any material deviation from the type, is inflammation of the intestinal mucous membrane. The symptoms indicating this complication are tympanitic distension of the abdomen and diarrhœa. After death, there is intense vascular engorgement of the mucous membrane with a variable quantity of the granular, croupose, or diphtheritic variety of lymph on its surface. In some cases the inflammation is limited to the mucous membrane of the colon; in some cases the inflammation passes the ileo-cæcal valve, and in others is said to be limited to the small intestine; but it never exhibits any tendency to affect Peyer's patches except in common with the mucous membrane of the whole circumference of the intestine. Typhous deposit, as it is called, is never found in typhus fever.

RELAPSING FEVER.—In relapsing fever the most common deviation from its type is produced by a functional disorder of the liver, which manifests itself by jaundice. I never saw jaundice in typhus or typhoid fevers, though this drawing of the ileum of a soldier, belonging to a native regiment at Sierra Leone, renders it probable that in some countries jaundice does occur in typhoid fever, and also that cases of that disease are confounded under such circumstances, with yellow fever.[1]

The hue of the skin when jaundice occurs in relapsing fever varies from slight sallowness to intense yellowness. At the same time that the skin is yellow, and bile is present in the urine, the stools contain an abundance of bile, and if death occur the gall-bladder is found full, and the cystic and common ducts pervious. Doubtless, some of the cases known in practice as jaundice from hepatic congestion, are in reality cases of relapsing fever, and a suspicion of this should always cross the mind when a patient is suddenly seized with febrile symptoms and yellowness of the skin, the stools being at the same time dark-coloured. In relapsing fever epigastric tenderness is often a prominent symptom. In the second variety of relapsing fever there are lividity and coldness of the surface; a feeble and frequent pulse; delirium of a low type; drowsiness, unconsciousness, and rapid death from asthenia. Jaundice may or may not be present in these cases.

ERYSIPELAS.—There are three great varieties of erysipelas in addition to the typical. I have twice examined fatal cases of erysipelas after death without detecting any marked departure from healthy structure when during life a little dusky redness about the nose and the most trifling redness of the throat had been the only direct evidence of the disease. The general symptoms were delirium at first active and then muttering, followed by somnolence and stupor.

The peculiarities in the other two varieties are dependent on the effects of the severity of the inflammation of the skin and subcutaneous tissue in the one case; and on œdema of the loose cellular tissue about the entrance into the larynx,

---

[1] The drawing referred to was kindly lent to me by Dr. Andrew Smith. It was made when at Sierra Leone by Dr. M'Diarmid, and is contained in the Museum of Pathological Anatomy at Fort Pitt.

especially that of the arytæno-epiglottidean folds, in the other.

In regard, then, to the deviations from the typical forms of the acute specific diseases, the extreme differences observed in the general aspect of the patient are most commonly due to the severity of the general specific disease in typhus fever and relapsing fever ; to the severity and extent of the specific local processes in small-pox and erysipelas ; to the presence of local complications in measles ; and as often to the severity of the general specific diseases as to the extent and severity of the specific local processes and their immediate effects in scarlet fever and typhoid fever.

Each of the acute specific diseases has preserved, for the last two centuries at least, its distinctive characters. Circumstances which have led to the confounding together diseases so opposite. Two great classes of cases received into a fever hospital as cases of fever which do not belong to the order of acute specific diseases: 1st, Diseases in which the constitutional disturbance is secondary to some local affection, e.g., pneumonia and intracranial inflammation—The diagnosis of these diseases. 2nd, General diseases not due to a specific cause—Febricula—Pyogenic fever or the acute purulent diathesis—Acute tuberculosis.

A GLANCE at the history of epidemics will render it evident, that each of the acute specific diseases we have now constantly among us, has maintained its identity through a lengthened series of years, in countries most distant from each other, and in climates most varied,—that each has presented, from first to last, the same group of symptoms, and the same order in their appearance,—that no one of them is a new disease.

That the symptoms of small-pox, the order of occurrence of these symptoms, its chief varieties and its complication, are to-day what they were two hundred years since, to go no further back, there cannot be a question. The same is true of scarlatina. In 1650, an epidemic prevailed in Saxony, characterised by general redness of the skin, sore throat, and desquamation of the cuticle, followed by anasarca; and from that time, at least, we have clear evidence of similar epidemics having every few years prevailed in some part or other of Europe and America:—sometimes arranged with other diseases, as with measles by Morton; sometimes having the mild cases described by one name, and the severe by another, as by Sydenham; sometimes, from one symptom having been very marked in an epidemic, called altogether by another name, as putrid sore throat by Fothergill, and malignant ulcerous sore throat by Huxham; sometimes having other diseases confounded with it, as the morbus strangulatorius, which was evidently diphtheritis rather than scarlet fever.

Now, having its connection with anasarca understood, as in the Saxony epidemic and in a Polish epidemic in 1664, and even having had the date at which the anasarca appeared fixed, as by Rosen von Rosenstein; then having the coincidence of the two in point of frequency of occurrence at the same period noted, the connection between them being overlooked, as by Huxham, who in 1753 described an epidemic, and mentioned that dropsies were frequent during the same constitution of the atmosphere; and then, again, by a third set of writers, having the coincidence in frequency even of the two overlooked. The same evidence of the preservation of its essential characters by measles, might be offered, by tracing accounts left us of epidemics that have visited Europe since that recorded by Forestus, in 1580, to the present time. But it would be useless; the description by Sydenham of the measles of his day will serve for that which we witness now. And yet, different as small-pox, measles, and scarlet fever appear to us—evident as it is, that the symptoms they now present were those which characterised them in times past, men whose powers of observation were of the highest order, viewing the phenomena of these diseases with the idea pre-occupying their minds that they were identical, long failed to discover any essential difference between them, so that it was only by slow degrees that the specific differences of small-pox and measles were admitted; and Morton maintained the identity of scarlet fever and measles, even when a perusal of his own histories of cases leaves no doubt on the mind, that he not only saw the scarlet fever and the measles that we now witness, but that, then as now, each disease had its specific cause, was generated by emanations arising from those suffering from the same affection, and not by emanations from those labouring under any other disease.

With reference to the steps of the process by which the separation of these three diseases into species was effected, they were the same as those by which typhus fever, typhoid fever, and relapsing fever have been in recent times separated into species.

At first, all three were confounded; then one of the three having prevailed for a while in its most perfect form, under the eye of a good observer, an accurate description of that one was obtained; then disputes arose as to the general applicability of the description to the disease in question. It was thought by some to apply to cases to be seen in one epidemic only; but, after a while, epidemics of each of the other two occurred, and good descriptions of these were given; then it was found that occasionally all occurred at the same place at the same time,—that exposure to the emanations of either one only produced the same group of symptoms, and ultimately, that neither disease affected twice the same individual; while, having suffered from one afforded no immunity to attacks of the other: and so the specific character of small-pox, of scarlet fever, and of measles was established.

Louis' work on *Typhoid Fever* was the first great step toward the separation of the continued fevers of Europe and America into species. In that most masterly production is a description of a definite disease, such as has never been given of any other disease.

Then the researches of Gerhard, Valleix, and Stewart proved the existence of a fever, having symptoms, anatomical lesions, and a course altogether different from that described by Louis as pertaining to typhoid fever,—and proved, moreover, that two patients might exhibit the symptoms of these two diseases, severally, during the same period of time. Fresh evidence of the same facts was supplied by other observers. In 1843, and again in 1847, Edinburgh suffered from an epidemic of fever. The cases presented the symptoms now commonly known as those of relapsing fever. A disease offering the same symptoms was seen in London at the same periods; but yet numerous cases, during the last-named epidemic, exhibited the characteristic symptoms of the disease known in this country and in America as typhus

2 F

fever; and of that known in France, America, and England as typhoid fever. It was next shown that an attack of typhus fever afforded no immunity against an attack of typhoid fever,—that an attack of relapsing fever did not secure the sufferer from an attack of typhus fever, or of typhoid fever; while, finally, it was shown that the specific cause of each of the three was different, because exposure to the emanations of either species produced only the symptoms of that species.

If, possessed with an idea of the specific individuality of typhoid fever, typhus fever, and relapsing fever, we review the histories left us of the various epidemics of fever that, from time to time, have swept over large portions of this and other countries, it is a task of far greater difficulty to determine to which of those diseases the descriptions of bygone writers apply, than it is to refer to their proper heads the descriptions given us by the historians of epidemics of small-pox, measles, and scarlet fever, when these three diseases were confounded, or imperfectly distinguished.

Nor shall we be surprised at this, when we reflect that the circumstances which favour the spontaneous origin, if such be possible, and the circumstances which favour the spread of all are the same; that the circumstances which favour the origin and spread of these diseases are just those circumstances which favour the development of the most grave varieties of each; and therefore the development of those symptoms which render their general physiognomy the most nearly alike,—low delirium, a black tongue, abundant sordes, and extreme prostration; symptoms which at once arrested the attention of those who described epidemics in general terms. Again, petechiæ, as is well known, may occur in any disease in which the vital depression is extreme, e.g. malignant measles, small-pox, scarlatina; and the circumstances which promoted the origin and spread of epidemics of fever in years gone by, were just those which cause it to assume a low type, and therefore to be attended by petechiæ; and, still further, the circumstances in question are just those which favour the occurrence of dysentery as a complication of typhus; and, as a consequence, we find descriptions of a fever in which abundant eruption, frequent and bloody stools and great prostration, were the most marked symptoms.

I may remark, that the chief difficulties experienced in determining the identity of the fevers of past years with those now common arise,—

1st, From authors having failed to define the meaning to be attached to the words they employed: *e.g.* petechiæ, miliary eruptions, and pustules, have been used to signify the most varied appearances.

2nd, From the very few examinations made after death, and the loose manner in which the lesions found were described.

3rd, From the description of the epidemics being couched in general terms, so that, if two or more diseases prevailed at the same time, the description was made broad enough to include both.

4th, From the frequency with which relapses escaped observation, *i.e.* from the patient falling under the eye of the physician during the first or second attack only.

5th, From the readiness with which differences actually observed were explained away by the supposed influence of remedies.

But, laying aside some epidemics which cannot, for the reasons just assigned, be referred to either of the species in question, there still remains enough evidence to prove that neither of these diseases differs from diseases which prevailed more than a century since, and strong reason to believe that all were witnessed two centuries ago. The symptoms of the new fever that prevailed in London from 1685 to 1690, as detailed by Sydenham, agree pretty closely with those of typhus fever; and from 1708 to our own times, more or less perfect pictures of the same diseases are contained in the writings of Rogers, O'Connell, Pringle, Rutty, Huxham, Hildebrand, Blane, Hecker, Cullen, Barker, Cheyne, and Armstrong.

In reference to typhoid fever, the histories of some of the epidemics of this disease that have visited Europe since 1697 have been collected by Ozanam. Huxham's Essays on the 'Slow Nervous Fever,' and on the 'Putrid Malignant Fever;' Dr. Gilchrist's (of Dumfries) 'Memoir on Nervous Fever;' 'The Letters to Dr. Lettsom,' by Dr. Vaughan, of Leicester, and Dr. Erasmus Darwin, leave no doubt on the mind of the prevalence of typhoid fever in England from 1734 to 1787; while the abstracts of memoirs and the details of cases collected by Gaultier de Claubry show the frequency with which typhoid fever prevailed, at the end of the last and the commencement of this century, in the hospitals and camps of every country which was the seat of war at that period.

Dr. Huck's account of the differences between the spots common in the cases of Vienna fever treated by De Haen, and called by him ' petechiæ,' and those present in the cases of the fever Sir John Pringle described, prove that the former was typhoid fever, and the latter typhus fever. It was in answer to the attacks of De Haen on the propriety of his treatment, that Pringle wrote: ' I have never considered the gaol or hospital fever and the miliary fever as similar; and, indeed, I may venture to say, that, as the symptoms of the two are so much unlike, they ought to be treated as different in species; and consequently, that neither the theory nor the practice in the one ought to be regulated by analogy from the other.'

At the present time there is an epidemic of fever at Croydon, a point connected with which illustrates the difficulty that may be experienced in fixing on the disease intended to be signified by the historians of the epidemics of past times, who speak in general terms. The disease prevailing in the town just referred to, has been said to be a new form of fever; and some of the medical practitioners of the town, at least, are of that opinion. Now, the fact is, that the Croydon fever differs in no single point from the typhoid fever which is, and has been for several years, so common in London and many other parts of England; in no point from the typhoid fever of Paris, as described by Louis; in no point from the typhoid fever of America, as described by Drs. Gerhard, Bartlett, Jackson, and Flint.

These preparations from the museum of the College, and these drawings, show the identity of the lesions found in the intestines in typhoid fever in years past and those now witnessed.

A few words will suffice to prove the existence for more than a century of a disease having the peculiar symptoms and course of relapsing fever.

Writing on the weather of 1741, Rutty says: 'There was frequently a fever, altogether without the malignity of the disease already described, of six or seven days' duration, terminating in a critical sweat (as did the other also frequently); but in this fever the patients were subject to a relapse, even to a third or fourth time, and yet recovered.' In 1800 and 1801 there was an epidemic in Ireland of a fever generally terminating on the fifth or seventh day by perspiration, and when that happened, very liable to recur. Barker and Cheyne's Reports, and Dr. Welch's work on blood-letting, prove the existence of a similar fever in 1816, 1817, 1818, 1819, and 1820, in Ireland and Scotland; while Dr. Christison's testimony goes to show the identity of the type of fever in the epidemic of 1826 with that described by Dr. Welch, and also the similarity of the fever in these epidemics to that prevalent in 1843 and 1847.

But, if these diseases be now, and have been for centuries, different in symptoms, course, and cause, how came it to pass that they were so frequently associated together? and wherein lies the difficulty now felt by some in admitting their individuality?

1st. From some marked characters being common to all, viz. those general symptoms and peculiarities which make it philosophical to combine them into one natural order, and from striking symptoms characteristic of one species being occasionally present in the others; thus, in typhus fever, we may have a blown belly and diarrhœa from the co-existence of inflammation of the intestinal mucous membrane: the rose spots in typhoid fever are sometimes so abundant as to simulate closely the mulberry-rash of typhus fever; while, on the other hand, the rash in typhus fever may consist of a few spots only; and, again, the skin may be free from spots in both the one and the other. In the rashes of typhus fever and typhoid fever, we see the same deviations from their types that we do in the rashes of measles and scarlet fever.

2nd. From certain varieties of these diseases simulating diseases of another class. When the general disease is not very severe or active in character, and one organ suffers severely, or when the constitutional disturbance and the local disease seem to be in proportion to each other, then the specific nature of the general disease may be overlooked, and the local affection raised to the rank of the primary disease. I have myself, I believe, committed this error repeatedly with regard to typhoid fever, having, accordingly as the cerebral, the thoracic, or the abdominal symptoms prevailed, held the cases to be meningitis, bronchitis, or muco-enteritis.

The third cause of the difficulty felt in admitting the specific differences of these diseases has been, that certain cases of other diseases resemble them generally, and so have been not infrequently associated with them. Just as certain forms of typhoid and of relapsing fever have been from their resemblance generally to some local diseases often ranked with them, so certain forms of other diseases have, from their general resemblance to some of the acute specific diseases, been confounded with them; and so long as the diagnosis of a case of fever is made *per viam exclusionis*,—so long as every case is held to be continued fever in which general febrile disturbance runs high, and no local affection to account for it can be discovered,—so long as acute cases with a hot skin and a quick pulse are termed continued fever *because* the physician can find no other name for them,—so long as the positive diagnosis rests on the presence of general adynamic symptoms,—so long, that is to say, as a brown tongue, a quick pulse, mental aberration, and extreme prostration, are regardéd as *the* characteristic symptoms of continued fever,—so long as *these* are the positive symptoms and *those* the negative symptoms on which the diagnosis rests, so long must a common name be assigned to diseases the most varied in their pathological nature and in their anatomical characters.

For as regards these positive symptoms, they are those of the severest forms of scarlet fever and of measles; they are the symptoms the most prominent in local inflammation in the aged, and in those persons the powers of whose nervous system have been shattered by excesses; they are the symptoms the most prominent in certain forms of acute tuberculosis, and of the so-called acute purulent diathesis; and they may be induced at will by the injection into the veins of certain foreign matters.

But to inquire more particularly into this point: if one

looks over a list of the diseases, other than the acute specific diseases, under which patients were labouring when received into a fever hospital with certificates from medical men that they were affected with fever, it is at once seen that these diseases are referable to two classes.

The one comprehends those local affections, the direct symptoms of which are masked or thrown into the shade by the prominence or peculiarities of the sympathetic or secondary constitutional disorder.

The other class includes those diseases in which a general febrile condition precedes the development of the local lesions; in which, in fact, the latter bear to the former the same relation that the local changes of structure bear to the general symptoms in small-pox and measles. Of the first class, pneumonia and intracranial inflammations are the most important; of the second, febricula, the purulent diathesis, and acute tuberculosis.

With reference to pneumonia and intracranial inflammation, time permits me only to observe, that it is to typhus fever alone that they bear any striking resemblance, and then only when occurring in persons of mature or advanced years; and in these persons typhus fever—if severe at least—is attended by mulberry rash. If this fact be considered, and the physical signs of pneumonia be sought for, an error of diagnosis in regard to that affection will indeed rarely be made, even though the patient come under observation in a state of insensibility, and at an advanced period of the disease. In typhus fever, when delirium sets in, headache ceases; and the occurrence of partial paralysis is extraordinarily rare in that disease. If these two facts be added to that just stated in reference to the rash, the differential diagnosis of typhus fever and intracranial inflammations, with general adynamic symptoms, will not present any great difficulty. But excluding these cases, there yet remain three general affections, probably blood diseases, sometimes confounded with the specific fevers, requiring more particular notice. These diseases are—febricula, the acute purulent diathesis or pyogenic fever, and acute tuberculosis.

The following are the characters of a moderately severe, typical case of—

FEBRICULA.

After fatigue, some slight excess, or without known cause; chilliness, with or without rigors; headache; sense of fatigue; pain in the limbs, very quickly followed by a hot and dry skin; the patient, however, rarely complains of a sense of heat; and, if in bed, when the clothes are removed, he quickly covers himself again from the discomfort produced by the cold air; the pulse is frequent, the heart often beating 120 or 130 times in the minute; the tongue is white; the appetite lost; the bowels sometimes confined; the urine scanty and high-coloured; drowsiness is sometimes present, but not infrequently the patient suffers from want of sleep. In young children a little wandering may be observed on first waking, or when about to fall asleep; and the little patient often talks while dozing. A physical examination of the thorax and abdomen demonstrates no deviation from health. The symptoms present on the first day continue, and sometimes increase in severity, for four or five days. About the end of the week a crisis occurs; most commonly an abundant perspiration, not infrequently a herpetic eruption about the lips; vomiting, diarrhœa, or hemorrhage from nose, uterus, or rectum; and then, in twenty-four hours or less, the patient is well.

As to particular cases, sometimes one symptom, sometimes another, is more marked than in the typical case I have so briefly sketched. I have seen the delirium or the vomiting give a character to the disease. The duration of this disease is sometimes less than forty-eight hours, and it is then called ephemera by some authors. In other cases it continues for nine or ten days, and such cases have been termed synocha, synochus, la synoque non putride, la synoque pléthorique, inflammatory fever, etc.

In some cases of febricula, an eruption of pale, bluish-coloured spots, neither elevated above the level of the surface nor affected by pressure, is observed; these are the *tâches bleuâtres* of Forget and other French writers. They bear no resemblance to the rose-spots of typhoid fever, nor to the mulberry rash of typhus fever. They are not confined to cases of febricula. I have seen them well marked in typhoid fever. They are therefore not characteristic of febricula.

Febricula is essentially a non-contagious and sporadic affection; however, now and then, it has reigned as an epidemic; thus, Ozanam refers to two great epidemics, the one described by Ingrassia, of Palermo, which occurred in 1557, and the other, the particulars of which were recorded by Hoyer, of Mülhausen, in 1700. Full descriptions of this affection are to be found in almost all writers, from Hippocrates to those who flourished at the commencement of the present century. About that time the influence of pathological anatomy on medical doctrines began more especially to be felt, and men hesitated to admit the existence of any essential fever, of any disease which the scalpel did not enable the anatomist to refer to some change of structure; and as febricula never proves fatal unless by complications established in its course, its existence was held to be apocryphal, and those who maintained its occurrence were regarded as bunglers in the art of diagnosis,—as men who overlooked the local lesion, and raised the sympathetic constitutional disorder to the rank of a substantive disease.

The recognition of the existence of febricula is, however, of considerable importance with regard to the advance of the science of medicine, for two reasons especially: first, because by an acquaintance with its phenomena the physician is prevented falling into serious errors in over-estimating the effect of remedial agents in the treatment of the acute specific fevers; and, secondly, because in its course local inflammations are very frequently set up which undergo, or appear to undergo, a more or less marked abatement when the general affection has run its course, and the physician is in these cases led to overrate the potency of the drugs administered; and as the supposed effects are striking in character, the impression produced on the mind is proportionably strong; or, he is led to under-estimate the severity, speaking generally, of the local inflammation, because it, in this striking case, did well without treatment, or under treatment singularly in opposition to received doctrines.

I remember a case of this kind I was once suddenly requested to see in the absence of the physician in attendance. The patient, a strong-made man, about forty-five years of age, was suffering, as I supposed at the time, judging from the signs and symptoms then present, from primary asthenic pneumonia. He was taking, under the direction of the physician, two ounces of sherry every six hours. No loss of blood had been practised. The skin was hot, the pulse quick, the cough troublesome. I did not, under the circumstances in which I was placed, feel justified in adopting any active treatment. A few hours subsequently the man sweated freely, and on the following day appeared, as far as his general symptoms were concerned, well.

The sudden cessation of the general symptoms in a case of pneumonia, on or about the seventh day of disease, by profuse sweating, would excite in my mind strong doubts in regard to its primary nature.

With reference to the symptomatological affinity of febricula, it is evidently closely allied to relapsing fever; but it differs from it etiologically, and, therefore, specifically. It has no power of generating a substance capable of reproducing its own phenomena in a healthy individual. Symptomatologically, again, it is more or less closely allied to the acute purulent diathesis or pyogenic fever and acute tuberculosis; but anatomically it differs from these in the most absolute manner.

PYOGENIC FEVER.

Acute purulent diathesis; or, as I would rather call it, *pyogenic fever*; or, to distinguish it from the specific fevers, *simple pyogenic fever*.

Immediately after the termination of the acute specific diseases, it is by no means uncommon for one or two small abscesses to form in the subcutaneous cellular tissue. A frequent seat of these collections of purulent-looking fluid is the subcutaneous cellular tissue of the scalp. More or less febrile disturbance may precede or accompany their development. Although more common, perhaps, in the situation referred to than elsewhere, they are by no means limited to it. Sometimes, instead of two or three, the number of these collections of purulent-looking fluid is considerable. If small, their contents may be absorbed; but this rarely happens if their size exceeds that of a walnut.

The signs of inflammation that precede the formation of

the pus are usually of the most trivial kind, the patient's knowledge of the existence of the local ailment being first derived from the presence of the swelling; the physician at the same time observes fluctuation. Sometimes, however, the signs of inflammation are more manifest, and, while pus is formed more or less rapidly at some spots, at others the inflammatory signs disappear, and neither before nor after their disappearance is any evidence of the presence of pus to be detected. The local lesion is limited to the first stage.

The disseminated abscesses in the subcutaneous tissue, after or during the progress of the acute specific diseases, are allowed pretty generally to have their origin in a diseased condition of the blood; only, by some they are held to be critical,—the evacuants of peccant matter: while by others they are regarded merely as local inflammations, excited by a diseased condition of the blood,—a diseased condition which gives to the local inflammation it excites a tendency to terminate in the exudation of a blastema susceptible only of evolution into an albuminous fluid and cells of low organisation.[1] The exudation of a blastema possessing the same properties in so many places at the same time, is held to indicate the existence of a definitely diseased condition of the fluid from which that blastema is formed, just as the deposit of many masses of cancer blastema in the same body at the same time is held to indicate the existence of a definite disease of the blood in the person who is the seat of them. The idea that these subcutaneous collections of purulent-looking fluid of small size, and the formation of which is attended with little constitutional disturbance, are due to any foreign solid matter, be it pus globules or any other, circulating in the blood, has never, as far as I know, been advanced;

[1] The cells found in the purulent-looking fluid are spherical, and about the size of pus corpuscles; as a rule, they have no nucleus, but contain only granules, composed partly of fat and partly of protein matter. The number of the granules varies; so that the corpuscles may be identical in appearance with the pyoid corpuscles of Lebert, or they may have in their interior so many granules as to resemble the ordinary granular corpuscle. Sometimes, however, the majority of the cells contain a single nucleus; and, now and then, pus corpuscles, with two, three, or four nuclei, are found to constitute the bulk of the cells.

it would be too untenable to be entertained for an instant.
But, instead of being attended by little constitutional disturbance, as in the cases to which I have just referred, we now
and then find that great constitutional derangement precedes
and accompanies the establishment of the suppurative action,
—that, instead of being situated in the cellular tissue immediately under the skin, the collections of purulent-looking
fluid are formed in cellular tissue more deeply seated.   Again,
in other cases, we find that they are not limited to the
cellular tissue, but that the pus blastema is exuded into the
joints; and yet further, that it is in rare cases disseminated
in masses through the viscera of the chest and abdomen.
Now, the transition from the first to the last described state
is by most insensible gradations; the circumstances under
which all occur are the same; and, if it be granted that the
first arises from a definitely diseased state of the blood or
system generally, I see not on what ground it can be argued,
that the others, which differ only in the more wide diffusion
of the local affections, may not also depend on the same
diseased state of the blood.   This disease seems very closely
allied to that condition of the blood in which purulent discharges issue at the same time from several of the mucous
membranes after some of the acute specific fevers, and to that
chronic state in which every scratch or abrasion 'festers,' as
the vulgar say.   The existence of this condition of the blood
or system generally, as a substantive disease, appears to have
been in modern times first recognised by Tessier in 1838.
He, however, associated with it the cases in which disseminated abscesses are excited by the circulation of foreign
matter in the blood.   Tessier described the state referred to
as a new pathological genus, under the name of the ' purulent diathesis;' and he defined it to be a modification of the
organism characterised by a tendency to suppuration in the
solids and coagulable fluids.

Amid much that is pathologically erroneous, the doctrine
of Tessier appears to contain an important truth, viz. that in
a certain number of cases of disseminated abscesses the febrile
disturbance is established before any local disease is set up,
and, consequently, before any pus is formed, and by inference,
that the abscesses are, in such cases, merely the effects of a

special alteration of the element from which that blastema is exuded out of which they are developed.

Although the morbid condition of the blood, which is thus manifested by its effects, is common as a consequence of the acute specific diseases, it sometimes arises without having been preceded by any other disease, *i.e.* as a primary substantive affection.

Of this the following case appears to me to offer some evidence :—

A man, aged thirty-one years, of temperate habits, and usually enjoying health, after feeling generally poorly for two or three days, became decidedly ill July 23rd. The symptoms were—heat of skin, headache, a furred tongue, and disinclination for all exertion. On the evening of the 24th, a red patch appeared on the outer aspect of either leg. On the 25th, there was induration of the same patches. On the 26th, there was redness of the left shoulder, and a red, indurated, elevated patch on the outer aspect of the left upper arm. The mind now became confused.

He came under my care in University College Hospital on the 28th. At that time his mind was confused, and occasionally wandered. His movements were rather tremulous, and there were now and then some twitchings of the muscles of the face. He was rather restless, and slept but little. There was no headache. The complexion was thick, and rather sallow. The tongue was moist and red at the tip and edges, and on its dorsum was a little dirty fur. The abdomen was rather full and resonant, but not tender. He passed, during twenty-four hours, one stool. The pulse was 96, moderately full, but rather weak. The heart's sounds were natural. Red patches,—the redness gradually shading into the hue of the surrounding skin, some indurated, others not,—were seated on the outer aspect of the right thigh, the calf of the left leg, the anterior aspect of the left tibia, the inner and anterior aspect of the right upper arm, and the centre of the right deltoid.

The whole surface was carefully inspected. There was not the slightest trace of suppuration at any spot; no redness nor tenderness in the course of any of the veins in the vicinity of the red spots, nor, so far as could be ascertained, elsewhere.

There was no cough. The respirations were 24 in the minute.

Time will not permit me to detail the daily notes of the case. Suffice it to say, that many other red patches appeared at various parts of upper and lower extremities,—that pus was evacuated from two seated on the anterior aspect of one tibia,—that fluid was effused into the knee-joints, and probably into one ankle-joint,—and that at no time was there reason to believe that any internal organ was the seat of purulent deposits. The patient recovered completely at the expiration of about a month from the first symptoms of illness.

The following is an abstract of a case of this disease, which occurred subsequently to measles :—

A boy, aged four and a half years, was admitted, under my care, into the fever ward of the Hospital for Sick Children, in August last.

About a week after the disappearance of the rash of measles, the child never having been free from symptons of illness, the wrists were observed to be swollen; then an abscess formed in the subcutaneous tissue of the back. Subsequently, collections of pus formed on the dorsum of the right hand, over the right wrist, in and over the left elbow-joint, under the right glutaeus maximus, in the cellular tissue about the right psoas, and in the left hip-joint; and there were purulent discharges from the ears. He died about five weeks after the swelling of the wrists commenced.

No purulent fluid was found in any internal organ. The examination of the body was made by my friend, Dr. Ballard. In these cases, as in *the majority of those belonging to the same order, the subcutaneous tissue and joints were exclusively the seats of the collections of purulent fluid.* In some such cases, however, abscesses are found in the lungs; but then they are generally small in size, few in number, and in a much less advanced state than those in the parts I have just mentioned; while it will be remembered, that when foreign solid matters, as pus corpuscles, etc., are thrown by the experimentalist into the venous current, it is the lungs which are alone affected in a large majority of cases; and when other parts suffer, the lungs are still the most extensively diseased.

Sedillot supports his doctrine, that the circulation of pus corpuscles with the blood is the sole cause of disseminated abscesses, by four orders of proof:—

1st, By the invariable pre-existence of a centre of suppurative action.

In the class of cases to which I am referring there is no pre-existing abscess or ulcer.

2nd, By the relation observed between the formation of pus in the veins, the passage of that liquid into the blood, and the development of pyæmia.

Of this relation there is no evidence in the class of cases of which I am speaking.

3rd, By the presence of pus in the blood, verified by observation.

There is no pus to be detected in the blood in those cases which I would class together under the name of pyogenic fever. Of this, repeated examinations enable me to speak with confidence.

4th, By the results obtained by the injection of pus into the veins of animals.

Now, as the symptoms and the *situation* of the disseminated abscesses are different in cases of pyogenic fever, and artificially induced pyæmia, it is improbable that the disseminated abscesses in the two have their origin in the same cause. And as the disseminated abscesses, artificially produced by Sedillot, were undoubtedly the effect of the circulation of pus with the blood, it is the more unlikely that the disseminated abscesses, in the class of cases I am describing, are the effects of the circulation of pus with the blood.

Thus, then, tested by Sedillot's four orders of proof, there are cases of multiple, or disseminated abscesses, which are not, or which cannot be proved to be directly or indirectly excited by the entrance of pus into the blood.

The acute specific disease, with which especially the acute purulent diathesis, or pyogenic fever, may be confounded, is, typhus fever. From this it is distinguished by the activity of the febrile symptoms at the outset, the early delirium, the absence of eruption, and the rapid formation of the numerous centres of suppurative action.

Pathologically, the affinity of this disease seems to be with erysipelas.

I ought not to quit this subject without stating, that, although I have spoken only of the two varieties of the acute purulent diathesis, which especially fall under the cognisance of the physician, viz. that which follows the acute specific diseases, and that which arises as a primary affection, yet Tessier considers, that phlebitis, phlegmonous erysipelas, and internal abscesses following operations, are consequences of the same general condition. The questions here raised are foreign to the object of these discourses.

ACUTE TUBERCULOSIS.

The third disease of this class, often confounded with typhus and typhoid fever, but especially with the latter, is acute tuberculosis; and, in many cases, the diagnosis, from the close similarity of the symptoms, is most difficult.

Like typhoid fever, acute tuberculosis rarely affects persons after the middle period of life.

The cases of acute tuberculosis I have myself mistaken for typhoid fever, or which I have seen others mistake for that disease, have assumed one of three forms—the insidious, the active febrile, and the adynamic.

The first form occurs almost exclusively in children ; the patient, often after measles, or scarlet fever, but not unfrequently without known cause, is observed to be languid; unwilling to make any exertion ; complains of headache; lies about; seeks quiet, leaving its companions; is heavy, dull, or irritable in temper ; the skin is hot and dry ; the pulse frequent; the tongue moist, and slightly furred; the appetite lost, or variable ; the bowels confined, or irregular ; the stools more or less clay-like, putty-like, or parti-coloured ; the abdomen free from tenderness, and of its normal form ; there is a trifling cough, and a little sonorous and sibilous rale, or the respiratory murmur is simply rough or harsh, and the expiration rather loud and prolonged, or, it may be, perfectly natural. Some time usually elapses before advice is sought, so indefinite are the symptoms of the illness; and after it is sought, the physician is occasionally some time in attendance before the gravity of the affection is comprehended; for the febrile symptoms often remit during the day, the skin being little above its natural temperature, and the pulse only a little quicker than natural, when he makes his visit. Thus the disease proceeds for two, three, or four weeks, when the functions of some one organ become disturbed in an extreme degree, and the patient dies with all the symptoms of tuber-onlar meningitis, bronchitis, pneumonia, or peritonitis.

After death in such a case, grey granulations, or yellow tubercles, are found in many organs; only, in the particular organ from the disorder of which the patient died, in addition to grey granulations, great vascularity, or the products, more or less abundant, of inflammation, serosity, lymph, or pus are discovered.

In the active febrile form, the symptoms are from the outset severe, the pulse is quick, and the heat of the skin considerable, and the patient, from an early period of the disease, confined to bed.

In the third, or adynamic form, the illness begins some-what suddenly, after a trifling sense of *malaise* of a few days' duration. The symptoms are, chilliness, hot skin, frequent pulse, moist furred tongue, headache, loss of appetite, confined bowels, vomiting, considerable sense of weakness, great un-willingness to be disturbed, with irritability of temper. After a week or ten days, the mind wanders occasionally, the bowels are generally confined, and the abdomen flat or con-cave; though the former are sometimes relaxed, and the latter full. The skin continues hot, dry, and harsh; the tongue becomes dry and brown; sordes collect about the teeth; prostration is extreme; and the patient sinks about three or four weeks after the outset of the disease.

The two last-described forms of acute tuberculosis are seen occasionally in adults; but, in them, the recent deposit of tubercle, the newly formed grey granulations, are almost always limited to one or two organs; in the cases that have fallen under my own observation, the pia mater, or the lungs, or both. Under these circumstances, more or less marked disturbances of the functions of the lungs or brain are observed. At the same time the general symptoms may be either those of the active febrile, or of the adynamic variety. In the *former* case,

2 G

the disease may be mistaken for idiopathic inflammation, and the general symptoms be regarded as symptomatic; in the *latter* case, the disease may be thought to be typhoid fever.

The diagnosis from typhoid fever, when the granulations occupy the pia mater, is formed *positively* from the frequency of the vomiting, the severity of the headache, and its continuance after the patient is delirious, the knitting of the brows, the frequent sighing, the dislike to light, the occasional and transient general flushings of the face, the slowness of the pulse, and evidence of paralysis. So long as it is very imperfect, the paralysis may escape observation, unless especially looked for. It is manifested thus :—Sometimes one pupil contracts rather less completely or less actively than the other when exposed to a strong light. Sometimes there is a slight deviation of the tongue. Sometimes the uvula is drawn to one side, and the opposite half of the velum pendulum palati drops. Sometimes one radial artery[1] is felt to be a little larger than the other, such differences not being natural to the patient. This last evidence of paralysis will occasionally precede any appreciable loss of voluntary muscular power.

There is this seeming peculiarity about these imperfect paralyses in the disease in question, viz. that when observed on the one side on any given day, on the following day the opposite side may be found to be the diseased side. This shifting of the disease is—in many cases at least—rather apparent than real; thus, the paralysis of the right side we will suppose to be very imperfect, but still sufficient to cause *comparative* sluggishness of the right pupil. On the following day, the left side is the more completely though still imperfectly paralysed; then there is *comparative activity* of the right pupil.

Negatively, the adynamic form of acute tuberculosis, with deposit of grey granulations in the pia mater, is distinguished from typhoid fever by the absence of diarrhœa, of distension of the abdomen, of enlargement of the spleen, and of rose spots.

---

[1] In several cases of hemiplegia I have observed the radial artery on the paralysed side to be larger than on the opposite side ; and, in two of these cases, no such difference in the size of the arteries existed the day before the fit.

But all the positivo signs may be wanting till near the close of the disease ; and, on the other hand, diarrhœa, tympanitic distension of the abdomen, and enlargement of the spleen may be present, sometimes with, sometimes without, the deposit of tubercles under the mucous membrane of the intestine, and in the spleen. As regards the rose spots, I have never seen them in a case of acute tuberculosis. But Dr. Waller, of Prague, states that he has observed them in cases of acute phthisis ; and Rilliet and Barthez say that very fugitive, imperfectly formed rose-spots are in rare cases present.

In reference to those cases in which the deposit of grey granulations is limited to the lungs, the positive symptoms for establishing the diagnosis are derived from the signs of oppressed breathing, the rough inspiratory murmur, with intense and prolonged expiratory murmur, and the general diffusion of these signs pretty uniformly over both lungs. Hæmoptysis occurs in some of these cases—rarely, if ever, in typhoid fever.

The affinity of acute tuberculosis with typhoid fever is shown by the general symptoms of the two being often undistinguishable, by the frequency with which particular parts are, in both, the seat of disseminated protein deposits, and by the tendency manifested in both to ulceration, not only of the mucous membranes generally, but of a part of the intestinal mucous membrane which is rarely the seat of ulceration in other diseases, viz. that covering Peyer's patches.

With reference to the close resemblance of the symptoms in some cases of local inflammation, with adynamic symptoms, and typhus fever, of acute tuberculosis, and typhoid fever, of measles and scarlet fever, of typhus and typhoid fevers, I would quote the following sentence by the author of the *Philosophy of Medical Science*:—' It is very important for us to bear in mind that great difficulties of diagnosis in individual cases are in no way incompatible with the existence of essentially and widely different diseases. Morbid affections, very unlike each other, and in most cases easily distinguishable, may, under certain circumstances, have many things in common ; and their symptoms may be so mixed up with each other, as to render, in the very imperfect state of our knowledge, a positive diagnosis very difficult or impossible, and this without throwing any doubt upon the general question of the radical dissimilarity between the diseases themselves.' —(Bartlett, p. 321.)

In conclusion, I may remark that it seems to me, from the survey we have taken of the symptoms of the typical cases of the acute specific diseases, of the deviations from those symptoms met with in practice, of the causes of those deviations, of the histories of epidemics of these same diseases, and of the diseases with which some of them are confounded, that, in adopting the division of them I have here advocated, and in grouping them as I have here grouped them, we avoid those errors to which I adverted at the commencement of these lectures, that we pay no homage to those *idola specûs* against which the voice of Bacon warned us,—that we should neither divide where Nature has drawn no line, nor generalise where Nature has bestowed no unity.

AN ADDRESS

ON THE

TREATMENT OF TYPHOID FEVER

DELIVERED BEFORE THE MIDLAND MEDICAL SOCIETY
AT BIRMINGHAM, NOVEMBER 4TH, 1879

ON THE TREATMENT OF TYPHOID FEVER[1]

WHEN the Council did me the honour of asking me to address the Society this evening I acceded to the request with the intention of bringing before its members some general subject; but subsequently I gathered that this Society has for its aim the dissemination among the members of practical knowledge rather than of medico-political opinions, and so I thought it wiser to follow the example of my predecessors, and fix on a purely practical subject.

Though I have nothing new on the matter to bring before you this evening, and have, therefore, in some measure to pray your pardon for occupying so much of your valuable time in the enumeration of common truth, I still think myself justified in selecting the Treatment of Typhoid Fever for my paper to-night (1) because of the intrinsic importance of the subject; (2) because some of the questions concerning the treatment of typhoid fever are considered by many to be still undecided; (3) because not only have I had, for a longer period, probably, than any of my hearers, much experience in the treatment of the disease, but I have also had during later years frequent opportunities of myself seeing the results of various modes of treatment as practised by others; (4) because, although I have written much and often on the etiology and pathology of the disease, I have never publicly expressed any opinion or written a line on its treatment.

In so complex a disease as typhoid fever—the mortality and symptoms of which vary not only with the age, habits, and family constitution of the patients, but also with the dose and mode of access to the system of the poison, the conditions which precede and those which accompany the disease during its incubative period and its earliest development, the epidemic constitution, the date at which the dis-

---

[1] From the *Lancet*, Nov. 15, 1879.

ease is first treated, and the early management of the patient
—it is scarcely possible to find two cases in all respects
identical, and quite impossible to collect records of a
sufficient number of cases practically identical to determine
by numerical analysis the best mode of treatment.   And
even of the specially prominent symptoms—*e.g.* temperature,
rapidity of pulse, diarrhœa—each one may owe its origin to
such different pathological conditions, and it is so often impossible to determine in any given case to which of these
several conditions it is due, that in the *present state* of pathological knowledge it seems to me that it is impracticable to
determine otherwise than by the opinions formed by individuals from personal experience what are the best means
to be employed in the treatment, not only of typhoid fever
itself, but also of each symptom, and how and under what
circumstances each remedy should be employed.   I do not
in the least degree under-estimate the immense importance
of numerical analysis for arriving at truth on medical subjects; and if it were possible to find the value of the several
remedies proposed for the treatment of typhoid fever, or of
its symptoms, by numerical analysis, the results of such an
analysis would be real steps in our knowledge, for facts would
replace opinions, and doubts in regard to the influence of
remedies be impossible.   Each special act of treatment would
then be based on firm grounds, instead of being, as it now is,
an experiment performed by the medical attendant.   The
sum of his own experiments constitutes each man's experience, to which, in proof of the correctness of his practice, he
appeals as to a judge whose decision is final and infallible.
And yet how different are the conclusions, all based on experience, drawn by different observers in regard to the effects
on any given disease or symptom of any given remedy.   The
physician orders a drug or a stimulant or employs a bath;
and then, according to the credulous or sceptical tendency
of his mind, his experience in the special disease he is treating, his knowledge of its natural course and history, his
powers of observation, and the general soundness of his
judgment, the *post hoc* is, in his opinion, a mere *post hoc*, or
a veritable *propter hoc*, and the remedies he employed have
been, in his opinion, of little consequence or all-important,

and so he builds up his experience on treatment. And the difficulty of building up treatment by the accumulation of the experience of many men, expressed by their opinions merely, is enhanced by the fact that, even when the conclusion is correct, and the good effect following the administration of the drug is a veritable *propter hoc*, it is for many men an impossibility to follow or define for themselves, much more describe to others, the several steps in the mental analysis of the facts before them which they have performed in arriving at their correct conclusion. Some men appear to be capable of performing this delicate mental analysis correctly without being able to follow the steps of the analysis in their own minds; they are no more capable of following their own mental efforts, or of telling another how they arrived at their correct conclusion, than are those children who solve complex arithmetical problems in a few seconds without themselves knowing by what steps they pass from the premises to the conclusion.

Believing, however, notwithstanding all these sources of serious error, that in the present state of pathological knowledge it is impossible to fix the treatment of typhoid fever on a more sure basis than individual opinions founded on experience, I propose to describe what my experience has taught me to be the most successful methods of treatment of the disease, and also of some of the symptoms which, by the severity they may attain, cause grave discomfort to the patient, or place his life in danger. I shall limit myself to those symptoms which may be considered to be the natural manifestations of the disease, for time will not permit me to pass, even briefly, in review all the symptoms common in the disease or the complications, although the patient often succumbs to these symptoms and to these complications.

To give a clear view of the treatment of these symptoms I shall be obliged to refer to the pathological conditions in which they severally originate.

I have never known a case of typhoid fever cut short by any remedial agent—that is cured. The poison which produces any one of the acute specific diseases (to which order typhoid fever as much as small-pox belongs) having entered the system, all the stages of the disease must, so far as we know, be passed through before the recipient of the poison can be well. If the patient can be kept alive for a definite time the specific disease ends, and then, if no local lesion remains to constitute a substantive disease, the patient is well. The treatment of typhoid fever is essentially rational. To treat a case with the best possible prospect of success the physician ought to be acquainted with the epidemic constitution of the period, the etiology of the disease, its mode of attack, its natural course, the order of appearance, and the natural duration of each of its symptoms, the way in which each symptom influences the termination, the several pathological lesions which produce or may produce each special symptom, and the complications to be watched for at each stage of the disease.

Certain facts have to be kept in mind when treating a case of typhoid fever and when estimating the effect of remedies:—First, that the disease, in the majority of cases at least, is produced by the action of a small portion of the excreta from the bowel of a person suffering from typhoid fever; that air from a drain, or air blowing over dry fæculent matter, may convey the poison to the patient, or his own fingers may carry it to his mouth, or that the vehicle for the poison may be a fluid—for example, water or milk; and that the poisonous properties of the excreta may be destroyed by boiling the fluid in which they are contained, though not by filtering the fluid. Secondly, that the natural duration of a well-developed case of typhoid fever is from twenty-eight to thirty days. Hence subsidence of the fever before that date should be regarded with suspicion, and the patient not treated as if the specific disease had ended, while the continuance of febrile disturbance after that date should lead to repeated and most careful examination of the patient, in order to ascertain if any local lesion is keeping up the febrile excitement. But not only is the duration of the specific disease limited, but the prominent symptoms have their regular order of sequence, and several their own natural limits of duration—that is, a time to begin and a time to end: and the natural termination of a symptom has often been attributed to the remedial agent last employed.

On what part of the system the poison exerts its earliest

influence, whether on the agminated glands or on the nervous system through the blood, must in the present state of our knowledge be doubtful; but that by the time the first symptoms of the disease occur the nervous system and the agminated glands of the small intestine are both seriously affected there can be no question. That the nervous system suffers at the outset is shown by the headache and the general nutritive disturbance, *i.e.* by elevation of temperature and loss of weight, due to waste of the tissues generally, and by the arrested or disturbed secretions generally; and that the agminated glands also suffer from the outset is shown by the pain in the abdomen and deranged action and secretion of the bowels, and also by rare post-mortem examination made within a few days of the beginning of illness.

In the earliest stage of typhoid fever the patient is prone to commit certain mistakes in treating himself, either of which may greatly add to the severity of the coming illness. (1) He may think that he has a common cold in his limbs, as it is called, and try to throw it off by strong exercise. A certain sense of weakness accompanies this early stage of the fever, but it is rarely so great as to prevent the patient, if stimulated by strong will, walking long and briskly. (2) He may consider that he is suffering from biliary derangement, and attribute to this the headache, disturbed nights, sense of malaise, want of appetite, and disordered bowels, and take a dose of drastic aperient. (3) He may think the weakness he feels is to be removed by food and wine. A dose of medicine, he says, cannot hurt; bed, he thinks, weakens; and food and wine, he knows, restore strength; therefore he prescribes a dose for himself which irreparably injures his bowel; he takes exercise which increases the waste material in his system, and he loads his stomach with food it cannot digest, and stimulants which heighten the fever and disturb the action of the eliminating organs, and then pays the penalty, perhaps, with his life, for the errors his ignorance had led him to commit.

The thermometer saves, or ought to save, the physician from the patient's mistakes. The temperature having rendered it even *possible* that the ill-defined and may be trifling symptoms are due to the poison of typhoid fever, the patient should be absolutely confined to bed. Exercise or fatigue immediately before or after the absorption of the poison, and especially when the action of the poison is manifesting itself, increases the gravity of the disease, partly by exhausting the nervous power, but chiefly, I think, by causing destruction of tissue, and so the presence of waste material in the system on which the poison can act; and at the same time, by disturbing the action of the eliminating organs, it leads to the retention in the system of the products of the destroyed tissue.

Some of the worst cases of typhoid fever I have ever seen have appeared to me to owe their gravity to the patient having travelled, after the commencement of the sense of illness, in order to reach home. I very rarely advise a patient's removal to his home if that be distant, so satisfied am I that the fatigue of travel, whether by rail or carriage, tends to make what would otherwise have proved a mild case severe, and to cause a bad case, which might after, perhaps, a struggle have ended favourably, to terminate in death. Not only is other tissue-destruction than that due to the fever process in a great degree prevented by rest in bed, but the nervous system is there less liable to disturbance, any tendency to moisture of skin is favoured, the elimination of the products of waste tissue is unchecked, and chances of error in diet diminished. The air of the room should be as pure as possible; the room in which the patient is placed be large enough to permit its being freely ventilated without draughts; if possible, the patient should occupy a different room at night from that used in the day.

From the first the patient should be restricted to liquid diet, with farinaceous food, and bread in some form if the appetite requires it. It is better to vary the broths, and to add to them some strong essence of vegetables. Sometimes a little strained fruit juice is taken with advantage, but skins and seeds of fruits and particles of the pulp are frequent sources of irritation of the bowels. Grapes are always dangerous, from the difficulty of preventing the seeds slipping down the throat. The value of milk as an article of diet in fever is generally admitted, but it requires to be given with caution. The indiscriminate employment of milk in almost unlimited quantities as diet in fever has led to serious troubles. Milk contains a large amount of solid animal food. The casein of the milk has to pass into a solid form before digestion can take place. Curds form in the stomach, and the digestive powers being weakened in fever, these curds may remain unchanged in the stomach, and produce considerable disturbance of system.

I have seen the patient restless, sleepless, or drowsy, his temperature raised several degrees above what it had previously been, vomit, eject a quantity of curd, and at once the restlessness cease, the temperature fall, the skin become moist, and the patient drop into a quiet sleep. All the threatening symptoms vanish with the ejection of the offending material. Or the undigested curds may accumulate in the bowel, inducing flatulent distension and pain in the abdomen, restlessness, and increased febrile disturbance. Under these circumstances, I have seen an enema of thin gruel bring away a large vesselful of offensive, sour, undigested curds. Or, again, the undigested curds may themselves (and this has not been an uncommon consequence of milk diet in my experience) irritate the bowels, and produce, keep up, or greatly increase diarrhœa. A distinguished chemist once remarked to me, ' Do not forget that a pint of milk contains as much solid animal matter as a full-sized mutton-chop ; ' and solid the casein of the milk must become before it can be digested ; and yet I have known a patient drink two quarts, and even more, of milk in twenty-four hours, i.e. solid animal food equal to four mutton-chops. Can anything approaching to such · an amount of solid animal food be digested, and if it could, is such an amount of animal food good for a patient suffering from typhoid fever ? He is weak because of the presence of the fever, and not from lack of food.

Patients suffering from typhoid fever should be allowed an unlimited supply of pure water. When pure water is freely absorbed, it passes away by the kidneys, skin, lungs, etc., and is of much service as a depurating agent. If it be *possible*, even, that the poison of the fever was conveyed into the patient by the drinking-water or milk of the district in which he is ill, then these fluids should be boiled till a different supply is obtained. All sources of foul air from drains

or cesspools should be sought for, and the air the pa
breathes be freed from all possibility of impurity ; disi
tants should be placed in the close-stool, and the de
buried if possible. If the bowels are confined in the
stage of the disease a simple enema should be given.]
stool retained in the bowel will produce irritation, and it
be catarrhal inflammation of the intestinal mucous r
brane, and so induce troublesome diarrhœa. Small dos
mineral acid, well diluted, are grateful to the patient,
may perhaps be useful.

The fever is thus met by rest, quiet, fresh air, ɪɪ
liquid food and bland diluents, and the exclusion of ,
doses of poison ; the intestinal lesion by the careful exclɪ
from the diet of all hard and irritating substances, anɪ
removal from the bowel of any local irritant.

Frontal headache and sleeplessness are two symptoɪ
the early stages of typhoid fever which may cause the pa
much distress. The headache is in some cases alleviate
cold, and in others by warm applications; but as the]
ache ceases spontaneously in about ten days from the o
of the fever, no active treatment is required for its
Local applications, the exclusion of light from the room,
absolute quiet, have been all the means I have seen necɪ
for its relief. Sleeplessness is a more important symɪ
for although it also usually disappears or diminishes ɪ
taneously during the second week of disease, still this ɪ
invariably the case ; and the nervous system may be gɪ
worn by the want of sleep, lasting as it does occasioɪ
unless treated night and day. The drugs I employ ■
from the continued sleeplessness, it seems absolutely ■
sary to relieve it, are henbane, bromide of potassium,
chloral. From a combination of the latter I have seen
good results, and, so far as my experience has gone, no ■
ill effects when its use has been limited to the earlier sɪ
of the disease, i.e. to the period anterior to signs of neɪ
prostration. If the patient's temperature be high, a ɪ
bath or sponging the surface will often at once induce ■
and no drug be required. In the earlier and also in the ﹗
stages of typhoid fever the sleeplessness has been treateɪ
opiates. Experience has convinced me that althougɪ

some cases, opium in sufficient doses to secure sleep has afforded relief, it is on the whole a most dangerous remedy. In the early stage of fever it disturbs digestion and checks secretion. In the later stages of the disease I have seen several cases fatal from its influence on brain, heart, and secreting organs. To my mind, the hoped for, and occasionally attained, good is altogether outweighed by the disproportionately possible evil and occasionally fatal effect resulting from the administration of direct sedatives, opium, and chloral in the later stages of fever.

Changes in the agminated glands are present from the earliest period of the disease, and to these progressing changes in Peyer's patches, in the mesenteric glands corresponding to the patches, and to the disturbances in the intestinal secretion and action consequent on these changes, the abdominal pains and laxness of bowels proper to the fever are due. So long as disease is limited to the specific changes in question there is probably little diarrhœa, but as local disease progresses catarrhal inflammation of the mucous membrane supervenes, and when this is extensive the stools become frequent, liquid, and more or less copious.

The changes preceding the ulceration, and the ulceration itself, of Peyer's patches are specific in nature, as much so as is the eruption on the skin ; and there are no drugs or other means of arresting or limiting these specific processes. But over the diarrhœa which usually accompanies these processes in their progress we can, in many cases, exercise a decided influence.

The chief causes of diarrhœa in excess of that due to the intestinal specific changes in typhoid fever are :—(1) Error in diet—e.g. the use of solid food,—the presence of particles of undigested food in the bowel, the abuse of milk, pure animal broths. My own experience has not satisfied me that one animal broth is more prone to produce diarrhœa than another. Excess of fluid, when there is inability to absorb the quantity drunk, passes through the bowel, and so stimulates excessive secretion from the intestinal mucous membrane. (2) Catarrhal inflammation of the mucous membrane and irritability of the bowel. These conditions are frequently the consequence of, or are greatly increased by, the unhealthy

intestinal secretions and contents, evidenced by their am-
moniacal, and especially offensive odour and strong alkaline
reaction, and by the passage through the bowel of undigested
food, whether liquid or solid. So long as the stools do not
exceed three to five of moderate quantity in twenty-four
hours, the looseness of bowels is rather advantageous than
injurious; but when, from their number or from their
quantity, there is risk of the strength of the patient being
reduced to a dangerous degree, then it becomes necessary to
restrain the diarrhœa. The treatment varies with the pathological condition which induces the diarrhœa. It is often
sufficient to examine the stools to detect the cause and
remove it—e.g. curds of milk. Inquiry may prove the great
excess of the fluid taken into the stomach over that passed
by kidneys and skin. When the stools are strongly alkaline,
diluted sulphuric acid sometimes affords marked relief.
When the stools are merely frequent, four ounces of starch
water thrown into the rectum night and morning will often
check the frequent action. Should this not prove efficacious,
from three to ten drops of laudanum in one ounce and a half
of starch water may be thrown into the bowel night and
morning *after* the passage of the stool. When very offensive, correctors of fetor should be given; a teaspoonful of
charcoal may be given two or three times a day. Under its
influence I have seen the stools lose their fetor and am-
moniacal odour, become less liquid, and in many cases the
irritation from the catarrhal inflammation of the mucous
membrane diminished. The greatest possible care should
be taken that the charcoal is an impalpable powder; animal
charcoal has, in this respect, some advantages over vegetable.
Other correctives of fetor, or antiseptics, will have as good
effects as charcoal; but this has given me such satisfactory
results that I have not resorted to other remedies of its class.
  Carbonate of bismuth, in twenty-grain doses every four or
six hours, is one of the best remedies I know for the catarrhal
inflammation of the bowel itself. If the fluid poured out be
very excessive, then a vegetable astringent, as catechu and
kino, may be given with the bismuth, and, should these
means fail, three to five drops of laudanum must be added
to each dose of the mixture. The use of opium, even in this

dose, by the mouth, should be avoided, if possible, as, by interfering with the action of the excreting organs, and its other effects on the nervous system, it may do more harm than the symptom for which it is prescribed. The administration of opium should, if possible, be limited to the bowel.

In place of being relaxed, the bowels are occasionally confined. Inaction of the bowels in typhoid fever may be due to torpidity of the large bowel, with free absorption of the fluid contents of diminished secretion of fluid by the mucous membrane of the bowel. Under these conditions the stools become hard and dry, and, if long retained in the bowel, may produce considerable irritation, and even catarrhal inflammation, of the mucous membrane of the bowel, with diarrhœa.

At the same time that solid stool accumulates in the rectum and colon, which may require removal, there may be extensive or deep ulcerations in the ileum. A small-sized enema of thin gruel repeated every other day, if necessary, is safer than a large enema at longer intervals. Laxatives, however mild, by the mouth, are liable to irritate the ulcerated surface of the bowel, and, if sloughs are separating, may forcibly hasten the detachment, and so produce hemorrhage, and turn the scale between recovery and death.

The most important, and a not infrequent, cause of inaction of the bowel in typhoid fever is *deep* ulceration of one or more Peyer's patches. Large superficial ulcers favour the occurrence of diarrhœa, and are often accompanied by catarrhal inflammation of the mucous membrane. A single *deep* ulcer will paralyse the action of the bowel, and so cause constipation, and this has to be kept in mind as a fact of the highest practical importance when it is proposed to relieve the bowels by an aperient. A deep ulcer is usually produced by the separation of a deep slough, and is often unattended by any catarrhal inflammation of the small intestine, or by any affection of the large intestine.

In all cases of typhoid fever there is some distension by flatus of the abdomen—the belly is more or less blown. The distension is sometimes so great as to interfere with the free play of the diaphragm, and so, by preventing the full expansion of the lungs, favours congestion of those organs and impede the circulation. Fluid will run through the bowels with little effort; air requires expulsion. Excess of flatus in the bowels may have its origin in deficient power of expulsion or excessive generation of gas. Sufficient paralysis of the bowel to cause accumulation of flatus may be the result of loss of nerve energy, or of local injury of the bowel. A single *deep* slough-formed ulcer will paralyse the action of the bowel, and lead to such an accumulation of flatus as produces enormous distention of the abdomen; the weaker the abdominal muscles, the greater, *cæteris paribus*, the accumulation of flatus. Want of power to expel the flatus, and excess in the quantity formed, reach their maximum as a rule about the latter half of the third, and during the fourth week of the fever, for then the sloughing and ulcerative processes of the walls of the intestine are at their height, the nerve-power is at its lowest, and the contractile energy of the abdominal and intestinal muscles is consequently at its minimum; while from the state of the stomach and the secreting glands generally, the antiseptic digestive processes are in a great degree arrested, and the food that finds its way into the intestines mingling with the fetid secretions from the diseased intestines, and with the sloughing particles separating from the solitary and agminated glands and from the floors of the ulcers, readily undergo the gas-generating decomposition. Of all the remedies proposed for the relief of flatulent distension of the abdomen, turpentine applied externally is the most extensively employed in practice. Now, I must say, with reference to the external application of turpentine, that I have never seen a diminution of the distension which seemed to me to be *propter hoc*.

The brief outline I have sketched of the pathological conditions causing the distension gives the key to what has seemed to me to be its most successful treatment. If the stools be frequent, and the distension is in part due at least to the excess in the gas formed, then to destroy this fetor and to arrest putrefaction and gas-generating decay of the contents of the intestine is for me the first object. Charcoal has proved a most efficient agent for effecting this purpose. It is of importance to select as food a substance which leaves no solid residue to undergo decomposition in the intestine. The administration of pepsin and acid at the same time as the food, and also the partial digestion of the food before it is taken, is often advantageous. The large intestine is occasionally so greatly distended as to lose from stretching its contractile power; the introduction of a long tube into the bowel, and the mechanical removal of some of the gas will occasionally be sufficient to enable the bowel to regain some of its contractile power. Alcohol in fit doses improves the nerve energy, and so increases temporarily the muscular power of the intestinal and abdominal walls.

In hemorrhage from the bowel in typhoid fever, the blood comes from the floors of the ulcers; the most copious hemorrhages occur at the time of the separation of the sloughs; by the separation of the sloughs a vessel of some size may be opened. Under such circumstances the hemorrhage is very copious, and the patient may even die on the chamber utensil. Much more frequently the blood, although considerable in quantity, escapes from minute vessels on the floor of the ulcers. I have never known it escape from the mucous membrane, though I have from the hemorrhoidal veins. Although in the majority of cases the bleeding is arrested by nature, the blood lost relieving the vascular fulness of the part; still, reliance should not be placed on this natural cure.

When blood in ever so small a quantity is observed in the stools, the patient is to be kept in the recumbent position. He should not be allowed to make any effort, and on no consideration to sit on close-pan, or raise himself or be raised by others to pass urine, etc. If the patient is unable to pass urine when in the recumbent position, the urine should be drawn off by catheter. All movement of the bowels should be restrained as far as possible and for as long as possible. An ounce of starch water with ten or fifteen drops of laudanum may be given at once as enema, and then a dose of acetate of lead every two or three hours by the mouth, with three to five drops of laudanum, or fifteen grains of gallic acid in a wine-glass of iced water every two or three hours with the laudanum. I think I have seen benefit from small doses of turpentine. It is a point of the greatest moment to keep the bowels empty, and therefore nourishment should be given in the most concentrated and absorbable form, *e.g.* essence of meat in tablespoonful doses frequently repeated. All nourishment which leaves solid residue—*e.g.* milk— should be avoided. Lumps of ice should be sucked, and all essence of meat, etc., be iced. When the loss of blood is sudden and copious, or is frequently repeated, the subcutaneous injection of ergotine may be employed, and an ice-bag applied over the region of the ileum. The faintness due to considerable sudden bleeding from the bowel should not be removed by stimulants unless it immediately threatens life.

Perforation of the coats of the intestine by the extension of the ulcer in depth, and finally by sloughing of the peritoneum is, so far as my certain experience goes, always fatal. I have recorded one case in which this lesion was supposed to have occurred, and to have been repaired, but, the patient dying some weeks after of erysipelas of the head and face, 1 found the perforation was not of the intestine, but of the peritoneum over a softened mesenteric gland. If adhesion occur over the perforated spot of intestine, my experience accords with that of Rokitansky, viz. that such adhesions are never permanent, *i.e.* permanent enough to permit the recovery of the patient. To give the patient a chance of recovery, absolute rest in the recumbent position must be maintained, and opium be given in quantity sufficient to stop all action of the bowel, and to subdue pain if pain be present. For pain, although in some cases most severe, is altogether absent in others, and this although the patient is perfectly sensible—not only conscious enough to feel pain, but able to tell those about him all he does feel. As any adhesions that form are so easily broken down, inaction of the bowels must be maintained as long as possible.

Tenderness of the abdomen is not limited to inflammation of the peritoneum from perforation of the intestine; there is often inflammatory vascularity of the peritoneum corresponding to the floors of the ulcers in the intestine, and even lymph may be found thickening the membrane or fixing it to adjacent parts. When death from other conditions has occurred I have not infrequently found this local preservative lesion to have been attended by very considerable tenderness of the abdomen. A like degree of tenderness arises from local peritonitis over the enlarged mesenteric glands, and also from the mesenteric glands themselves being inflamed from the absorption of irritating matter from the intestinal coats or contents. Warmth and moisture afford relief in the majority of cases, but if the temperature be high, and the tenderness superficial, an ice-bag to the part may be more beneficial, and more grateful to the patient. But the chief indication is to keep the tender part at rest, and to correct the fetor of the stools.

Tenderness in the left hypochondriac region, due to the state of the spleen, is not uncommon in typhoid fever. Enlargement of the spleen is one of the symptoms of most, perhaps of all the acute specific diseases; tenderness of the organ is only occasionally present. It is during the third week of typhoid fever that tenderness of the spleen usually reaches its maximum. When the tenderness is considerable it is a symptom of grave import; the tenderness is not due to local peritonitis, but to the condition of the proper substance of the spleen. For the relief of the state of the spleen indicated by tenderness, although a symptom of great significance in prognosis, I know no remedy of much importance: the application of warmth and moisture over the organ has sometimes seemed to be of service.

From the commencement of typhoid fever the temperature of the patient is elevated. This elevation of temperature is the direct result of excess in destruction of all the tissues of the body. The patient loses weight, and continues to lose weight so long as he is the subject of the fever, so that Zimmerman fixed the duration of typhoid fever by ascertaining how long after the onset of the disease the patient ceased to lose weight. In local inflammation, the temperature of the inflamed part is greatly in excess of that of the body generally. In uncomplicated typhoid fever the elevation of temperature is practically uniform in all parts of the body. Local inflammation, blood infection, and nerve disturbance are common causes of great increase of the temperature above that *proper* to any given case of typhoid fever—*i.e.* due to the action of the fever poison on the system generally. Thus, inflammation of the mesenteric glands is frequently excited by fetid or acrid matters conveyed to them by the lymphatics from the raw

and inflamed intestine, and blood infection may owe its origin
to the same cause. Congestive nephritis and pneumonia are
common lesions in typhoid fever, and are common causes of
increase of temperature. The power of the nervous system
to raise the temperature, or to produce sudden changes which
raise the temperature, in typhoid fever, is well illustrated by
the sudden rise which frequently follows mental emotion. I
have known the temperature start from this cause from
102° to 106°. In the progress of typhoid fever local inflammation causes more or less permanent elevation of temperature; blood infection,—rapid and sometimes temporary,
always varying, elevations of temperature; nerve disturbance,
—rapid and often transient elevations of temperature.

The treatment of typhoid fever by cold baths, when the
temperature reaches 104°, or even less, is very generally
adopted in Germany; but neither my own limited experience
nor the evidence adduced by others in its favour has carried
conviction to my mind of its advantage. At the same time
I entertain no doubt that the direct cooling of the body is in
some cases essential to the preservation of the life of the
patient—gives him, so to say, his only chance of recovery;
while in others it alleviates the severity of a symptom which
increases the danger of the patient.

A certain degree of elevation of the body is incompatible
with the favourable progress of the case. Thus, a temperature of 106° rising to 107°, and still advancing, will, unless
lowered by treatment, speedily end the life of the patient;
for these, fortunately very rare, cases, the direct and rapid
depression of the patient's temperature by the cold bath is
essential—is the only source of hope. Again, a temperature
of 105° if continuous for forty-eight hours, or broken only
by a slight fall of short duration, may itself, by the degenerative changes it favours or produces in the heart and other
organs, cause the fatal termination; for these cases, a tepid
bath gradually cooled down is sufficient to bring down the
temperature; the bath has to be repeated as the temperature
rises. Persons at an age when degenerative changes of tissue
naturally occur suffer more from continued high temperature than do younger persons. If the disease be advanced,
the skin dry, the patient prostrate, and the internal organs

congested, especially the kidneys, a tepid or warm pack is often followed by marked improvement in temperature and in the other symptoms. When the temperature is for some time $103\frac{1}{2}°$ to $104\frac{1}{2}°$, and even higher, cold effectually applied to the head (*e.g.* by the indiarubber tubing cap) will often suffice for its reduction—reduction, that is to say, not only of the temperature of the head, but of the body generally: when the temperature falls the cap should be removed, but be reapplied as often as it rises again. Tepid sponging will reduce the temperature a little, and soothe and quiet the patient if he be restless and sleepless.

Thus limiting the employment of direct means of lowering temperature, I have seen none of the ill effects which are said occasionally to follow its vigorous use—viz. collapse and failure of the heart's power; while I have seen what has appeared to me to be indisputable good follow its employment.

Other means are used to reduce temperature. When the high temperature is conjoined with rapid feeble heart's beat, when the patient is advanced in years, or when the extremities feel cold, though the temperature of the body generally is high, a fall of temperature frequently follows the administration of alcohol. Quinine, in occasional large doses, or in smaller doses repeated at intervals, has been followed by a reduction of the temperature in typhoid fever. Salicylate of soda is also said to have a like effect. When judging of the effects of these and other drugs for reducing temperature, one must not lose sight of the fact that sudden fall of temperature when no drug is given is not of infrequent occurrence, and also that the temperature varies daily. This natural fall of temperature I have seen attributed to the drug. I must say that I have been disappointed in the effects of the two drugs I have named as reducers of temperature, while I have seen both occasionally do much harm by disturbing the stomach and interfering with digestion. In a disease which runs a limited course like typhoid fever, the greatest possible care should be taken to preserve the powers of the stomach, as the life of the patient may depend on his power to digest nourishment towards the end of the disease.

Typhoid fever cannot be cured by perspiration, but the patient suffers much less discomfort, and is lest restless when the skin is gently moist. The most certain means for producing gentle perspiration I know is the application of a large, warm, and moist flannel, covered with oil-silk, over abdomen and chest, and the administration of warm bland fluids. In the later stages of the disease profuse and most exhausting perspiration sometimes occurs. The perspiration is kept up and greatly increased by the heat of the patient's body and the moisture of the perspiration itself. To prevent chill, the nurse carefully covers the patient; thus, with a relaxed skin disposed to sweat, he is kept, so to say, in a prolonged vapour bath. I have seen lives lost from the asthenia thus produced. To restrain this profuse perspiration, the patient's skin should be dried with a warm napkin every few minutes if necessary, and dry cloths placed between the wet linen and the skin. Alcohol should be given at the same time to stimulate the nervous system and increase the force of the heart's action. Sponging with tepid vinegar and water is sometimes of much service.

The state of the heart, as indicated by the frequency of its beats and the strength of its impulse, has always been considered of the greatest significance in determining the treatment to be pursued at any moment in a case of typhoid fever. As a rule, the weaker the more frequent are the heart's beats. This feebleness and rapidity in excess of that proper to the fever may be due:—(1) To changes in the muscular tissues of the heart, e.g. softening with granular degeneration passing into fatty metamorphosis of the muscular fibres. No doubt the occurrence of these changes is favoured by long-continued high temperature of the blood. (2) To the circulation of poisoned blood through the vessels of the walls of the heart, the poison being produced in the system under the influence of the fever, or of its effects. (3) To nerve influence.

Feebleness of the heart's action due to either of these conditions may cause the death of the patient directly by asthenia, or indirectly by enfeebled *vis a tergo* producing local congestions. Although the two first-named causes of cardiac weakness are the most serious and the least affected by treatment, the third is the most common, and very frequently greatly exaggerates the effects of the other two.

To avert death from failure of heart-power alcohol is the great remedy. Over defective cardiac action, due altogether to changes in the muscular tissue, when once established, or to the circulation of poisoned blood through its vessels, alcohol exerts comparatively little influence; but when the weakness and frequency of cardiac action are due to nerve influence in part or altogether, then alcohol exerts a singularly beneficial effect on the rapidity and feebleness of the heart's action.

When the patient is, from natural temperament and the effect of the fever poison, in a state of nervous trepidation, or either directly from the mental state or from some appreciable accidental circumstance giving a colour to his hallucinations or his dreams in a state of fright, a little abdominal pain or disturbance will cause him to start from sleep or awake in fear. In these circumstances the temperature rapidly rises—I have known it mount to 106°—the pulse becomes extremely frequent, 150 or more, and feeble or irregular. The effect is so great in the patient's state that death has, I believe, from cases I have seen, not infrequently happened. A free use of stimulants removes all the gravest symptoms, the temperature falls, and the heart's action becomes steady; it falls in frequency and increases in power.

Mental disturbance in typhoid fever varies from trifling wandering—from which the patient is readily recalled by directing his attention to some common object, or by requesting him to perform some simple act—to the most violent delirium. Delirium due to fever is never conjoined with headache; headache in typhoid fever may be most intense, delirium most violent, but the headache ceases before the delirium begins. If the delirious patient complains spontaneously of headache, then we should doubt the accuracy of our diagnosis; or if that is beyond question, then we must conclude that there is present that infinitely rare complication of typhoid fever, intracranial inflammation. Delirium is, as a rule, one of the symptoms which are influenced for good by alcohol, but it is one in which the effects of the alcohol should be most closely watched. When alcohol is contra-indicated or proves useless or injurious, the head should be shaved, and cold applied either by an ordinary ice-bag or by the cold water tubing cap, or the head may be kept cold while the force of the heart's action is maintained by alcohol.

There is one nerve symptom to which I attach great and grave significance, and which is a guide to treatment—it is tremor.

Tremor is sometimes so great that the patient is unable to protrude his tongue; his jaw trembles, and his voice quivers, and if he attempts to hold any vessel he spills its contents, not from weakness or drowsiness, but from shaking of the hands. Tremor out of all proportion to other signs of nervous prostration is evidence of *deep* destruction of the intestine. A small *deep* slough will be accompanied by great tremor; a large extent of superficial ulceration may be un-attended by symptoms. Now, it is deep ulcers following separation of deep sloughs which are especially liable to give rise to severe hemorrhage and perforation. In these cases of tremor alcohol should always be given to increase nerve energy, and so to limit the sloughing and ulceration to what is the direct consequence of the specific process.

I may sum up my experience in regard to the use of alcohol in the treatment of typhoid fever thus. Its influence is exerted primarily on the nervous system, and through it on the several organs and processes; for example, the heart and the general nutritive processes—changes on which the rise and fall of temperature depend. In judiciously selected cases it lowers temperature, increases the force and diminishes the frequency of the heart's beats; it calms and soothes the patient, diminishes the tremor, it quiets delirium, and in-duces sleep. It should never be given in the early stage of the disease, or with the hope of anticipating, and so prevent-ing the occurrence of prostration and debility, but should be prescribed only when the severity of special symptoms, or the general state of prostration, indicates its use. Hence a large number of cases of typhoid fever end favourably with-out alcohol being prescribed from the beginning to the ter-mination. It should not be prescribed when a sudden gush of blood has induced faintness, unless the faintness is so great as to threaten life immediately.   Nor should it be given when, after the first few doses, the temperature rises, the heart's action becomes more frequent or more feeble, delirium increases, sleeplessness supervenes, or drowsiness deepens, so as to threaten to pass into coma.   When the urine contains a considerable quantity of albumen, alcohol should not be prescribed, unless absolutely necessary for the relief of some symptom immediately threatening life, and then it should be given with the greatest caution, and its effects on temperature, the circulation, and on the urinary and other secretions, both as to quantity and quality, be carefully and frequently noted.   The quantity of alcohol prescribed should be as much only as may be necessary to effect the object for which it is prescribed.   In the fourth week, to tide the patient over the concluding days of the disease, it may, as a rule, be given more freely than in the second or the beginning of the third week of the disease, but it is in exceptional cases only that more than twelve ounces of brandy in the twenty-four hours can be taken without inducing some of the worst symptoms of prostration.   Nearly all the good effects of alcohol, when its use is indicated, are obtained by four, six, or eight ounces of brandy in twenty-four hours.   Taken in excess—even when in smaller quantities it would do the patient good—it dries the tongue, muddles the mind, or induces delirium or drowsiness approaching to coma, and diminishes the action of the secreting organs, on the healthy action of which the elimination of the materials destroyed by the action of the fever poison depends.   For the last thirty years I have made it the rule of my practice in the treatment of typhoid fever to abstain from giving alcohol if, in the case before me, I *doubted* the wisdom of giving it; when in doubt I do not give alcohol in typhoid fever, and when there is a question in my mind of a larger or smaller dose I, as a rule, prescribe the smaller.   The reverse of the rule I laid down for myself in the treatment of typhus fever.

In conclusion, I will briefly sum up the chief points that my experience has taught me in regard of the treatment of typhoid fever:—

Typhoid fever cannot be cured; but more lives may be saved by the judicious treatment, and more lives lost by the improper treatment of typhoid fever than of any other acute disease.

For a very large proportion of cases no other treatment is really required from beginning to end than rest in bed, quietude, fresh air, pure water, and regulated diet, although most cases are benefited by a little wine in the third and fourth weeks. If medicinal, in addition to hygienic, treatment is required, it is because special symptoms by their severity tend directly or indirectly to give an unfavourable course to the disease. At the same time it must be remembered that the gravity of some symptoms is in certain cases due to lesions of structure beyond the possibility of successful treatment—*e.g.* primary deep sloughs of Peyer's patches; and that other grave symptoms pass away spontaneously, although no special treatment is prescribed for their relief. When drugs *are* required to hold in check a special symptom, their use should be discontinued when the gravity of the symptom for which they are prescribed has subsided.

Temperature so high and continuous as to be a cause of danger, either directly or indirectly by favouring serious degenerative changes of structure, is present in exceptional cases only, and for such cases alone is the direct application of cold to the general surface required.

Alcohol, by the influence it exerts on the nervous system, is of the greatest value in the treatment of typhoid fever, but it should only be given for the purpose of attaining a definite object; its effects should be watched, and the dose so regulated as to attain the desired effect from as small a quantity as possible. As the treatment in reference to many symptoms is in the present state of our pathological knowledge tentative, it may have to be varied frequently both as regards continuance and dose of drugs, of stimulants, and of cold. My experience has impressed on me the conviction that that man will be the most successful in treating typhoid fever who watches its progress, not only with the most skilled and intelligent, but also with the most constant care, and gives *unceasing attention to little things*, and who, when prescribing an active remedy weighs with the greatest accuracy the good intended to be effected against the evil the prescription may inflict, and then, if the possible evil be death, and the probable good short of the saving of life, holds his hand.

While admitting without reserve that heroic measures, fearlessly but judiciously employed, will save life when less potent means are useless, the physician whose experience reaches over many years will, on looking back, discover that year by year he has seen fewer cases requiring heroic measures, and more cases in which the unaided powers of nature alone suffice for effecting cure; that year by year he has learned to regard with greater diffidence his own powers, and to trust with greater confidence in those of nature.

DIPHTHERIA:

ITS

SYMPTOMS AND TREATMENT

Originally published in 1861.

PREFACE TO THE ORIGINAL EDITION

THE Two Lectures which form the greater part of this little book, were delivered to the medical clinical class at University College Hospital. Thinking that even an imperfect and incomplete account of the present epidemic of Diphtheria in London, by a practitioner who has seen most of its severer phases, would be acceptable to the profession, I determined to publish my experience. The symptoms of diphtheria, during the present epidemic, agree in all essential particulars with those observed in past epidemics. Indeed my study of the histories of epidemic and other diseases, leads me to the conclusion that diseases preserve their essential characters and natures from age to age, while the opinions of the profession respecting them and their treatment change from year to year. This change seems to be sometimes the result of the personal sway of some influential teacher—sometimes the result of real advances in pathology and therapeutics.

The Lectures are dogmatical in tone, because they were addressed to students; and I believe dogmatism to be essential for successful student-teaching. I endeavoured to make them practical in regard of diagnosis and treatment, because they were delivered to a clinical class. The details of the cases are few, partly because the majority of the patients were seen in private, and partly because I have found that students are more confused than instructed when copious details of a case are placed before them.

Since the Lectures were delivered, several other cases of Diphtheria have come under my observation. Some of these having presented special points of interest, or peculiarities illustrating general statement in the Lectures, I have added materially to the text, and slightly modified its arrangement.

LONDON, 1861.

DIPHTHERIA

ITS SYMPTOMS AND TREATMENT

LECTURE I

GENTLEMEN,—On the table are several pieces of 'false membrane,' coughed up by a young gentleman twenty-one years of age, while suffering from diphtheria; also the pharynx, larynx, and lymphatic glands connected with those parts, from two children who died a few days since from the same disease.

Diphtheria is one of the acute specific diseases; that is to say, it is a general disease, runs a quick and definite course, and has a specific cause. Its anatomical character is—spreading inflammation of the mucous membrane of the pharynx, attended by exudation of lymph.

About three years since, diphtheria became epidemic in London. Since the early part of 1858, I have seen about fifty-eight cases, of which thirty-four have proved fatal.[1] And these cases have, with few exceptions, been scattered over the district bounded on the south by Holborn and Oxford Street, on the north by the Highgate and Hampstead hills, on the east by Hackney, and on the west by Shepherd's Bush: they may be considered to represent the general characters of the epidemic in its severer forms in the north of London. As several of the cases occurred within the last three weeks, and as they differed in no essential particulars from some of the cases I saw three years ago, I conclude that the epidemic preserves its original characters.

As in the other acute specific diseases, so in diphtheria the general or the local symptoms may predominate, and give its special feature to the case. The patient may die

---

[1] From these numbers it is not to be concluded that half the cases of diphtheria prove fatal, seeing that a very large proportion of the fifty-eight cases came under my observation solely because of their extreme gravity, many of the patients being in a dying state.

from the severity of the general disease, or he may die from the severity of some one of its local consequences. In this particular, diphtheria bears a closer affinity to typhoid fever than to any other of the acute specific diseases; for in typhoid fever, as you know, the patient may die of the general affection: i.e. of the fever; or, the symptoms of the general disease being trifling in the extreme, he may die of a local consequence of the fever, e.g. perforation of the bowel. Diphtheria is by no means new to England. I have seen cases of it every now and then, as long as I have practised medicine, and the writings of the older English physicians prove that, from time to time, it has been epidemic, or very common, in many parts of England. You will understand, however, that I am to-day describing diphtheria as it presented itself in the cases from which the preparations on the table and under the microscope were obtained, and from the other cases of the disease which I have seen during the past three years. I have told you that the anatomical character of diphtheria is spreading inflammation of the pharynx, attended by exudation of lymph. It may be that the mucous membrane covering one of the tonsils is the primary seat of the exudation, or it may be that the arches of the palate, the posterior surface of the soft palate, the uvula, the nares, or the mucous membrane of the pharynx itself is the starting-point of the local lesion. At first there is redness and some swelling of the parts, and perhaps a little excess of mucus on them; then a white or grey patch, due to the presence of a layer of lymph, is seen on the reddened surface. Usually the redness involves the whole mucous membrane within reach of the eye, posterior to, and inclusive of, the anterior arches of the palate, before any lymph is exuded. Sometimes you see at once many little points of lymph: sometimes only one. Thus starting from one or many centres, the exudation spreads anteriorly on to the soft palate, upwards to the posterior nares, and downwards to the upper suface of the epiglottis, and, if not arrested by nature or by art, it descends into the larynx, the trachea, and the bronchi. I have seen, though not during the present epidemic, the lymph extend into the œsophagus and stomach.

Tear off, during life, the lymph from the mucous membrane of the pharynx, and you expose a raw, bleeding surface, which in a few hours is covered by a new layer of lymph.

I have spoken of lymph, but included under the word lymph are a variety of very different-looking substances. Sometimes the lymph has a granular appearance and very little consistence or tenacity; sometimes the part is covered with a thinner or thicker coating of a white or grey pulpy substance; so thin, soft, and separated from each other may be the little particles which together form the coating of lymph, that we cannot apply to it, correctly at least, the term membrane; for no shred of lymph can be stripped from the surface. At other times the layer of lymph is very tough, elastic, and as much as one-eighth of an inch in thickness. In the one case, the lymph resembles cream in appearance and consistence; in the other, it resembles wash-leather. Between the two extremes we meet with all intermediate conditions as regards consistence and tenacity.

Pus, granular corpuscles, oleoprotein granules, and epithelium constitute the bulk of the softer forms of the so-called lymph; such fibres as we see in the buffy coat of blood coagula constitute the bulk of the toughest varieties of 'lymph.' Now and then ulceration, and even sloughing, of a superficial layer of the subjacent mucous membrane occurs; and blood and pus, and semi-detached pieces of lymph may form fœtid shreds of some size.

As to the presence of vegetable growths in the diphtheritic exudation, no doubt they have occasionally been seen: but I am sure they have not been present in several cases I have carefully examined; consequently I feel satisfied that epiphytes have played no essential or important part in the cases of diphtheria I have seen.

At the bed-side, and in this room, I have seized every opportunity of impressing on you the general fact, that when a part is severely or deeply inflamed, the lymphatic glands to which the lymphatics of the inflamed part lead, become the seat of active congestion, and ultimately of inflammatory exudation. In diphtheria we have an illustration of this general law, for the lymphatic glands, to which the lymphatics of the pharynx, etc., lead, are found to be larger, redder, and moister than natural; and, if the disease has continued long to have that peculiar brittleness, and pale, but brightish red colour, which are characteristic of the presence of inflammatory exudation in the glands. During life we feel the enlarged lymphatic glands behind the angle of the lower jaw on either side, as well as down the neck by the sides of the larynx when that organ is involved in the inflammation. When the discharges from the pharynx are fœtid, and the mucous membrane is sloughy, not only are the glands behind the angles of the jaw enlarged, but the cellular tissue in which they are placed is the seat of effusion of serosity, and even of exudation of lymph, and very great general swelling of the part is the result.[1]

After death from diphtheria, too, we find that the inflammation of the pharynx has not been limited to the mucous membrane, or even to it and the submucous tissue, for the deeper parts are thickened and toughened. The contraction of the exudation poured into those parts is sufficient, in many cases, to diminish considerably the capacity of the pharynx, its mucous membrane being thrown, partly from this cause and partly from its own swollen condition, into longitudinal rugæ. Acute pulmonary vesicular emphysema, the result of the obstacle to expiration produced by the imperfect occlusion of the larynx and trachea; collapse of lung tissue from the combined effects of lymph or mucus in the smaller bronchial tubes leading to the collapsed tissue, and of the impediment to deep coughing offered by the state of the larynx; pneumonia, lobar or lobular, primary, or, as is more commonly the case, secondary to collapse of lung tissue: some congestion of the spleen, of the liver, and of the kidney, induced mechanically by the state of the lungs; and enlargement of lymphatic glands at a distance from and no ways

---

[1] Trousseau attaches much diagnostic value to the enlargement of the lymphatic glands of the neck in diphtheria. I cannot agree with him on this point. The enlargement of the glands has been—in the cases of diphtheria which I have seen—in proportion to the severity and depth of the local, nasal, pharyngeal, laryngeal, and tracheal disease. I have never seen it greater in proportion to the local primary mischief, than in other forms of cynanche pharyngea. In children generally, the swelling of the glands, other things being equal, is greater than it is in adults; and in strumous children the enlargement is always greater, other things being equal, than it is in rickety or in healthy children.

related to the pharynx ;—are all the lesions additional to those constituting its anatomical character, which I have found after death from diphtheria during the present epidemic.[1]

The specimens on the table illustrate much of what I have just told you.

In one (Specimen I) we see the reddened mucous membrane of the pharynx, larynx, trachea, and larger bronchi. On the mucous membrane of the pharynx and larynx is a layer of the granular or pulpy variety of lymph ; as we reach the trachea, the lymph gains in consistence, so that, towards the middle of the trachea, it can be raised as a distinct membraniform layer; where it can be so raised, its under surface is, here and there, crimson, from a little blood. The uvula is all but *gone* from sloughing, and there is a minute slough on one tonsil. On removing the lymph from the epiglottis, we see a little ulceration of its mucous membrane. The whole tract of mucous membrane covered by lymph is bright crimson and thickened. The microscope shows us that the softest lymph is composed of pus corpuscles—the pyoid corpuscles of Lebert, and other smaller and larger granular corpuscles, epithelium, and oleoprotein granules ; and, though we have used re-agents to render the animal matter transparent, no vegetable growths can be detected.

In the second specimen we have a good example of the thick, tough, elastic variety of lymph. In both these cases the local disease extended from the pharynx to the larynx, trachea, and bronchi. If you examine the lungs on the table, you will see that the mucous membrane of the first, second, and third divisions of the bronchi is coated with lymph. The largest piece of the tough lymph (Specimen 2) is in the form of a hollow tube, and is evidently a cast of the inside of the trachea. Extending from some of the larger portions are branches, which appear to have been formed in the bronchi. I have placed a little of this tough variety of lymph under the microscope, and you will note the imperfectly fibrous appearance it presents.

In the third specimen on the table, the lymph coats many

---

[1] I have seen (though not during the last three years) the exudative inflammation spread down the œsophagus and the stomach, and the mucous membrane of those parts, as a consequence, covered with lymph.

even of the very smallest bronchi, as well as the larynx, trachea, and large bronchi. The presence of the lymph and mucus in the smallest bronchial tubes, dependent partly on the state of the larynx and trachea, preventing deep coughing, has led to the collapse of the lung tissue: pneumonia, lobar and lobular, has followed. The child from which this specimen was removed was the subject of rickets. Its trachea was opened during life. You will observe that there is neither collapse nor pneumonia of the lung in the first case; the false membrane, as it is called, does not extend beyond the larger bronchi, and the lungs are the seat of acute vesicular emphysema.

As the lymphatic glands connected with the pharynx and larynx are still attached, you see that they are considerably larger, as well as redder and more brittle, than they should be. In neither specimen are the tonsils much larger than normal; but all the tissues of the pharynx and soft palate are thickened in the first specimen; while in the third specimen there is a point worthy of your note, of the highest importance, viz., that, while the larynx, trachea, and bronchi are coated with lymph, there is but a small patch on the pharyngeal mucous membrane; that patch is limited to the posterior wall of the pharynx, and is not in the least degree continuous with the lymph in the larynx. There were here, then, two separate centres of exudation, and the laryngeal exudation occurred for some time before the pharyngeal. The exudative inflammation did not spread from the larynx to the pharynx. The laryngeal symptoms were urgent before the pharynx was in any way affected, and you see most clearly that there is no continuity between the lymph in the larynx and that in the pharynx; that the latter is situated at some distance from the former. In the first case the exudative inflammation began in the pharynx, and spread to the larynx; and we see that the layer of lymph in the pharynx is continuous with that on the larynx, the continuity being well seen on the arytæno-epiglottidean folds. Observe for yourselves the differences in this particular in the two specimens.

The most practical way of making you acquainted with the symptoms of diphtheria, including those which were present in the cases parts of which are before you, will be, I think, to group the cases I have seen, so as to constitute varieties.

FIRST VARIETY.—*The mild form of diphtheria.*—There are cases in which the general symptoms and the local lesions are trifling, and no sequelæ follow. Of these mild, but unequivocal cases of diphtheria, I have seen only seven; viz. three out-patients at the Hospital for Sick Children, and four cases in private practice.

Here are the particulars of a case of this kind I saw with Dr. Hawkesley.

The patient was six years of age. She had long had chronic enlargement of the tonsils, and suffered occasionally from acute inflammation of the tonsils. In the attack of diphtheria, inflammation of the mucous membrane covering the tonsils and arches of the palate, but very trifling in degree, preceded for some days the exudation of lymph. When the exudation occurred, it was seated between the uvula and the tonsils, on the anterior arches of the palate. In addition to the exudation of lymph, trifling febrile disturbance, the least possible soreness of the throat in swallowing, and a little more swelling of the glands near to the angle of the jaw that is always present in this child, were all the ailments in the case. Dr. Hawkesley examined the urine daily, but no albumen was present, and no affection of the nervous system followed. [1]

SECOND VARIETY.—*The inflammatory form of diphtheria.*

[1] This variety of diphtheria is doubtless more common than my personal experience would lead me to suppose. It is probable, also, that there are many inflamed throats which have their origin, when diphtheria is epidemic, in the diphtheria miasm, whatever that may be, just as many cases of diarrhœa originate in cholera miasm, when that disease is epidemic. And it is as difficult to say in some cases that an inflamed pharynx is not due to mild diphtheria, as it is to say that a serous diarrhœa is not cholera. Of course one or more members of a family having exudation on to the pharyngeal mucous membrane, and others at the same time having merely inflamed throats, would be strong presumptive evidence that the latter had diphtheria without exudation. As when two children of a family have scarlatina with rash, and a third, at the same time, just before, or just after, has sore throat without rash, we consider there is strong presumptive evidence that the latter was a case of scarlatina *sine eruptione.* In describing diphtheria in these lectures, however, I have drawn my description from those cases only in which exudation has occurred.

—Symptoms of severe cynanche pharyngea precede the exudation of lymph in what may be called the inflammatory form of diphtheria. There is, in this variety of the disease, redness, and swelling of the mucous membrane covering the arches of the palate, the uvula, and the tonsils. The redness is in some cases vivid, in others dusky. The swelling of the uvula is frequently considerable, and it often has, from effusion of serosity into the submucous tissue, a jelly-like transparency and aspect. The pain in the act of swallowing is great, so that occasionally deglutition is, from this cause, almost impossible. The febrile disturbance may be extreme, or moderate; the pulse is frequent, but soon becomes weak; there is considerable sense of weakness and of illness. From twelve to forty-eight hours from the first symptoms of throat affection, a layer, more or less extensive, of tough lymph coats the inflamed surface, and when death follows, it does so from extension of the exudative inflammation to the larynx, trachea, etc.

Let me give you an outline of some cases of the inflammatory form of diphtheria.

Dr. E. called on me one morning, complaining that he felt extremely ill and weak, and that his throat was very sore. I found his pulse rapid, but not strong; his skin hot. On examining his throat the arches of the palate and all the parts visible beyond were deep but dusky red and swollen,—the uvula was œdematous, the effort to swallow caused severe pain. In three days all the previously red parts were covered by a thick layer of tough lymph, having the colour and general appearance of wash-leather. The disease did not extend to the larynx, and Dr. E. recovered.

Mr. A., who expectorated the cast of the trachea on the table, was a patient of Mr. Pearse, of Tavistock Square. Feeling poorly Mr. A. left home on last Thursday fortnight, for two or three days:—on the Monday following Mr. Pearse examined his throat, found it dusky-red, and the uvula to have that peculiar gelatinous aspect which indicates submucous serous effusion. On the next day Mr. Pearse observed patches of lymph on the right tonsil and on the uvula. On Friday, not only was there a layer of lymph covering the uvula, arches of the palate, part of the soft palate, and the pharynx, but, by depressing the tongue, we could see the erect epiglottis covered with the same tough lymph. That the patient's larynx was affected was shown by his husky whispering voice, the necessity he was under of sitting erect in bed, the recession of the soft parts of the chest walls when he inspired, the lengthened inspiration, the lividity of his lips, the fulness of his eyes, and the venous injection of his conjunctivæ.

His urine was loaded with lithates; it contained a considerable quantity of albumen, and a very few granular casts of tubes. There is a specimen of the urine on the table, and I have placed some of it under the microscope. A large number of crystals of uric acid have formed in it since it was passed. On Saturday night he coughed up the cast of the trachea on the table, with temporary relief to the breathing. Many large pieces of membraniform lymph were coughed and hawked up the next day, but on Sunday afternoon he died somewhat suddenly. His pulse on Friday was 120; on Saturday 130; and on Sunday midday as frequent. Of seven cases I have seen referable to this variety, three proved fatal; one forty-eight hours from the first symptom, and one (Mr. A.'s) so late as the eleventh day of illness,[1] and all three by extension of the exudation to the larynx.

The following is a mild case of the inflammatory form of diphtheria :—Eliza R., aged 20, had been in constant attendance on Dr. E. On March the 13th, 1858, she began to feel ill, with sense of weakness and general lassitude. Her throat at this time was slightly sore; her skin was hot, her pulse quick, her bowels confined: she was thirsty, without appetite, and had constant nausea. I saw her on the 18th, when there was, in addition to these symptoms, a patch of lymph on the left tonsil, which was red and swollen. On the 20th she was admitted into this hospital. On this, the eighth day of illness, her skin was still hot, and her pulse frequent but not particularly weak. There was some swelling and tenderness just outside the angle of the jaw on the left side, the lymphatic glands down each side of the neck were enlarged and tender, deglutition was painful, and the voice was hoarse.

[1] If diphtheria began on the Monday, then Mr. A. died on the seventh day of illness.

The patch of lymph noted on the enlarged left tonsil on the 18th had increased in size; it was removed by a pair of forceps, and a raw, red, bleeding surface was exposed. The arches of the palate were very red; and the tongue was covered with a white fur; there was no albumen in the urine.

When rapidly convalescing from the diphtheria, she had, on the 24th of March, an attack of acute rheumatism, from which she recovered in little more than a week, and left the hospital well.[1]

I must add yet one other case of this form of diphtheria, the constitutional disturbance in this case being even less than in Elizabeth R.

Thomas C., aged 33, a night railway-porter, a strong-made and generally healthy man, was admitted into this hospital on Sunday, April 4th, 1858.

This man awoke at nine o'clock on the morning of his admission into the hospital (having felt quite well on going to bed a few hours before) with a sensation of 'swelling in his throat.' The effort to swallow caused intense pain. The surgeon, whom he at once consulted, touched his throat with nitrate of silver. At one o'clock he was seen by my assistant, Dr. Pougnet; the uvula was then so enormously enlarged, 'as thick as the little finger,' that he could not see into the pharynx.

I saw the man on Monday, i.e. the second day of his illness. The uvula was as large as on his admission; its anterior surface was covered with lymph, and when it was raised, on its posterior surface was found a transparent whitish layer of lymph which could be peeled off with a pair of forceps. There was a small patch of lymph extending from the uvula on to the soft palate, which was generally of a bright red colour. The pharynx and tonsils were free from lymph. The lymphatic glands at the angles of the lower jaw, and down the neck on each side of the larynx, were larger than natural, and tender. On the next day the uvula was unchanged in appearance, but the arches of the palate were very red, and dotted over with small patches of opaque white lymph. On Wednesday, i.e. the fourth day of disease, the

[1] In one case several joints were swollen, hot, and tender during the attack. The patient recovered.

uvula had diminished in size, but the exudation on it formed a thick tough layer. There was a small patch of lymph on the right tonsil. The pain in deglutition was still very great.

On the sixth day the man's general state and local lesion had considerably improved; he looked much better.

Up to this time his pulse had ranged from 88 to 96, and on the fourth day it was noted to be full and hard. The temperature ranged from 99° to 100° Fahrenheit, and on the fourth and fifth days the skin was noted to be hot and dry: before and after that it felt cool to the hand.

On the tenth day the man was almost well, only his uvula was rather redder and larger than natural.

THIRD VARIETY.—*The insidious form of diphtheria.*—In the cases referable to this head there is no severity in the general symptoms, no marked soreness of throat, no notable swelling of the lymphatic glands, but suddenly and, if the pharynx has not been examined, unexpectedly, laryngeal symptoms supervene, and death rapidly follows from suffocation. If the pharynx be not examined the disease is confounded with primary croup.

A child, aged about six years, living in a villa near the Brecknock Arms, had suffered for some days from slight sore throat, but was not thought to be sufficiently ill to require medical advice, or even to be kept in the house, when the sudden occurrence of 'croupy' breathing excited alarm. Mr. Baly, of Kentish Town, was called to the child. He found that the pharynx was covered with lymph, and that the larynx was deeply involved in the disease. About two P.M., within an hour of Mr. Baly's first visit, I saw the child with him; the friends declined to allow tracheotomy to be performed; the same afternoon the child died.

Ten days since I saw a similar case a few hours before death, with Mr. Noyce, of Brecknock Crescent. Several children of the family had just suffered, and recovered without treatment, from sore throat. They had been, in the parents' estimation, worse than was our little patient (æt. 6), when her croupy breathing excited their alarm. The friends declined to allow tracheotomy to be performed, and the child died within forty-eight hours from the supervention of the first laryngeal symptoms.

A child, aged about six years, had suffered for two or three days from sore throat. The surgeon who saw the child before the father left home in the morning assured him that the disease was trifling. On the father's return, late at night, the croupy breathing excited his alarm. I saw the child, with the surgeon, about midnight. There was then rapid pulse, husky whispering voice, shrill respiration, and great dyspnœa. Before seven o'clock in the morning the child was dead.

The infant child, aged eleven months, of a surgeon, had for a day or two slight symptoms of sore throat. The father's fears, although he is an anxious parent and a most intelligent and experienced practitioner, were not excited till between ten and eleven at night when he noticed for the first time laryngeal breathing. The extreme recession of the softer parts of the chest walls during inspiration proved the impediment to the passage of the air through the larynx. There was a little lymph on the pharyngeal mucous membrane when I saw the child about eleven P.M. Before morning it was dead. These cases will impress on you the importance of examining carefully the pharynx in every case, even the most trifling, of sore throat.

FOURTH VARIETY.—*The nasal form of diphtheria.*— Another set of cases constitute what has been termed the nasal form of diphtheria. After some febrile disturbance of low type, a sanious discharge from the nose attracts attention: then the glands about the angles of the jaw swell; the arches of the palate and the tonsils are found to be red and swollen: muco-purulent fluid bubbles in quantity from the narrow isthmus faucium, and prevents you obtaining a clear view of the pharyngeal mucous membrane. After a few days the disease subsides, and you remain in doubt as to its nature; or it spreads to the larynx, and the diagnosis becomes easy, and death enables you to verify it; or some other member of the family or an attendant sickens with unmistakable symptoms of diphtheria. Or the disease begins with trifling sanious discharge from the nares; the lymphatic glands are scarcely at all affected, and the nature of the disease is not even suspected till death is imminent from suffocation; or again, when the exudation reaches the pharynx, the pharyngeal symptoms may be most distressing, and lead to inspection of the part and the detection of the disease.

In November, 1859, I saw, with Dr. Carlill of Berners Street, a very interesting case of nasal diphtheria, remarkable especially for the difficulty of the diagnosis, even at a time when serious symptoms were present. The patient was a girl aged two years. The parents first observed that the child had a little sanious discharge from the nose, and was very decidedly out of health. The discharge from the nose had ceased when I saw the child. There was no enlargement of the lymphatic glands of the neck. The great feature in the case at that time was frequent vomiting. Almost every attempt to swallow was followed by efforts of vomiting, and the forcible ejection of fluids through mouth and nose. As the vomiting seemed sometimes to come on before the fluids could have reached the stomach, the throat was inspected by both Dr. Carlill and myself; nothing wrong in it could, however, be detected. Although the nature of the case was obscure, the whole group of symptoms present led us to the opinion that they were the consequence of disordered innervation from cerebral disturbance, rather than the result of any throat affection. 'Two days,' Dr. Carlill wrote me, 'after you visited her, I saw a thin pellicle partly covering the velum pendulum palati, and partly detached and hanging down into the mouth. She died the next day, never having been able to swallow more than a small part of what was given her for about six days.' The immediate cause of death was the extension of the exudation to the larynx ; the child died from suffocation, as in primary croup.

The following case of nasal diphtheria possesses special interest from the chief evidence in favour of the diagnosis being the communication of the disease to another—just the kind of evidence which we consider conclusive in regard of the nature of some obscure cases of scarlet fever.

Master P., aged about two years, suffered some febrile disturbance of low type, and profuse muco-purulent discharge from the nares, and redness and swelling of the velum pendulum palati, uvula, arches of the palate, and tonsils; the posterior wall of the pharynx was not very clearly to be seen, in consequence of the large quantity of muco-purulent fluid that bubbled in the pharynx. Dr. Carlill, whose patients this little one and his brother, less severely but similarly affected, were, thought the cases were true diphtheria. I had considerable doubt on the point. At any rate, as we could see no lymph, and the larynx was not affected, I hesitated to admit it. Dr. Carlill was in attendance from the 15th to the 28th of March 1860, and a lotion was injected into the nares and throat by Dr. Carlill daily, from the 15th to the 25th. On two occasions Dr. Carlill remembered distinctly that the child coughed some sputa into his face. On April 2nd, Dr. Carlill was himself attacked by diphtheria.

Had the child whose case I am now about to relate recovered, and had not the child in the next bed suffered within a few days from unquestionable diphtheria, doubts as to the nature of the disease under which it suffered might have been felt.

William W., aged two years and three months, a delicate child, the subject of rickets, was admitted into the Hospital for Sick Children on the 31st of December 1860, the rash of measles having appeared on that day. The rash came out full and well; from the first there were abundant sonorous and mucous ronchi audible over the whole chest. On the 3rd of January, that is, the fourth day of the eruption, there was much discharge from the nose, and a little ulceration of the orifice of the nares. His appetite was good, there was no difficulty in swallowing; the skin was very hot.

By ten o'clock the same night a marked change had taken place in the child, and the following notes of its state were made by Mr. Sydney Ringer, the very able Medical Registrar to the Hospital :—

'Child prostrate; pulse 160, weak; respirations hurried but not laborious; no lividity of the face or body. Abundant dirty muco-purulent discharge from the right nostril. Fauces, uvula, and tonsils red, and very much swollen, and covered with thick tenacious mucus. No exudation can be seen, but then the thick mucus in the pharynx prevents a perfect inspection of the parts.' At nine A.M., the fifth day of eruption, the child was weaker, but could still swallow solids and fluids, and apparently without difficulty. The eruption was well out.

About one P.M. the nurse raised the child's head, in order to give it some food—it fell back and died without a struggle.

The body was examined the next day. The lungs were the seat of extensive acute emphysema, and of a little collapse. The lymphatic glands along the trachea were not enlarged; those behind the angles of the lower jaw were only just perceptible to touch before the integuments over them were divided. The whole substance of the *velum pendulum palati* and uvula was considerably thickened and toughened. The cavity of the pharynx was smaller than natural, the mucous and sub-mucous tissues thickened; the mucous membrane was bright red, and elevated into rugæ. Here and there, on the surface of the mucous membrane at the upper part of the pharynx in the vicinity of the posterior nares was a little lymph, granular in form, very soft, and easily removed by scraping with the knife, nowhere forming a continuous layer. The *arytæno-epiglottidean* folds were greatly thickened, the epiglottis also decidedly but less thickened. The mucous membrane of the larynx was less smooth and polished, and at the same time redder than it should be, and the *chordæ vocales* were more spongy-looking than natural. The abnormities of the larynx were all insignificant in degree—perhaps such as are often present in measles. The lesions of the upper part of the pharynx were decided, although still trifling; they were the result of nasal diphtheria, complicating the measles. The child probably died at so early a period of the diphtheria, in consequence of the weakness resulting from the severe attack of measles under which it was suffering at the time the diphtheria supervened, and its natural delicacy of constitution (it was not only rickety but also tubercular). The cause of death was asthenia.

As if to prove to us the nature of this case, the child in the next bed sickened with well-marked diphtheria within twelve hours of William W.'s death. In twenty-four hours from the first symptoms of illness, its trachea was opened by Mr. Berkeley Hill, death by suffocation being imminent. I shall describe this case at some length in my next lecture when speaking of the value of tracheotomy.

FIFTH VARIETY.—*The primary laryngeal form of diph-*

theria.—I have seen three cases in which the exudation seemed without doubt to occur first in the larynx, the pharynx being subsequently affected. We may call this— primary laryngeal diphtheria. In one of these cases the patient was a medical man, about forty-five years of age. The disease began with pain in deglutition, and redness and swelling of the mucous membrane of the pharynx, arches of the palate, uvula, and soft palate. Laryngeal symptoms rapidly supervened; then a little lymph was seen on the arches of the palate, the exudation being more abundant at the base of the arch than above, and equal on the two sides; it looked as if it had spread upwards from the larynx. The patient would have died from apnœa had not the larynx been opened on the third day of illness. During the second week of illness, he almost died from asthenia.

Another case was that of the child whose pharynx, larynx, trachea, etc., are on the table (Specimen 3). I described the parts to you early in the lecture (p. 501).

In all the varieties of diphtheria I have described, the disease when fatal proved so in consequence of exudative inflammation affecting the larynx. The patient dies in such case from the impediment to the entrance of the air into the lungs. In the variety of which I am now about to speak the patient, when the disease proves fatal, dies from the general disease.

SIXTH VARIETY.—*The asthenic form of diphtheria.*—In this form the disease begins sometimes with general and local symptoms of moderate severity. Soon, however, the pulse is rapid and feeble; the sense of weakness and of illness extreme; the skin is not very hot, but there is a peculiar feverish pungency in its heat as appreciated by the touch; the complexion has that dirty-looking, pallid, and opaque aspect which we see in so many general diseases. In some cases, from an early period of the disease, the brown tongue, the sordes on the teeth, etc., and the muttering delirium which are characteristic of the so-called typhoid condition, are present. On examining the throat, more or less lymph is seen on the pharyngeal mucous membrane. The lymph in these cases has always, in my experience, been of the granular, pulpy, or softer form. The patient may swallow with perfect facility and the throat symptoms be trivial in degree, and this even when the pharyngeal mucous membrane is covered with lymph. In other cases the pain in deglutition is extreme. The extension of the exudative inflammation to the larynx, when it occurs, is shown by a little huskiness and want of power in the voice, and imperfectly marked laryngeal breathing. The patient usually dies in about ten or twelve days, death being the result not of apnœa, but of asthenia.. It is failure of the heart's action and not want of breath that causes death.

I saw a case referrible to this head with Dr. Turle, of St. John's Wood. The patient, a little girl aged eight years, lived at the extreme verge of London in that direction. She had been poorly for a few days when seen by Dr. Turle. The friends said there was only slight sore throat and weakness.

Dr. Turle noted, on the 6th of October 1859, 'skin not only hot, but feverishly pungent, slightly furred tongue, some enlargement of the glands behind the angles of the jaw, and all the parts of the pharynx visible to the eye covered with lymph.' On the 12th the urine contained a good deal of albumen. On the 15th I saw the patient; there was then evidence of extension to the larynx, but the laryngeal symptoms were not at all urgent. On the 18th death occurred, as Dr. Turle says in his notes of the case, 'from exhaustion, and not from asphyxia.'

The following case is remarkable for the rapidity with which the disease ran its course, the early delirium, and the severity of the general symptoms. Although the larynx was severely affected, it was manifest that its lesion played but a small part in causing death. Had the general derangement been less, no doubt the affection of the larynx would soon, however, have formed a prominent feature in the case, and even have led to a fatal termination in another twenty-four hours.

Henry M., aged seventeen years, was in good health on Friday night, February 12, 1858. He had spent the evening in society, and sung a good deal. The next morning he had sore throat and difficulty in swallowing; slight cough; he vomited, and felt cold and shivered. By noon he was unable to swallow; at night his breathing became difficult, his breath offensive, and he was delirious. On the 14th he was still

2 K

unable to swallow, could not get out of bed without assistance, and was delirious. At two P.M. on the 14th, he was
carried to my ward in this hospital.

Soon after his admission, Dr. Pougnet found him in a
very prostrate condition, lying on his back, and muttering
deliriously. He could not be made to answer questions, or to
protrude his tongue; and as he resisted all attempts to open
his mouth, the state of his pharynx could not be seen. But
as there was swelling about the angles and under the rami of
the jaw and down the neck, the breath had a gangrenous
odour, and there was profuse discharge of yellowish offensive
fluid from the mouth, and no rash on the skin, and as he had
not been exposed to the scarlet-fever poison, the diagnosis of
diphtheria, although not absolute, was highly probable. His
face was puffy, his lips blue, his pulse frequent, small, and
weak. He died the same night; thirty-six hours only from
the first symptoms of disease.

After death the mucous membrane of the pharynx was
found dark crimson grey in colour, and covered over its
greater extent by a layer of the granular variety of lymph.
The capacity of the pharynx was less than natural, in consequence of œdematous thickening of the submucous tissue
and corrugation of the mucous membrane. The *velum
pendulum palati* was greatly thickened, and the posterior
surface of the uvula was covered with lymph.

The upper and under surfaces of the epiglottis, the
arytæno-epiglottidean folds, and the mucous membrane
covering the larynx above and below the vocal cords, the
trachea, and the first division of the bronchi were covered by
the soft form of lymph. The lungs were the seat of acute
emphysema.

In a case I saw with Dr. Part, of Camden Road Villas, the
young lady, about eighteen years of age, exhibited no laryngeal symptoms. When Dr. Part first saw her on December
17, 1858, there was very trifling sore throat, with little or no
constitutional disorder. The febrile disturbance throughout
was extremely trifling, and although the mucous membrane
of the pharynx was soon covered with a creamy-looking layer
of lymph, the patient swallowed both liquids and solids without difficulty. The pulse was from the first very rapid and

weak. At our last visit, on the afternoon of the 26th December, Dr. Part and myself were accompanied by a surgeon who had seen little of the disease in this epidemic. The patient had eaten some chicken for dinner; she sat up in bed, and, though very anxious about her own state,[1] laughed, and talked to us without difficulty.

Dr. Part and I agreed that she had not many hours to live, so rapid and so feeble was her pulse, notwithstanding the quantity of support she was taking. The surgeon, who had not felt her pulse, and judged alone from her aspect and voice, said, 'I should have had no idea she was in great danger.' In twelve hours she was dead. The illness in this case lasted ten days.

There is yet another set of cases in which death appears to result from the evils consequent on the absorption of foetid matters from the pharyngeal tissues. The pharynx is covered with lymph, the mucous membrane below sloughs, the breath is very offensive, the glands about the angles of the jaw swell extremely, the cellular tissue in which they are imbedded is the seat of the effusion of serosity, the skin assumes that dirty-yellowish tint which it has in septicæmia, the mind wanders, and the patient rapidly sinks.

I trust you will not fail to understand that although I have described to you several varieties of diphtheria, there is no sharp line of distinction between them, any more than there is any sharply defined line of demarcation between scarlatina simplex, scarlatina anginosa, and scarlatina maligna. You may say this is a case of inflammatory diphtheria, and this of nasal diphtheria, and this of asthenic diphtheria; but you will meet with all intermediate shades of the disease; cases which you cannot refer with certainty to one or the other variety. So we meet constantly with cases of scarlet fever which cannot be referred to either variety, but which combine in themselves the essential characters of two. The acute specific diseases are really different one from the other. Each variety of each acute specific disease passes insensibly into the other varieties of the same disease; and these several varieties of each exhibit the most Protean combinations. Still, for those who desire to draw a picture of these

---

[1] Her sister had died just before of diphtheria.

diseases for others' use, the division of each acute specific
disease into varieties is a necessity, however artificial and
imperfectly defined the varieties may be.

The duration of the cases of diphtheria I have seen has
varied from forty-eight hours to fourteen days. When fatal
within a week from the first symptoms of illness, death has
always been preceded by extension of the exudative inflammation to the larynx. I have never known laryngeal symptoms commence after the expiration of the first week of the
disease. As I have pointed out to you, laryngeal symptoms
are sometimes present from the outset; at least they are now
and then the first symptoms to attract the attention of the
patient and his friends. I have twice seen death occur
within twelve hours from the time the laryngeal symptoms
were first noticed, and I have never known death delayed
more than five days from the time when symptoms indicated
clearly that exudation had occurred in the larynx. In rather
more than half of the fatal cases of diphtheria I have seen.
death resulted directly from the disease of the larynx; and
in rather more than half of the remainder, laryngeal disease
was present, although death resulted apparently from
asthenia. When death has occurred from asthenia the fatal
result has usually taken place during the second week of the
disease, unless the patient has been greatly weakened by previous disease; thus, I have just seen diphtheria occur in a
girl aged ten years, who had long suffered from hip-disease
with profuse foetid discharge, etc. She died from asthenia
with rapid feeble pulse on the fifth day of the disease. In
the very remarkable case of Henry M., aged seventeen years,
you will remember the disease terminated from the severity
of the general affection in thirty-six hours after the occurrence
of the first symptoms of illness.

The specific disease in the not-fatal cases I have seen has
terminated between the eighth and fourteenth day of illness.

NOTE.—An examination of the cases recorded in Bretonneau's
Memoirs on Diphtheria fully confirms the conclusions I have arrived
at from my own experience, as to the proportion of fatal cases in
which the larynx suffers so as to lead to death; as to the period of the
disease at which the larynx becomes affected; and as to the duration

of the fatal cases when death occurs from laryngeal complication. Thus, in Bretonneau's 1st, 2nd, and 4th Memoirs, are contained the details of forty-five cases; of these, four are wanting in data, or have no bearing on this subject. In twenty-nine of the remaining forty-one cases, the larynx was the seat of disease, and three only of the twenty-nine ended in recovery.

Of the twenty-six cases—fatal from the laryngeal complication—one terminated on the second day of illness, one survived till the sixteenth day of illness—tracheotomy having prevented death on the fourteenth day. In no case did the patient survive the sixth day of the laryngeal symptoms unless an operation retarded death, and in five only of the twenty-six cases did the patient survive the third day of the laryngeal symptoms.

In all of the twenty-nine cases, excepting one, the laryngeal symptoms supervened before the end of the first week, and in sixteen of the twenty-nine cases on or before the third of illness.

The emphysema of the lungs seen after death from diphtheria is that which is so commonly found in young children. It is a mere over-distention of healthy air-vesicles. Gluge terms it Insufflation. We can produce it by inflating the lungs after their removal from the body; or, by compressing one part of a lung, we can drive enough air to other parts to over-distend their air-vesicles, and so produce a condition identical with acute vesicular emphysema. As there is no damage to the texture of the lungs in this form of pulmonary emphysema, the air-vesicles recover their normal size when the over-distending force is removed. Bretonneau describes a case of diphtheria in which, not only were the air-passage and the air-vesicles over-distended, but one or more gave way, and air was found extravasated into the subcutaneous tissue. Trousseau has recorded a similar case. The latter distinguished pathologist attributes the subcutaneous emphysema to violent inspiratory efforts. This is manifestly an incorrect explanation of the facts. There is no power brought into play during inspiration to draw the air into the subcutaneous tissue. It is during the expiratory efforts that the air, unable to escape freely through the larynx, is driven with such force into the least compressed and least supported parts of the air-passages and vesicles as to over-distend them, to rupture them, and to inject the air into the cellular tissue. The same accident, as is well known, sometimes happens, from the same cause, during the violent efforts of parturient women. Doubtless the extreme inflation of the lungs when false membrane exists in the larynx and trachea, is partly the result of accumulation of air in them; the false membrane acting, as Bretonneau says, as a valve, permits air to enter but none to escape.

LECTURE II

GENTLEMEN,—In a certain proportion of cases after the termination of the diphtheria, symptoms of a very remarkable kind occur, referrible to deranged innervation. There can be no doubt that the latter are the consequence of the former—that the patient would not be suffering from the nervous symptoms if he had not just had diphtheria.

I will briefly describe the various kinds of deranged innervation consequent on diphtheria, which have fallen under my observation during the present epidemic. I mentioned, you will remember, in my last lecture, the case of Dr. E., who suffered from the active inflammatory form of diphtheria, accompanied by the exudation of wash-leather-like lymph. On recovering from the diphtheria, he was annoyed to find that his voice was singularly snuffling—he talked through his nose, as it is called. He was troubled very soon after by occasional irregular action of the pharyngeal muscles, causing fluids to return through the nose; there was also now and then while swallowing solids a choking sensation, accompanied by violent irregular action of the pharyngeal muscles.

This condition of voice and of impaired power of deglutition continued for several weeks; gradually, however, the voice regained its normal quality, and the pharyngeal muscles their healthy action.

This is the most common form in which derangement of the nervous system shows itself after diphtheria. Trousseau has shown that in these cases there is loss of sensibility in the *velum pendulum palati.*

The organ which next in frequency to the pharynx gives evidence of disordered innervation is the heart. Treasure this case in your mind; it is an instructive one:—

In July last I twice saw, with Mr. Adams, of Harrington Square, a young gentleman about ten years of age. There was nothing to excite alarm in one less aware than Mr. Adams of the grave nature of even mild cases of diphtheria. The local and general symptoms were very slight. The exudation on the pharyngeal mucous membrane was limited in extent; deglutition was easy; the general symptoms were, with the exception of a feeble pulse, trifling. The local disease quickly improved. On one day only was there even a trace of albumen in the urine, and even on that day, so small was the quantity that its very presence was not beyond doubt. The intellect was unaffected throughout.

The boy was considered by his friends convalescent, when vomiting occurred. Still, there was nothing to alarm the bystander. But Mr. Adams, at his visit, found the heart's beats, which had been falling in frequency for two days, thirty-six in the minute, and at the same time weak. He at once appreciated the gravity of the boy's situation. When I met Mr. Adams an hour after, the lad's countenance was not indicative of any very serious affection; it spoke only of a sense of languor; vomiting was said to be frequent, but the tongue was scarcely furred; the mucous membrane of the throat looked healthy; there was no albumen in the urine; the air entered freely to the bases of both lungs (we could not of course sit the boy upright, but we turned him on to his side); the heart's beats were rather feeble, the first and second sounds free from murmur, and of normal duration; the period of rest—the long silence—was longer than it should be, that is to say, the heart's beats were infrequent, not slow.

The infrequency and the feebleness of the heart's beats and the vomiting alone told that the boy's life was in danger The next morning Mr. Adams informed me that the pulse notwithstanding the freest use of stimulants, had fallen tc 32, in the afternoon it was 24 only, and soon after he died apparently from cessation of the heart's action.

The return of fluids through the nose, the fall in the frequency of the pulse, and the vomiting, sometimes occur before the local and general symptoms have subsided. Thus, in one of the two fatal cases I saw with Mr. Jay, in July 1858 : some days before the little girl's death, which occurred a fortnight after the first symptoms, Mr. Jay noted that there was stertorous breathing, diminution in temperature, relaxation of the skin with free perspiration, return of fluids through the nose, with so great a fall in the frequency of the pulse that for some time before death there were not more than sixteen beats of the heart in the minute. The heart's sounds were natural. At no time was there any notable quantity of albumen in the urine.

That a fall in the frequency of the heart's beats before death is not constant, is proved by the case of the child whose pharynx, larynx, etc., are on the table. Its pulse, five minutes before it breathed its last, while it was yet conscious, was 140 in the minute.

There are again a class of cases in which the nervous symptoms are far more striking, the paralysis more widely spread—not limited, as in the cases I have hitherto mentioned, to parts to which the par vagum is distributed. Here is the brief outline of a family group of cases of diphtheria, some of which I saw with Mr. Adams.

On the 26th January 1859, Master Cl., aged three years and six months, died of diphtheria, having been ill thirteen days. Two days before his death, his sister, aged eight years, sickened with the same disease; in her case the local lesion was not grave, and was confined to the pharynx; and the general symptoms were of moderate severity. At one time there was a little albumen in her urine. I saw her on the 31st of January, and for the last time on the 9th of February, when she was considered convalescent, though weak. Mr. Adams informed me, that instead of gaining she lost power. She was removed to the country on the 23rd, but grew less and less able to support herself, and died, so far as Mr. Adams and I could gather, from general loss of nervous power on the 4th of March. The day before her death, she had been taken out of doors.

On the 1st of March, another boy of the same family, aged five and a half years, began to suffer with his throat; he died on the 6th of March from extension of the exudative inflammation to the larynx. This boy was attacked, and died in the country, where he had been sent with his elder sister on the 31st of January.

Miss Cl., aged twelve years, the eldest of the same family,

sickened from diphtheria, on the 8th of February, while with her brother in the country. She was considered to be convalescent on the 22nd, and returned to London March 7th. At this date her parents thought her quite well. She gradually, however, fell into the state in which I saw her on the 17th of March; at that time she looked in tolerable health ; there was no emaciation, and only moderate pallor of the skin and mucous membranes. To walk, however, a step, she required the aid of two persons. She had very little power in her lower extremities, and still less control over their movements. There was some loss of power in the hands and arms, so that she could not cut her food.

Solids were swallowed without difficulty, but fluids frequently returned through the nose. It was manifest that she exercised very little control over the muscles of the pharynx. Her mind was perfect, her tongue clean, her appetite good ; she was taking most nourishing diet ; there seemed to be no derangement of the digestive organs. I saw her again on the 23rd,—there was no improvement ; and Mr. Adams informs me that she became more and more powerless, and died shortly after her visit to me on the 23rd.

The following interesting case I saw with Mr. Sillifant, of Thornhill Square, last September. Master S., aged one year and ten months, began to suffer from diphtheria on August 16th, 1860 (his brother having died shortly before of the same disease). In three weeks the child had recovered, ran about, resumed its usual habits, and seemed well.

On the 16th of September, his mother noticed that he staggered in walking. Paralysis gradually increased, until he was in the state I saw him with Mr. S. on September 26th. I then noted :—'He is very pale, anæmic-looking, thin, muscles small and flabby; but he is not emaciated to any extreme degree. He is intelligent, and eats and sleeps well. There is no evidence of paralysis of any of the muscles of the face, tongue, or eyes. When in his mother's arms, his head falls on one side,—backward or forward, according to the position in which he is accidentally placed. When he sits, there is posterior and lateral curvature of the spine, such as occurs from want of muscular power, e.g. in rickets. The arms can be moved at pleasure, though their movements are performed slowly and languidly. The legs are almost powerless; he is quite unable to stand, but when sitting in a chair, supported by pillows, he can move his legs a little. His voice is weak. The respiratory movements are performed feebly. He swallows without difficulty. Fluids do not return through the nose. His pulse is weak—seventy-eight in the minute. There are no evidences of rickets, albuminoid disease, or tubercle. Mr. Sillifant had tested the urine,—it was free from albumen.'

Mr. Sillifant informed me that the child lived only two days after I took these notes.

'He grew weaker each day; and while sitting propped up in his chair taking some nourishment, he suddenly fell back, apparently in a fainting condition, and died.'

He lived thirteen days only from the supervention of the first noted symptoms of deranged innervation.

For an opportunity of seeing the following case I am indebted to Dr. Baly, who kindly sent the patient to me, knowing I was interested in the subject. It affords an example of another form of deranged innervation.

Mr. M., aged twenty-two, a medical student, had an attack of diphtheria while staying in Bedfordshire. The exudation of lymph was limited to the pharynx. The disease began on the 12th of January 1860. He was ill three weeks. At the end of the illness part of the fluids attempted to be swallowed returned through the nose.

He recovered; was in health for a fortnight; then he had recurrence of the sore throat, and fluids again returned through the nose, and his voice was snuffling. To relieve these symptoms, part of his uvula was removed, and he thought with benefit to his powers of deglutition and voice. Loss of vision of the right eye followed, and he fancied the eye was more prominent than the other: he regained his sight while taking quinine. As the power of vision returned, he began to suffer from tingling and a slight want of power in the feet, the right foot being first affected. I saw Mr. M. first on the 1st of May; the upper extremities below the elbows were then chiefly affected. He had a difficulty in cutting his food, and experienced a constant tingling in the hands, and a sensation as if something were placed between the fingers and the objects they touched.

There was no albumen in his urine; no manifest derangement of his circulatory or digestive organs. He was strong and healthy-looking, only he had, perhaps, a little less colour in his mucous membranes than he should have had.

This gentleman, Dr. Baly informs me, regained his health after some months.

The symptoms of disordered innervation have commenced in the cases I have seen within three weeks from the date of convalescence. Where the disorder has been limited to the parts supplied by the branches of the par vagum, it has supervened earlier than when it has been more generally diffused. The longest period after the first symptoms of diphtheria at which I have known death occur from disordered innervation is about two months.

Before considering the pathology of the disease—its nature, as it is called—there are some points connected with its etiology and progress which the cases I have seen have strongly impressed on my mind.

1st. That the disease is infectious.

2nd. That the infection-element does not require for its development any of the ordinarily considered anti-hygienic conditions.

3rd. That it is very doubtful even if any of those anti-hygienic conditions favour its development, or give to it a more untoward course when it occurs.

4th. That family constitution is one of the most important elements favouring the development of the disease, and determining its progress.

1st. Dr. E. lived in Euston Road. He was attending a child ill from diphtheria, when he sickened with the same disease. As he recovered, his attendant was attacked with it, and admitted into ward 3. No one in his house, although there were other inmates, suffered excepting Dr. E. and the young woman who was in constant attendance on him. The child from whom Dr. E. appeared to have caught the disease resided some distance from Euston Road.

Mr. B.'s infant had diphtheria; three of the other five children and the nurse who held the infant in her arms the greater part of the time it was ill took the disease. The nurse was the only adult in the house who suffered.

Miss C. had diphtheria. She went to the country a fortnight after the commencement of her attack, and within a fortnight after her arrival, her brother, some time resident in the country, had an attack.

Miss and Master B. visited at a house where a child was ill from some disease of the throat, of which she died shortly after. Miss and Master B. sickened with diphtheria a few days after their visit.

A boy, aged about five years, was sent from home in consequence of two members of his family having diphtheria; shortly after a third suffered from the same disease. Two of the three who had diphtheria recovered; they were sent to the country, but to a residence some miles distant from that of the little boy. Three weeks from the time the boy left his home, he was allowed to go to the house to which his sisters had been removed on their recovery, and where they were still staying. Ten days after his arrival there, the boy sickened with diphtheria. In this case either the poison was in the child's system when he left London, and remained latent for a month, a supposition highly improbable, or he caught the disease from his sisters after they met in the country.[1]

2nd. Of the cases of diphtheria I have seen the last three years, twelve only occurred in hospital practice. Now of all other diseases I have seen many more in hospital practice than in private practice. And, speaking generally, it may be said that people who seek medical assistance at a hospital are placed in much more unfavourable hygienic conditions than are private patients. These facts are strong evidence in favour of the opinion that the ordinarily reckoned antihygienic conditions are not especially favourable to the development of diphtheria.

3rd. As to the influence of these conditions unfavourable to health in inducing a fatal termination. Of my hospital patients, half died; of my private cases, rather more than half. With reference, however, to this point, I should observe

---

[1] See also the cases of Wm. W. and G. O., pp. 510 and 540.

that as the large majority of the cases I have seen in private houses have been in consultation, they indicate a greater mortality than the average in the rank of life in which they occurred, a second opinion being sought usually because the case is severe.

4th. As in all the other acute specific diseases, the influence of family constitution in favouring the occurrence of the disease, and in disposing to a fatal termination, is very remarkable. You attend a case of typhoid fever, the patient dies; other members of the family sicken, your anxiety for them should be the greater because one of the family has already succumbed. For we often meet with families who have lost several members from typhoid fever, or from scarlet fever, from whooping-cough or from measles, and that not only during the same epidemic and in the same locality, but at long intervals and at far-off places. There seems to exist in some families, though to appearance healthy, an inability to resist the injurious influences of certain specific poisons. This influence of family constitution in favouring the occurrence and determining the ending of diphtheria has, I think, been manifested during the present epidemic.

Thus I have seen one or more of four cases in one family of four children, of which two proved fatal;
of two in another family of three children, both fatal;
of two cases in another family of small size, both fatal;
of five cases in a family of six children, one fatal;
of four cases in a family of six children, all fatal;
of two cases in a family of small size, both fatal;
of two cases in a family of (I think) five children, both fatal;
of two cases in a family of (I think) four children, one fatal;
of two cases, an uncle and nephew, one year between, and in
    different localities, both fatal;
of two cases in a small family, both fatal;
of two cases in a family of six children, both fatal.

In all these cases the hygienic conditions were good; there was nothing patently bad as regards drainage, ventilation, overcrowding, water-supply, food, or work. All the patients were in the middle rank of life, and resided in good-sized houses, and in fairly open situations.

These facts, of course, speak strongly in favour of contagion, as well as in favour of the influence of family constitution.

As to the pathology of diphtheria; the want of relation in severity between the local and general symptoms, the differences in the characters of the general symptoms, the albumen in the urine,[1] the definite course, the nervous symptoms which follow in some cases, the specific origin, and the frequency with which it occurs as an epidemic, all point to the same conclusion, viz., that diphtheria is primarily a general disease. On the more intimate nature of the disease, my cases throw no light, they afford no clew to its blood or nerve origin.

Diphtheria has been supposed to be modified scarlet fever, but the fact that it attacks indiscriminately those who have and those who have not had, proves that it is altogether a different, though it may still be a closely allied, disease.

The child I saw with Dr. Turle, at St. John's Wood, as well as his sister, subsequently attended by him, had both suffered from scarlet fever two years and a half before.

Of five children in one family at Kentish Town, who were attacked by diphtheria, I had attended three a year before, when they were suffering from scarlet fever. A child I saw, a few hours before it died from diphtheria, with Mr. Baly, had been attended nine weeks before by that surgeon for scarlet fever. A second child in the same family, who had had scarlet fever at the same time, sickened from diphtheria a few days after the first died.

Diphtheritic inflammation of the pharynx sometimes complicates scarlet fever. I have seen two well-marked cases of this during the present epidemic. One of the patients was a child, whose sister, shortly after, was under my care for scarlet fever without the diphtheritic inflammation of the throat—the other was a man aged twenty-two, a patient in the hospital. In neither case was the throat affection very severe; both ended favourably.

The diagnosis of the scarlet fever rested in both cases on the presence of rash: desquamation followed in both.

Are diphtheria and croup essentially the same disease?

[1] For a knowledge of the highly important fact that albumen is present in the urine of the great majority of fatal cases of diphtheria, we are indebted to Dr. Wade of Birmingham.

I think not; because there is no evidence to show that croup is anything more than a local disease, that it is contagious—that it occurs as a widespread epidemic—that it affects a large proportion of adults—that there is albumen in the urine—that symptoms of disordered innervation follow recovery from the primary affection.[1] We must not confound diphtheritic exudations with diphtheria, any more than we must confound the acute specific disease erysipelas, such as the physician sees, with erysipelatous inflammation of the skin so common in the surgical wards.

A girl named O'Brien, five years of age, was lately an in-patient at the Hospital for Sick Children. She was suffering from severe chronic pemphigus. She had been in the hospital several weeks, when a large excoriated surface on the side of her chest was noticed to be covered with a thick layer of the wash-leather-like variety of diphtheritic exudation; in a day or two little patches appeared on the conjunctivæ. The child died suddenly and unexpectedly the day after the conjunctivæ were observed to be affected. The parents were Irish, and no examination of the body could be obtained; there were no pharyngeal or laryngeal symptoms. In scarlet fever it is not uncommon to have a little diphtheritic exudation on the tonsil and arches of the palate and pharynx; and I have seen it extend to the larynx. In my first lecture are the details of a case of diphtheria supervening towards the decline of measles.

There were lately in the hospital two cases of ulcer of the leg, when several cases of diphtheria were admitted. The ulcers became covered with diphtheritic exudations. No severe constitutional disturbance accompanied the exudation, and local remedies (nitrate of silver) sufficed for the cure.

Of the pathology of the disordered innervation we know but little. In some of the cases it is probable that the par vagum is chiefly affected. This is shown by the irregular action of the pharyngeal muscles, by the vomiting, and by the failure in the heart's action. I need only mention Weber's experiments, to recall to your minds the influence that nerve exerts on the frequency of the heart's beats. Let the par vagum be exposed and divided in the neck, and then

[1] This opinion was subsequently modified by the author. See Lecture on Croup, p. 563.

the poles of a galvanic battery be applied to the cut extremity
of its distal portion, the heart's action is instantly arrested;
remove the wires from the nerve, and the beating of the
heart is resumed; re-apply the wires, and the action of the
organ ceases; and so, for some time, you can at pleasure stay
and set going again the action of the heart.

The only other acute specific disease in which I have
noted such fall in the frequency of the heart's beats is relapsing fever.   In that disease, however, the singularly infrequent
beating of the heart, which follows the profuse critical perspiration, indicates the return of health; in diphtheria it
tells of approaching dissolution, and that even when the mind
is clear and the senses acute.

Diagnosis.—You will have gathered from all I have told
you, that the absolute diagnosis of diphtheria in any given
case must rest on the detection by the eye of lymph on the
mucous membrane of the pharynx.   But you may often suspect that the disease is diphtheria before the exudation
occurs; and sometimes may be almost certain that it is so;
just as in measles or scarlet fever, you may venture on a
diagnosis before the anatomical character of those diseases,
i.e. the eruption, has appeared.

Thus, when diphtheria is epidemic or prevalent in the
neighbourhood, or has recently occurred in the same house,
and the whole mucous membrane of the pharynx is red and
swollen, the uvula thickened, and the parts covered with
tough mucus, and the glands behind the angles of the jaw
enlarged, you would have strong reasons for apprehending
the disease to be diphtheria, and especially so if there was
epistaxis or sero-purulent discharge from the nose.   Bleeding
from the nose is occasionally an early symptom of diphtheria.
The general aspect of the patient in some cases adds weight
to the local evidence.   For in a few cases of diphtheria, the
skin has a dirty opaque appearance, and in many a pallid
pasty aspect, very peculiar, though by no means diagnostic.
If the patient has had scarlet fever, or if the papillæ of the
tongue be neither enlarged nor redder than natural, the probability is still higher that the case is one of diphtheria.
When the inflammation has spread to the larynx, all doubt
ceases in regard of diagnosis.

French writers describe an herpetic eruption on the mucous membrane of the pharynx, which may be mistaken, they say, for diphtheria. It is commonly associated with herpes of the lip; and, as a rule, is much more painful than diphtheria, the pain being limited to a single spot in the pharynx. Several cases of this kind have fallen under my observation; in none has there been any great difficulty in separating them from cases of diphtheria.

Prognosis.—No case of diphtheria is unattended by danger. However mild the case may seem at the commencement, death may end it. Never be off your guard.

During the first week of the disease, the great danger to life is from the extension of exudative inflammation to the larynx. If it does reach the larynx, death is the result in a vast proportion of cases. There cannot be in diphtheria the least laryngeal quality in the respiration heard at the bedside, without there being grounds for the greatest anxiety as to the final result. Suppose the first week of illness to have passed without the inflammation extending to the larynx, then death is to be apprehended from exhaustion and loss of nervous energy; and I beg you to bear in mind that death from these causes may follow even when the pharyngeal inflammation and exudation has been trifling in degree and extent.

An extremely rapid and feeble pulse is of grave import; a very infrequent pulse is of fatal significance. Vomiting is another unfavourable symptom, especially if repeated many days in succession. Bleeding from the nose and other organs not only weaken the patient, but are indications of profound blood change; if profuse, the patient's life is in great jeopardy.

Even a trace of albumen in the urine is an unfavourable symptom; when very abundant, a fatal termination of the case is most probable. The albuminous urine probably indicates rather an abnormal state of the blood than disease of the kidney. At least, after death, I have never seen more than congestion of the kidneys. When the albumen is abundant and the urine scanty, some of the symptoms of uræmia may be conjoined with those of exhaustion; *e.g.* extreme drowsiness, a little wandering of the mind, and a rapid and feeble pulse. All the cases in which I have known delirium occur have ended fatally.

My experience not only justifies the conclusion that diphtheria is more common in childhood than in adult age, but also that the danger is in proportion to the youth of the patient: thus, while seventeen of twenty-two cases ten years of age and under proved fatal, only six of thirteen cases fifteen years of age and over proved fatal.

In the child, death is generally the result of the extension of the disease to the larynx; after puberty, death more often occurs from the general affection: thus, of the seventeen fatal cases ten years of age and under, twelve died from exudation in the larynx; while of the six fatal cases fifteen years and over, only one proved fatal from the laryngeal complication.

Treatment.—We have no specific remedy for diphtheria. It is to be treated on the same general principles as the other acute specific diseases. We have no specific remedy for any of the acute specific diseases. We save by medical aid many lives that would be lost from scarlet fever, from typhoid fever, from typhus fever, from measles, etc.[1] We save such lives, however, only by from time to time averting special modes of death. The specific disease is not cut short—it is not cured by our remedies; it runs its course, do what we may to prevent it.

To avert death in any given acute specific disease, we must know and bear in mind how it kills. Thus scarlet fever kills, first, by the severity of the general affection; secondly, by the local throat disease and its consequences; thirdly, by the kidney affection and its consequences; fourthly, by accidental complications, as pericarditis, pleurisy, etc. And in treating a case of scarlet fever, we are always on the watch lest any one of these should attain a fatal degree of severity. And by treatment we can do much to moderate the severity of the general disease, and still more for the

---

[1] ' Tendencies accompany or conditions survive the fever,' says the most judicious English writer on medicine of the present day, ' which remedial measures, opportunely and judiciously applied, avail to oppose and control. Our object must be, when the fever is once established, to conduct it to a favourable close, to " obviate the tendency to death."'—*Lect. on Princ. and Pract. of Physic.* By T. Watson, M.D. 4th ed. Vol. ii. p. 843.

throat affection, etc. In the present epidemic of diphtheria, I have seen patients die from the general disease—from the local throat disease and its consequences—from derangement of the nervous system.

With reference to the general disease, I would advise you to be guided by the same rules that would guide you in treating a case of erysipelas or of typhoid fever, modified only by your knowledge of the special tendency of each to be complicated by certain local lesions of structure, e.g. you would not purge in typhoid fever. So long as there is heat of skin and firmness of pulse, you should abstain from alcoholic stimulants, and give simple febrifuges, as they were once called, viz., saline medicines, which exert a slight action on the skin and on the kidneys, or on both. Acetate of ammonia and citrate of potash are agents well suited for the purpose. At the same time, the bowels should be well cleared out by a dose of calomel and jalap, or calomel and colocynth pill, followed in the inflammatory form of the disease by a saline aperient, e.g. infusion of roses and sulphate of magnesia. In this stage of the disease the inflammation of the throat should be treated by warm fomentations externally, and the inhalation of water vapour with acetic acid. A wine-glass full of vinegar to a pint of boiling water is a good proportion—Squire's inhaler is the best I am acquainted with. You may frequently see it in use in the wards. A lead gargle—one drachm of the solution of the diacetate of lead to eight ounces of rose-water—may occasionally be useful; but if gargles cause inconvenience or pain from the muscular exertion of the throat in gargling, their use should never be persisted in. The patient should be confined to bed, the temperature of the room kept at about 68° Fahr., and its atmosphere made moist by placing a kettle with a long spout on the fire. The form of kettle devised by the late Dr. Pretty is very good for the purpose,[1] and very simple. The young child can neither gargle nor inhale, and at this stage of the disease painting

---

[1] This is a tin kettle, with a small aperture at the top closed by a screw instead of a common lid. From the front of the kettle project two spouts of about three feet in length ; one spout springs from the upper part of the kettle and passes forward in a straight line,—the other spout springs from near the bottom of the kettle and passes obliquely upwards. The lower spout ends in

the throat with nitrate of silver, etc., is worse than useless. But you can envelop the young child in a warm moist atmosphere much more perfectly than you can an adult; make a tent with blankets over its little bed, and pass the spout of your kettle under the covering of the tent. The kettle need not be on the fire; fill it with boiling water, and then keep it boiling by spirit-lamps. The diet, so long as the febrile disturbance lasts, should be mild. At the same time do not forget that diphtheria, like erysipelas and typhoid fever, is a disease of low type.

When the disease begins with marked feebleness of pulse, dusky redness of throat, and extreme sense of general weakness, wine in full quantities is required at an early period. From six to eight ounces of sherry or port for an adult, and as good a diet as the patient can take must be given from the first. In the course of the disease, much larger quantities of wine, or a proportionate quantity of brandy, may have to be given. Of course the quantity of stimulant must be regulated by the age and habits of the patient, as well as by the character and the stage of the disease; but remember that, as a rule, young children bear and take with advantage, in diseases of depression, much larger quantities of stimulants than you would probably suppose. A child of three years of age now under treatment at the Children's Hospital for diphtheria, is taking with apparent advantage one to two drachms of brandy every hour, i.e. from three to five ounces of brandy in twenty-four hours. Under all general conditions attention must be paid to secure efficient action of the bowels, and the urinary and intestinal secretions must be examined daily.

The presence of blood or of albumen in the urine shows that diuretics are contra-indicated. Mustard poultices, followed by warm linseed-meal poultices, may be applied to the loins under such circumstances. The presence of a large amount of lithates in the urine should cause us to weigh the propriety of giving a mercurial aperient; that is to say, to inquire into the state of the biliary excreta.

a spoon-like projection, just under the slightly curved down open mouth of the upper spout. The steam passes out of the upper spout, and the condensed vapour drops into the little spoon, and is returned by the lower spout to the bottom of the kettle.

As to the value of local applications after the most acutely inflammatory stage has passed, when exudation is occurring, I have formed, from the cases I have seen treated by others, and have treated myself, two decided opinions:

1. That the single efficient application of a strong solution of nitrate of silver—a scruple to a drachm of water—frequently stays the spread of the exudative inflammation; but that, on the whole, hydrochloric acid and water in equal parts more frequently attain that object.

2. That the repeated application at short intervals of these strong local remedies is injurious; I think I have seen serious evil result from their application two or three times a day.

To apply any substance efficiently to the throat of a child, the little one must, before any attempt even to look into its throat is made, be firmly fixed, so that all sudden movements of its hands and head are completely prevented, and held so that the light may fall directly down its throat. Then the moment must be seized when the child in crying opens its mouth, and a firmly made tongue depressor or a broad-handled table-spoon be passed to the back of the tongue. Having the spoon or depressor in that situation, it is your own fault if you do not have a full view of the pharynx, and, unless much mucus be present, of the epiglottis. Depress the further extremity of the instrument and bring the tongue at the same time a little forward, and all the parts are within sight. If you use a small teaspoon or a very weak instrument, or do not fix the child firmly, or put the extremity of the instrument on the centre of the dorsum of the tongue, the result will probably be that after a struggle, more or less prolonged according to your own, the child's, and the parents' temper, you will fail altogether in attaining your object, or attain it most incompletely.

Having a good view of the part, the exudation, but especially the surface around the exudation, is to be painted with a camel-hair pencil dipped in the solution, the brush being passed over the surface two or three times in quick succession. The efforts to vomit, which your manipulations may excite, offer no real impediment to your proceedings. The application having been effectually made, you are to wait till the consequences of the application have passed away. Bear in mind, that both the acid and the strong solution of nitrate of silver produce white discoloration of the parts to which they are applied, and do not confound this discoloration with the spread of the diphtheritic exudation. I am sure I have seen severe inflammation of the pharynx kept up by the repeated daily application of irritants, used to cure the disease which they themselves were occasioning. The discoloration from the acid passes away in about thirty-six hours; that from the nitrate of silver somewhat quicker. The ordinary sponge probang is a very clumsy instrument for the application of powerful agents to the pharynx. You know not where the fluid from it goes; but a curved piece of whalebone, with a *very* small piece of sponge attached, must be used when you desire to apply fluid to the pharyngeal openings of the posterior nares and back of the *velum pendulum palati.*

The solid nitrate of silver carefully applied around the spreading diphtheritic patch, has appeared to me in some cases to have at once arrested its spread. I have never seen these powerful topical remedies of use while the parts were much swollen, bright red, and covered with mucus. Nay, under such conditions I have seen them do harm. In a case I saw with Dr. Schulof the frequent injection of cold water into the pharynx, which he had employed before I saw the patient, seemed to afford much relief: the patient recovered.

Do not tear off the false membrane; to do that is to commit a decided blunder. I have seen it done repeatedly, but never with good effect, and sometimes with decidedly bad results.[1]

Chlorate of potash, in doses of four grains dissolved in two drachms only of water, has seemed to me of some use in

[1] 'The authors of the sixteenth century agree in reprobating the forcible removal of the false membranes, and also scarifications, together with all roughness of frictions and applications. I have had occasion several times to convince myself of the justice of these precepts, and I have seen the pellicular inflammation aggravated by all kinds of mechanical irritation. When the disease is not arrested in its progress by two energetic applications made at intervals of twenty-four hours, and the signs of the affection of the air passages begin to be manifested, this local treatment offers very uncertain chances of recovery.'—*Dr. Semple's Translation of Bretonneau's 'Memoirs on Diphtheria,'* p. 106. The accuracy of these statements of Bretonneau is confirmed by my experience.

allaying the laryngeal inflammation. I have had no experience of powdered alum, of which Trousseau speaks very highly.[1]

In treating the local pharyngeal disease, you will note that the objects to be attained are the prevention of the spread of the exudative inflammation to the larynx, and the prevention of the occurrence of such an amount of local mischief as may lead to septicæmia; the latter is infinitely rare, the former is very common. By topical applications you do no good to the general disease, i.e. to the diphtheria. The end you have in view in the employment of the acid and nitrate of silver solutions is merely to avert death by the extension of the disease to the exudative inflammation of the larynx, and death by septicæmia.[2]

On the table are the pharynx, larynx, trachea, and lungs of a child who died recently in the Hospital for Sick Children. You will note that the exudative inflammation has extended low into the bronchi; that there is extensive collapse and scattered pneumonia of both lungs; and that the pneumonic solidification is of that kind which so often follows on collapse. You will see that there is an opening in the trachea; this was made, and well made, during the life of the child by my friend and former pupil Mr. Berkeley Hill, lately house-surgeon at this hospital, and now residing at the Hospital for Sick Children.

With reference to the propriety of performing laryngotomy or tracheotomy, when the larynx is invaded by the exudative inflammation, there can be no doubt that some lives have been saved in this country by an opening being made into the larynx or trachea, when death from suffocation in croup and in diphtheria was imminent.

A most unequivocal case of this kind was that of Dr. C. There is not a shadow of a doubt on my mind that he would have been dead in two minutes had his larynx not been opened at the moment it was by Mr. Quain. I never saw

[1] Fifteen grains of powdered alum are mixed with a little sugar, placed on the end of a straw, and blown from it into the pharynx several times a day. Tannin and other astringents have been applied in the same way.

[2] Trousseau, the most recent, and, after Bretonneau, the best writer on diphtheria, expresses a very different opinion as to the value of local remedies in diphtheria. See note, p. 551.

any one so manifestly brought back from the threshold of death. His complexion had that bluish pallor that precedes immediate dissolution. My hand was on his wrist. I felt his pulse failing under my finger, until at last it was imperceptible. His eyes closed, and his diaphragm was making those convulsive contractions which indicate that respiration is about to cease, when the knife entered the larynx, and the air was drawn by what really seemed the last effort of the diaphragm into the lungs. The natural hue of his face returned; his pulse was again perceptible; his eyes opened; consciousness was restored; and the patient was alive again. He finally recovered. Now a thousand failures of the operation in saving life cannot, after seeing this case, prove to me that tracheotomy ought not to be performed when suffocation is imminent from the presence of lymph in the larynx or trachea; for here is a man, whose life was invaluable to his family and most useful to society, restored to health, who, but for the operation, would have been dead.

In France, tracheotomy in children—putting aside those cases in which it is unnecessarily performed—is more successful than it is in England. Why is this? It is said that the operation in England is performed too late; that the patient is allowed to be weakened to an extreme degree before tracheotomy is resorted to. I doubt the correctness of this explanation. I have seen too many children die who were operated on before they were worn out by disease, to admit it. To answer the question, we must examine the facts bearing on it a little more closely. What lesions of structure, not directly due to the operation, do we find after death where tracheotomy has been performed, and what symptoms, explicable by these lesions, are noted during life?

Muco-purulent fluid, in quantity in the bronchial tubes, collapse of lung-tissue, and solidification of lung-tissue from inflammation—the inflammation being commonly secondary to collapse—these are the lesions we find to account for death after tracheotomy in cases of diphtheria and croup. These are the lesions to be seen in the lungs on the table, to which I just now directed your attention. During life we hear mucous and submucous râles over the lungs, and it may be that we find here and there a little dulness on percussion.

The increased difficulty to the entrance of the air into the lung-tissue, occasioned by the mucus accumulating in the bronchial tubes, may be measured from hour to hour almost, by the increasing recession of all the softer parts of the thoracic walls during the inspiratory efforts.

The sequence of events then seems to me to be as follows: —formation of irritating muco-purulent fluid in the trachea and largest bronchial tubes; the advance of the mucus, at each inspiration, further and further into the ramifications of the bronchial tubes; irritation by its presence of the bronchial mucous membrane, and the pouring out of fresh muco-purulent fluid. There is, as a rule, no active inflammation of the bronchi, there is little swelling, little tenacious mucus; hence there is during life little or no sonorous rhonchus. But why, you may ask, does not the patient get rid of the muco-purulent fluid by coughing? The answer is easy. He can cough but imperfectly, on account of the state of his larynx and trachea.

Remember the mechanism of cough and of expectoration. How often have I, and how often shall I again recall it to your mind? To cough freely and deeply, so as to remove obstructions from the bronchial tubes, you take a deep inspiration and then close the glottis; next you compress the air-distended lungs by violent expiratory effort, and then suddenly opening the larynx you drive out of the bronchial tubes by the force of the expelled air all matters contained in them; you expectorate. The child who has a tube in his trachea, or whose larynx is so diseased that he cannot close it firmly, is necessarily unable to cough deeply. He cannot compress the air-containing tissue of the lungs with force enough to drive out by the current of expressed air any excess of mucus, or other matters, from the bronchial tubes. You may excite cough as often as you desire by closing the tube for an instant, and some expectoration will follow; but unless a deep inspiration has preceded the closure of the tube, the quantity of air driven out by the expiratory effort must be small, and the force of its current feeble, consequently the cough will be ineffectual for the clearance of the bronchial tubes; the next inspiratory effort draws the mucus and the secretions from the larynx, trachea, etc., still lower into the tubes. After a short time collapse of lung tissue necessarily follows, and too often the collapse has for its sequences congestion and exudation, *i.e.* pneumonic consolidation. In diphtheria there is irritating and abundant secretion from the larynx and trachea. In order to cough effectually, you understand, a preliminary full inspiration is essential. Whatever, therefore, prevents such an expansion of the chest-walls or lungs as shall perfectly distend the air-cells of the latter with air, prevents effectual cough, and so favours the accumulation of mucus, and of the acrid secretions from the larynx, trachea, etc., in the bronchial tubes, and therefore favours the occurrence of pulmonary collapse, congestion, and inflammation.

Flexibility of the chest walls is a condition which prevents full inspiration of air when there is the least obstruction to its free passage through the bronchial tubes. The greater the flexibility of the chest walls, the greater is the mechanical difficulty to the inspiration of air. It is because of the flexibility of their chest walls that little children, constitutionally healthy, more often die from an attack of bronchitis than do adults, and that children whose ribs are softened from disease commonly die from pulmonary collapse when they are the subjects of trifling catarrh.

Trousseau remarks that he has seen only three children under two years of age recover after tracheotomy for croup. The principal reason for the mortality in children of this age is, that their chest walls are so flexible that mechanical power is wanting to draw air beyond the fluid which from any cause finds its way into the bronchial tubes. Supplementary causes are the susceptibility of young children to capillary bronchitis, and to the supervention of pneumonia or pulmonary collapse.

But why do a larger proportion of older children die after tracheotomy in England than in France? The cause of this difference is, I think, to be found in the greater frequency of rickets in England, and consequently in the greater flexibility of the chest walls in proportion to the age of the children. You will observe that many children who are not decidedly rickety are still the subjects of slight softening of the bones. There is no sharp line of demarcation in regard of consistence between the bones of a healthy child and the bones of a rickety child.

As to the early or late performance of tracheotomy in diphtheria, be sure before opening the trachea, first, that the exudative inflammation has extended to the larynx, and secondly, that it is advancing in severity. In judging on these points do not omit to look at the chest, and be guided to a considerable extent by the degree and increase of the recession of the soft parts of the parietes during inspiration. Being satisfied on the two points I have just mentioned, the sooner the operation is done the better. The mortality under any treatment is frightful, but tracheotomy will save a small proportion of cases. Then why refuse life to those few? As you grow older you will know the satisfaction it is to have a well-founded conviction that in even a single case you have been the means of saving life. In the adult, laryngotomy is to be preferred to tracheotomy; the larynx is large enough to admit a tube; in children it is too small, especially when narrowed by swelling of its mucous membrane and exudation on its surface. In children, then, you must open the trachea; open it, however, as near to the larynx as possible. It is said, open below the seat of disease; I think the reverse should be the rule. If you open into the healthy part you establish a new centre of irritation and inflammation.

The child whose trachea, etc., is on the table, and of which I have before spoken, was only a year and ten months old, and the subject of rickety softening of the ribs. Observe that there is no increase of the disease at the spot where the opening was made, though Mr. Hill opened into the diseased part. Had such a case as this occurred in private practice, the friends of the child should have been informed that death was certain unless an operation was performed; that an operation would give no more than the shadow of a shade of a chance of recovery. And even under more favourable circumstances, i.e. when the patient is older, and not rickety, you should fully explain to the friends the small proportion of operations that terminate in ultimate recovery. In all the cases, save one, that I have seen operated on, temporary relief and prolongation of life has been the result.

After tracheotomy, I have seen children die from two lesions of structure, directly due to the operation. One is injury (ulceration, etc.) to the trachea, from the mechanical irritation of the tube, and the other, suppuration in the anterior mediastinum, inflammation extending downwards from the lower border of the wound in the neck, through the cellular tissue in front of the trachea to the loose cellular tissue in the anterior mediastinum.

Against these as well as other dangers you must guard. I will describe to you a case lately under my care in the Hospital for Sick Children; and from that description you will learn the symptoms which I consider indicate the propriety of opening the trachea, and all the precautions I thought desirable to favour a successful termination of a case of tracheotomy for diphtheria.

The child (George O.) was three years and two months old; its ribs for its age were remarkably firm; its mother had had hæmoptysis.

This child was in the hospital, rapidly convalescing from measles, accompanied by very severe bronchitis, for which ammonia and brandy had been required. When about one a.m., *January 5th*, 1861, *i.e.* twelve hours after the death of William W.,[1] who lay in the next bed, it was observed by Mr. Hill to be hoarse, and breathing rapidly and stridulously. The cough had assumed a croupy character. There was no lividity of the surface, no recession of the soft parts of the thoracic walls. The mucous membrane of the fauces was very red and swollen. There was no lymph on it. The child had been seen by Mr. Hill at ten p.m. in his ordinary round, and at that time the breathing was not noisy; in fact, the boy seemed to be progressing towards health most satisfactorily.

The child was at once placed in a bed, to each corner of which is attached a rod, three feet in height; the four upright rods being connected at their tops by four transverse rods. Blankets were thrown over this framework, and into the circumscribed space so formed, hot water vapour was introduced from a long-spouted kettle. At the same time the bed was drawn near to the fire, and bottles of hot water placed in and on the bed; the object being to envelop the

[1] See p. 510.

child in a pure, moist atmosphere, having a temperature of about 70° Fahrenheit; subsequently a current of hot dry air was passed in a tube through the tent. Fifteen minims of tincture of sesquichloride of iron in water were ordered to be given every two hours, and half a drachm of brandy every hour. The child slept at intervals during the night, and at nine o'clock on the morning of the 5th, Mr. Ringer noted the child lying on its back asleep; in breathing it made a loud snoring noïse. On waking, the child coughed; the cough was hoarse, metallic, and ringing in character; it was followed by stridulous inspiration, the ordinary breathing had the laryngeal quality; the voice was thick. The child swallowed without pain or difficulty, it did not look oppressed, its skin was warm and free from lividity. The pulse was frequent and weak. There was, during inspiration, considerable recession of the lower part of the sternum, and of the margin of the thorax, as well as deepening of the supra-sternal and supra-clavicular regions, and of the intercostal spaces.

At two p.m. of the same day I made the following notes:—

" The inspiratory and expiratory sound as heard at the bedside are both laryngeal in quality.

" The pulse is 132, small and weak.

" The respirations are 48 in the minute.

" The child breathes through its open mouth, at the same time the nares dilate during inspiration.

" There is occasional cough, laryngeal in quality.

" The recession of all the softer parts of the thoracic parietes during inspiration is considerable, the lateral regions being flattened.

" On percussion both sides of the thorax are hyper-resonant.

" On auscultation the inspiratory murmur is very faintly audible. No abnormal sounds are heard in any part of the chest.

" The tonsils, uvula, arches of the palate, etc., are red and swollen. Much mucus obscures the view of the pharynx. The mucous membrane of the nose is dry. The lymphatic glands behind the angles of the jaw and down the sides of the larynx are somewhat larger than natural, but not tender."

The dose of the brandy was increased from half a drachm

to a drachm every hour. I expressed a wish that the trachea should be opened, in case the impediment to the entrance of the air into the chest increased.

At ten p.m. Mr. Ringer noted that the child looked more oppressed, that the lips were slightly livid, that inspiration was more difficult and prolonged, that the sound accompanying inspiration was more strongly laryngeal, that the soft parts of the chest walls fell in very greatly during inspiration. It was obvious that the impediment to inspiration was rapidly increasing. The pulse was frequent, but of pretty good power. No time was to be lost, every quarter of an hour was of moment, and therefore tracheotomy was at once performed by Mr. Berkeley Hill. I again use the notes of our accurate and able Registrar, Mr. Sydney Ringer.

Much blood was lost in the operation (this is sometimes unavoidable); the trachea was opened as near to the larynx as possible. After the tube [1] was introduced there was some blood and mucus in the trachea, which caused the child much annoyance and excited frequent efforts to eject it. In about an hour these efforts ceased, and the child fell into a calm sleep, lying on its back and breathing quietly. There was now no falling inwards of the softer parts of the chest walls during inspiration. The colour of the lips was good, there was no pallor of the face, no lividity. There was still a little dilatation of the nares during inspiration. When the tube became clogged, but then only, was there recession of the softest parts of the chest walls. The pulse was 108, and of tolerably good power. The respirations were 42 in the minute, but very irregular.

The skin, as judged by the hand, was of normal temperature, and moist. There was much moist râle at the bases of both lungs.

On January 7th, the second day from the operation, and the third day of the disease, the breathing was very tranquil, but occasionally hurried. There was no lividity of the surface. The boy had some colour in his cheeks, he looked calm. The pulse was 132, soft, not particularly weak.

---

[1] The tube used was a common double silver canula, as large as the trachea would receive. The canula, with an aperture on its dorsal surface, seems to me, however, better than that here used.

On January 8th the pulse was 132. The respirations were 38; there was no lividity, the lips were of good colour.

Mr. Hill placed his finger on the tube, then in a second or two withdrew it; the child necessarily took a deep inspiration. Seizing the moment when the chest was distended by air, Mr. Hill again placed his finger on the tube, waited until effort to cough was made, and then suddenly withdrew the finger; by this manœuvre he succeeded in making the boy expectorate much muco-purulent fluid.

The wound was freely cauterised with nitrate of silver.

On January 9th, the fourth day from the operation, the child's general condition had greatly improved; he sat up in his bed and played with his toys. The nurse reported that he had slept well at night. The bowels had acted once during the last twenty-four hours, as they had daily from the outset of the disease. The urine had been 'tested daily, but *on this day, for the first time, it was found to contain albumen. The albumen was always to be detected in the urine from this date till the child's death.*

Some muco-purulent fluid was coughed past the tube through the larynx into the mouth. The child ate a little dry sponge-cake. Mr. Hill took out the tube in the evening and closed the aperture in the trachea with his finger, to test the child's ability to breathe through the natural passages. The child struggled so much for breath that the finger was soon removed; a good deal of dirty-looking, fœtid, muco-purulent matter escaped from the trachea through the wound. The tube was reintroduced.

On January 11th, *i.e.* the seventh day of disease, the child's general condition was very good; the pulse 136, the respirations 42. It ate and slept well, and displayed more irritability of temper than it had previously done. The wound, however, looked in a bad state, its edges being sloughy and offensive. Mr. Athol Johnson, who saw the patient with me, advised that the wound should be washed with a solution of chlorinate of soda.

On January 12th, *i.e.* seventh day after the operation, the child at the time of my visit in the afternoon was sleeping so tranquilly that its respirations were inaudible, the frequency was only to be determined by the hand placed on the abdomen. The respirations were 40, the pulse 136. The skin was soft and normally cool. The wound was looking more healthy, but the opening into the trachea was wide and ragged-looking. In the evening the child sat up in bed and played lustily with a drum.

In the course of the evening Mr. Hill removed the tube for a few minutes; a violent fit of coughing was the result, during which some mucus was ejected through the opening in the trachea, but it hung around the wound, so that it was drawn into the trachea again at the succeeding inspiration. When the tube was in the trachea the mucus was expelled from the tube, and so removed from the influence of the next inspiration. As the child became livid and the pulse very feeble from the obstruction to the ingress of air offered by the mucus drawn into the trachea, the tube was replaced.

On January 13th, the pulse was 138 and rather irregular in force and frequency. The child breathed calmly, and was cheerful. Its skin was cool, its appetite excellent.

Every day, however, that anæmic pasty look so often seen in diphtheria had increased.

From the day of the operation the child had not been allowed to drink, but all his food had been soaked in milk, wine and water, or beef-tea. The importance of giving all fluids in the form of sop is to be impressed on the nurse, because two or three days after the operation the glottis has been observed to lose some of its irritability, and fluids have passed into the larynx and even caused the death of the patient. A friend of mine told me that he lost a very promising case, apparently from this accident, on the fourth day after the operation.

The boy having declined the tincture of the sesquichloride of iron on the second day, it was omitted, and a few grains of the ammonio-citrate of iron were given in its place.

From the 13th to the 17th January the pulse rose daily in frequency. On the 16th it was 160 in the minute. All this time, however, the child continued cheerful.

On the 18th January, i.e. the fourteenth day of illness, the child took its breakfast as usual; at noon it was evidently sinking; its pulse was 176, its respiration 76, and there was great recession of the chest walls during respiration.

At five P.M. the pulse was too rapid and feeble to be counted, and the respirations were 86 in the minute. At nine P.M. the child died.

The child had never been removed from the bed for the purpose of examining its chest from the time of the operation. Much injury might have resulted to the child from the exposure and exertion, while no good end could have been attained by the knowledge that a little mucous or sub-mucous râle, or a little fine crepitation, existed here or there.

After death, the wound showed no signs of attempt at repair. It was sloughy-looking, and at places on it was some granular lymph. The lungs were acutely but highly emphysematous, so that they met in the middle line and almost covered the heart. The most depending part of the inferior lobe of the left lung was collapsed. The collapse affected about one-third of the lobe. The bronchial tubes leading to the inferior lobe contained a large quantity of very thick air-less purulent fluid. The smallest tubes running through the collapsed tissue were filled with fluid of the same character. The collapsed portion broke down too easily on pressure, and was less flabby than is merely collapsed lung-tissue; it was evidently the seat of incipient secondary pneumonia. On cutting across the emphysematous parts of the lung, i.e. all the lung not collapsed, a good deal of aërated muco-purulent fluid escaped. The inferior lobe of the right lung was scarcely if at all collapsed. The posterior third of the superior lobe was solid, chiefly from pneumonia. Here and there, around and mingled with the lobules, solid from pneumonia, were little portions of collapsed lung-tissue; and the small bronchial tubes running through the collapsed and solid-from-pneumonia lobules were filled with thick airless purulent fluid. The lymphatic glands behind the angles of the jaw, down the neck, beside the larynx, and at the bifurcation of the trachea, were large, red, moist, and brittle.

The uvula and the *velum pendulum palati* were thickened. On the posterior surface of the velum was a patch of tough lymph about the size of a sixpence, and from this a layer of tough lymph extended upwards, even into the posterior nares. The coats of the pharynx itself were thickened and somewhat contracted. The epiglottis seemed healthy, except that its under surface was covered with thick mucus. The arytæno-epiglottidean folds were scarcely thicker than natural. Below the root of the epiglottis, the mucous membrane, as low as the bifurcation of the trachea, was covered with a continuous layer of tough lymph. On removing this, the mucous membrane beneath was found to be intensely red. The opening from the trachea into the larynx was completely blocked up by lymph.

The wound internally looked healthy. Over the ring of the trachea next below the opening, the mucous membrane to a small extent was abraded or superficially ulcerated. The kidneys and other abdominal viscera contained an excess of blood, but seemed otherwise healthy.[1]

You will note in the account I have given you of this case, as especially worthy of remembrance in regard to the operation for tracheotomy—

1. That the operation was performed as soon as it was evident that the laryngeal disease was progressing, and was seriously interfering with the entrance of the air into the thorax; the excess in the falling in of the chest walls over that of health during the child's ordinary inspirations being regarded as the measure of the impediment to the passage of the air through the larynx.

2. That the opening into the trachea was made near to the larynx. It was so, first, in order that there might be as little chance as possible of the inflammation extending to the cellular tissue of the anterior mediastinum; secondly, in order that the air might have as long a passage as possible to pass through before reaching the lungs; and thirdly, and especially, in order not to excite inflammation lower down the trachea than already existed when the operation was performed.

3. That no fears respecting the evil consequences of opening the diseased part of the trachea exercised any influence in determining the spot for the operation.

4. That the tracheal tube was of good size.

5. That the edges of the wound were freely cauterised after the operation.

---

[1] They were examined with the aid of the microscope.

6. That the air the child breathed was kept as nearly as possible at 70° Fahr., and was moist. These conditions were secured by the arrangements of the bed I have described to you, and by covering the openings of the tube by a neck-comforter.

7. That measures were taken from time to time to excite deep cough, and so to favour expectoration of the morbid matter drawn into the bronchial tubes from the trachea, and formed in the bronchial tubes from the irritation of that matter, etc.

8. That the child was well supported by food and stimulants from the first,—fluids being always supplied by soaking sponge-cake, bread, etc., in them; baked apples and grapes were given freely.

At the time of the operation two facts were in favour of the child's recovery, viz., it being more than two years old, and its ribs being firmer than is usual at its age. But then, on the other hand, the child was weakened by the attack of measles and bronchitis, from which it had scarcely recovered when it began to suffer from the diphtheria; it was still at an age when capillary bronchitis, collapse, and pneumonia, secondary to collapse, are very common; and the diphtheria, the general disease, had yet to run its course.

The death of the child was the consequence of the general disease, hastened probably a little by the state of the lungs.

The operation was successful so far as concerns the attainment of the object for which it was performed. The child would have died on the 5th of January had the trachea not been opened; it lived till the 18th. Slow suffocation is one of the most distressing modes of death; death from asthenia one of the least. So that twelve days of life were gained and much suffering was avoided by the operation.[1] You will

---

[1] If tracheotomy did no more than substitute the easy death from collapse and pneumonia, or from asthenia, for the painful death from obstruction in the larynx, it would in many cases be a justifiable operation. Trousseau has drawn, with a master's hand, so faithful and graphic a picture of the terrible suffering in death from slow suffocation, in acute laryngeal inflammation, that I cannot refrain from quoting his words and his description at length :—

'Cependant les accès se rapprochent en devenant de plus en plus violents; et jusqu'au moment de l'agonie il n'y a bientôt plus entre eux d'intervalles de

reinember that I told you, that the laryngeal affection all but
always kills within a week from its outset, and usually within
three days, and that the general disease more commonly
causes death during the second week.

The sequence of events in this case, and the relation and
importance of those events, seem to me to have been as
follows :—

Diphtheria late in the night of January 4th; the exudative
inflammation affecting the larynx and pharynx. Exudation
of lymph into the larynx early on the 5th. Death by suffocation averted on the night of the 5th by opening the trachea.

Continuance of the diphtheria. Extension of the exudation downwards to the bifurcation of the trachea; and
upwards to the posterior surface of the *velum pendulum
palati*, and thence forward to the anterior nares.

Diphtheritic inflammation of the wound. Expectoration
through the opening in the trachea, facilitated by the firm
state of the ribs and the management of the tube, and thus
death by collapse averted.

The progress of the general disease shown during life by
the occurrence, for the first time, of albumen in the urine on
the fourth day of disease, and the continuous and gradual
rise in the frequency of the pulse, and, after death, by the
exudation on the pharyngeal and nasal mucous membranes.

The little collapse and the small amount of pneumonia
probably supervened during the last day of life, the patient

tranquillité; le sifflement laryngo-trachéal est continu. De temps en temps,
les pauvres enfants, dans un état d'agitation impossible à décrire, se dres-
sent brusquement sur leur séant, saisissant les rideaux de leur lit qu'ils dé-
chirent dans leurs mouvements de rage convulsive; quelquefois ils écorchent
avec leurs ongles les papiers tendus sur les murs; ils se précipitent au cou de
leur mère et des personnes qui les entourent, les embrassant, et cherchant à
s'accrocher sur ce qui se trouve à leur portée pour y prendre un point d'appui.
Dans un autre moment, c'est contre eux qu'ils tournent leurs efforts impuis-
sants, portant violemment leurs mains à la partie antérieure de leur cou comme
pour en arracher quelque chose qui les étouffe. La face bouffie, violacée, les
yeux hagards et brillants, expriment l'anxiété la plus pénible et une profonde
terreur; puis l'enfant tombe accablé dans une espèce de stupeur durant
laquelle la respiration reste difficile et sifflante. La face, les lèvres sont alors
pâles, les yeux abattus. Enfin, après un effort suprême de respiration,
l'agonie commence, et la lutte se termine sans qu'il y ait eu, à partir de ce
moment, autant d'accès de suffocation qu'auraient dû le faire prévoir ceux
qui ont eu lieu jusque-là. Chez l'adulte, le tableau est plus effrayant encore.

no longer expectorating the irritating matter drawn into the bronchi from the trachea.[1]

Death from asthenia at the end of the second week of the disease.

With regard to the remedies that have been praised as specifics in diphtheria, or as all but meriting that high name, I have seen nothing like unequivocal specific good from any of those of which I have had experience. I have either given myself, or seen given by others, the tincture of the sesqui-chloride of iron, in doses of twenty drops every two or three hours; sesquicarbonate of ammonia, in doses of four or five grains every two or three hours; bark in various forms, with and without ammonia; and calomel; but by none of these have I seen any specific influence exerted. From all, some benefit has accrued, when their exhibition was specially indicated,—just the kind of good we see from them when judiciously administered in other diseases.

As the septicæmia results from the absorption of fœtid matters from the throat, local applications are indicated—solid nitrate of silver should be applied freely to the fœtid surface, as soon as the glands behind the angles of the jaw begin to increase quickly in size, and to become tender, and gargles or washes of chloride of soda, or of Condy's fluid, used; by cauterising the surface from which the infection is proceeding, and by the use of these antiseptics we may prevent that which, when fully established, we are impotent to cure.

La violence des accès de suffocation, l'espèce de rage qui s'empare du malheureux mourant, étranglé par cet obstacle dont il ne peut se débarrasser, sont impossibles à dépeindre. À la fin, lorsque les lèvres sont devenues livides, lorsque le visage est bouffi, violacé : au dernier terme de l'asphyxie, l'adulte tombe, comme l'enfant, dans cette sorte de stupeur et d'enivrement, et meurt ordinairement dans un état de prostration.'—*Clinique Médicale,* 1861, p. 322.

Those only who have witnessed the sufferings so described, and the instant relief from them that follows on the opening of the windpipe, can appreciate fully the palliative value of tracheotomy.

[1] It will be gathered from the account I have given of this case that I cannot agree with Trousseau in the following statement :—

'It seems as if the disease, having reached the air-passages, exhausted there all its force, and *if by giving passage to the air into the respiratory apparatus by tracheotomy we prevent the patient dying, the cure will occur naturally.'—Clinique Médicale,* 1861, p. 424.

With reference to the treatment of the nervous disorders which follow diphtheria, as all the symptoms of those disorders indicate loss of power, and are accompanied by pallor and other anæmic symptoms, nourishing animal and stimulating diet, fresh air and exercise, and steel and quinine, seem especially to be indicated. Where the paralysis has been limited to the pharyngeal muscles, to tingling in some parts, to affections of the special senses, or to slight want of power in the extremities, those measures have proved successful; but when the paralysis has been widely spread or extended to the heart, the cases have ended fatally, notwithstanding the employment of the remedies I have mentioned. In any case of the kind I again see, I shall certainly give strychnine, in small doses, a fair trial, in addition to general tonic remedies. Perhaps stimulation by blisters over the upper part of the spine might be of use.

In the treatment of the diphtheritic throat affection I have seen blisters applied, and it has seemed to me that their effects were injurious.

The vomiting is best allayed by iced stimulants internally, and mustard poultices to the epigastrium. Vomiting often continues notwithstanding all our remedies, and by exhausting the patient hastens the fatal termination. Restlessness and delirium are to be treated by opiates. The doses of these remedies must of course vary with the ages of the patients.

To conclude, the great facts I desire to impress on your minds are—

1st. That diphtheria is a general disease, having exudative inflammation of the pharyngeal mucous membrane for its anatomical character.

2nd. That it attacks persons of all ages, from early infancy to old age; but is most common and most fatal in childhood.

3rd. That it is contagious, but requires for its propagation either complete exposure to the contagious principle, or predisposition on the part of those receiving it, and that the latter is probably by far the more important of the two conditions of development.[1]

[1] There is not the shadow of ground for the belief that the disease can be carried by the clothes, etc., from one house to another.

4th. That the general disease varies in its character from sthenic febrile to typhoid febrile, but always has a tendency to assume an asthenic type.

5th. That the local nasal, pharyngeal, and laryngeal disease is inflammatory in nature, the inflammation varying in character from sthenic to asthenic, but always showing a tendency to become asthenic.

6th. That, as we have as yet discovered no specific remedy for the general disease, we must treat it in accordance with general principles, bearing in mind its tendency to assume an asthenic character.

7th. That *all* we are to expect from the topical employment of active agents, such as nitrate of silver, is the arrest of the exudative process before it has extended to the larynx, and the prevention of the absorption of fœtid matters.[1]

8th. That in opening the windpipe, the sole object we have in view is the prevention of death by suffocation; that by so averting death, time is gained for the general disease—the diphtheria—to run its course.

9th. That the muco-purulent fluid in the smaller bronchial tubes, which by its presence in them necessitates pulmonary collapse, is partly drawn into them from above and partly secreted in them; the secretion being due chiefly to the irritation of their mucous membrane by the morbid matter drawn into them from the trachea, etc.

10th. That death so often follows tracheotomy for

---

[1] Trousseau thinks that the general disease is curable, or at least that it is capable of being arrested by remedies applied to the throat.

'There is, however,' he says, 'an essential difference between diphtheria and the diseases I have just named (*i.e.* small-pox, measles, syphilis), viz., that greater account is to be taken of the local affection in diphtheria than in those diseases. If in small-pox, for example, we do not occupy ourselves with the pustules, if we occupy ourselves with them, at least, only for diagnosis and prognosis, if we do not occupy ourselves with them in regard to treatment, it is not so in diphtheria. We may compare, indeed, what happens here with what happens in malignant pustule, where, in attacking directly the local affection, we check (*enrayons*) *the progress of the general disease* of which that affection was a first manifestation. *So in diphtheria, by interposing energetically to combat the first manifestation, we may sometimes arrest the progress, prevent the ulterior manifestation.*'—*Clinique Médicale,* 1861, p. 363.

The doctrine taught in the text, founded on my own experience, is quite opposed to these views.

diphtheritic inflammation of the larynx and trachea, because
of the mechanical facility which exists for inspiring the morbid
secretions of the larynx, trachea, and larger bronchial tubes
into the smaller bronchial tubes and air-cells, and of the
mechanical difficulty of expectorating matters from the
smaller bronchi when there is an opening in the windpipe, or
when the chest walls are very flexible.

11. That death from the laryngeal complication occurs,
with very rare exceptions, during the first week of disease;
that death from asthenia more commonly occurs during the
second week of disease, and that the youth of the patient is
a predisposing cause of the laryngeal affection.

12. That in exceptional cases (as in the lad M.) diphtheria
proves fatal in a few hours from the severity of the general
disease, just as happens now and then in scarlet fever.

13. That disordered innervation is an occasional consequence of diphtheria; that the parts of which the innervation
is most commonly disordered are some of those to which the
par vagum is distributed, viz., the pharynx, the stomach, and
the heart; that the disorder may affect all or some of the
motor and sensitive nerves, or the motor or the sensitive
nerves of the trunk or of the extremities, as well as the
nerves of special sense.

14. That these disorders of the nervous system are to be
treated on general principles, and that as anæmia (sometimes
even a high degree of it) is a common concomitant, restora-
tives, including steel, are indicated.[1]

15. That an extreme fall in the frequency of the heart's
beats during the disease, or as a result of one of the nervous
derangements succeeding it, is a fatal sign; and that decidedly diminished power in the inspiratory muscles is
probably of equal significance.

16. That delirium, frequent and uncontrollable vomiting,
considerable hæmorrhage from the nose or other parts, a very
rapid and feeble pulse, and albumen in the urine, are most
unfavourable symptoms.

[1] I have not had an opportunity of examining, after death, a case in which
disordered innervation was a prominent symptom; but, judging from the
character of the symptoms, I should not expect to find any appreciable
change in the structure of the brain, spinal cord, or nerves. In the few cases
that have been examined by others, no change has been detected.

ON CROUP AND THE DISEASES THAT RESEMBLE IT: A CLINICAL LECTURE,

1875.

CROUP, AND THE DISEASES THAT RESEMBLE IT.

GENTLEMEN,—There are no cases more trying to the young practitioner than those the chief symptoms of which are due to impediment to the passage of air through the larynx. There is no time to think over such a case; the patient needs to be relieved at once. The friends are alarmed, and properly so; for death is, in every such case, imminent. The degree of danger, the probability of a fatal termination, varies, however, with the nature of the cause of the impediment.

The acute diseases which I have seen thus impeding the passage of air through the larynx I may enumerate as follows:—Œdema of the arytæno-epiglottidean folds; rapidly developed inflammation, terminating in suppuration, of a cyst in the immediate vicinity, or in the substance, of one arytæno-epiglottidean fold; suppurative inflammation of the cellular tissue external to the larynx, compressing the larynx; catarrhal inflammation of the larynx; membranous inflammation of the larynx; paralysis of the larynx; spasm of the larynx.

You will at once see that the relief possible to be afforded in these cases varies considerably, and that the mode of giving the relief must also vary. To confound, as I have seen confounded, a collection of matter external to the larynx with membranous inflammation of the larynx itself, is to cause, if I may say so, the death of the patient; for the means which it would be proper to use in membranous inflammation of the larynx would, I need not say, be impotent as a remedy for the difficulty of breathing due to a deep-seated collection of matter in the cellular tissue. Hence I am about to-day to describe the means of distinguishing from each other these various forms of difficulty of breathing, and at the same time

¹ Published in *The Lancet*, January 2, 1875.

to point out to you the mode of affording relief to the patient in the several special affections.

I think we shall best clear the way, so to speak, by considering first the two diseases which, in the above enumeration, I have placed last—spasm and paralysis of the larynx.

'Laryngismus stridulus,' 'spasmodic' or 'false croup,' is limited to infants, especially affecting children during the period of dentition. It is supposed by many to be a reflex action, the source of irritation being the teeth. This idea is favoured by the fact that the majority of children who suffer from laryngismus stridulus have, for their age, too few teeth. We shall see presently, however, that it is doubtful whether the relation between the two conditions is one of direct causation.

The symptoms of laryngismus stridulus are so marked that, once aware of the existence of such a disease, you can hardly confound it with any other. He who had never seen a case before would know it at once if he were acquainted with its symptoms. It needs no experience to make the diagnosis.

You will see a great many children who, from the description of their attacks by their nurses, you know to be the subjects of laryngismus stridulus, before you see the child in the attack itself, and for the reason that the attack rarely lasts more than a few seconds. It is often brought on by trifling causes, and the nurse may be able to tell you what will bring it on. So, if disposed to witness the symptoms of laryngismus stridulus, you may be tempted to induce an attack. But remember that a child not very unfrequently dies in an attack; and I myself, twice, in my comparatively inexperienced days, nearly killed a child by bringing on an attack—once that I might myself witness the attack, and once, years after, that I might show it to my class.

I will describe to you, briefly, the characters of a severe attack of laryngismus stridulus. The child is seized suddenly with an inability to inspire. It seems as if about to die from inability to get the breath through the larynx. At this time there is no noisy breathing, no 'croupy' sound. The larynx seems absolutely closed. The face and lips are slightly livid.

but pale, often very pale. There is no movement of respiration, and the child, as in one of the cases to which I have just referred, that in which I was displaying the case to my class, may seem dead. I thought it was dead; the mother thought it was dead, and flew from the room, leaving the child in my arms. The students around thought, of course, with the mother and myself. Then comes a crowing inspiration. The larynx is evidently partly open, and entering air produces a crowing sound. The child gets its breath, its colour returns, and in a few minutes it is as well as it was before. In the case to which I have alluded, when the mother returned in a few minutes with her husband to take the child away, it was sitting up and laughing at one of the students. When this occurred I had never seen a fatal case, and did not know the dangerous nature of the trial, for, instead of getting its breath, the child may die—may die in an instant. The rapidity with which death occurs is remarkable. Not long since I saw a child who had had many attacks, but was supposed to be having them much less severely. I saw the child in its room, well, as I was assured, and as it seemed, so far as its breathing was concerned. It had had fewer and less severe attacks than it had been in the habit of having. But I had not reached the door when the child was dead.

The attacks are not at first so severe as that which I have described to you. Usually the mother or the nurse notices a little crowing inspiration, perhaps on first waking, perhaps only when the child is danced, when something startles it. In the intervals the child is, as regards its breathing, and maybe in the opinion of the friends, in tolerable health. It is said perhaps to be quite well in the intervals of the attacks. We shall see presently that it is not well.

When the attacks are severe the friends will often bring the child to you, saying that it has 'fits.' So beware, when you hear that a child has had many fits, that you inquire a little into the case before you conclude that such fits are ordinary convulsions. The crowing inspiration, so peculiar and characteristic, will always enable you to separate this laryngeal affection from convulsions commonly so called. At the same time, remember that it is not uncommon to have

contractions of the thumbs and great toes, and not very rare
to have contractions of all the fingers, of the wrists and the
ankles, so that the hand may be flexed and rigid, and the
soles of the feet turned inwards, and the feet extended,
between the attacks, and sometimes the child has attacks of
general convulsions.

This affection of the larynx, this spasm which closes the
larynx, and so interferes with the entrance of air into the
chest, never lasts long enough to produce extreme lividity.
The appearance of a child is rather that of fainting, with
slight blueness as well as pallor. The child either dies, or,
the spasm relaxing, air enters, and it recovers. There is no
period of imperfect aëration of blood, i.e. of lividity, but
sudden and absolute closure of the passage through the
larynx.

This spasm of the larynx is said to be due, in some cases,
to cerebral congestion. Formerly it was supposed that the
great bulk of such cases depended on this, and I remember
that when I was a young practitioner the first question one
asked oneself concerning such a case was, Is it dependent on
cerebral congestion? As the great bulk of the cases were
held to be due to that cause, leeching was common, and I,
unfortunately, was the unhappy cause of the death of a child
by leeching. The leech divided imperfectly a twig of the
temporal artery, and the loss of blood killed the child.

Now, I may say that for the last twenty-five years I have
not seen a single case of laryngismus stridulus depending on
cerebral congestion, and therefore I have strong misgivings
whether I ever did see one. There is no doubt that laryngismus stridulus is occasionally conjoined with hydrocephalus,
but whether in such cases the laryngismus is due to the
hydrocephalus is in my mind a matter of very grave doubt.
I am inclined, and very decidedly inclined, to the opinion that
the two are due to a common cause, to the constitutional
state to which I am about to refer, as that which is all but
invariably present in laryngismus stridulus—namely rickets.
Laryngismus stridulus is exceedingly common in rickety
children, and, where the larynx is in other particulars healthy,
is almost limited to rickety children. Now you will understand why it is that these children, the subjects of laryngismus

stridulus, are so often supposed to be the subjects of difficult dentition; for you know, I trust, that rickety children are very late in cutting their teeth, and that the retarded dentition is not the result in these cases of any difficulty in the passage of the tooth through the gum, but is due to a want of developmental power. So, in these cases, the large head so often present is due, remember, to that peculiar condition of the white matter of the brain, especially of the anterior lobes, which is common in rickets. And, again, the wide fontanelle is the result, not of the accumulation of fluid within the cranial cavity, not to excess of blood there, but to defective bone growth, and is part of the local manifestation of the rickety cachexia.

All this will lead you, I think, to the conclusion that laryngismus stridulus occurs in those of weakly constitution, as it is termed. You know how sensitive the nervous system of the child is, how easily convulsive affections are induced in children. Even in the healthy child the nervous system is, as some one has expressed it, ' always at full-cock, ready to go off like a hair-trigger.' You know, moreover, that whatever weakens any one renders their nervous system more irritable, more sensitive, and such a person is liable to be thrown into a convulsion by trifling causes. I mean by ' trifling causes ' that the exciting cause need be but trifling. In all intermitting convulsive affections—epilepsy, hysteria, for example—we have the two conditions to consider: the general state of the nervous system and the excitant of the attack. Here, in laryngismus stridulus, the excitant may be the stomach, bowels, teeth—in fact, at any part of the system. In treating such a case we look for the excitant; but this is often out of our immediate reach—sometimes, often, not to be found. We have seen how trifling it may be—a draught of cold air, a start, may suffice. When we know it we cannot in the majority of instances guard the patient from the direct excitant; but we may in almost all instances render the child's system so strong—remove, that is, the extreme excitability of the nervous system—as to render the child insusceptible to the attacks.

In treating laryngismus stridulus, therefore, you must endeavour so to strengthen the child that its nervous system may be less sensitive. We do this first by attention to the child's diet. In a large number of cases the child is being underfed, or fed with food unsuited to its years—rather, perhaps, one should say, unsuited to its stage of development. As I have told you, these rickety children are developed below their years.

We endeavour to strengthen the child's constitution, also, by careful general management. Many of these children are kept in the house. They are said to be subject to attacks of croup, and they are kept in-doors that they may not catch cold. You must insist upon their getting fresh air. You must attend likewise to the various other points proper for the treatment of rickets and the constitutional cachexia from which the child is suffering, by the administration of iron, cod-liver oil, and generally of that class of remedies. Cod-liver oil is, as you know, considered by some to be a specific in the treatment of rickets. Attention must be given especially to the state of the bowels. But remember that you will do harm by attempting to correct disordered secretion by courses of alterative treatment. The mildest aperients occasionally are all that is required—a little rhubarb or rhubarb-and-soda. I cannot tell you the horror with which I regard the excessive use of grey powder in these cases.

Lastly, the bromides of potassium and ammonium have a special effect in rendering the nervous system less sensitive to reflex irritation, and are of great service in preventing the attacks of laryngismus stridulus till such time as the constitution is strengthened by other means. Bromide, according to my experience, should be given in rather large doses at infrequent intervals. Full doses night and morning are, I think, better than small doses frequently repeated during the day.

I have referred to paralysis of the larynx. There are persons who maintain that laryngismus stridulus itself is a paralysis of the larynx; but the disease to which I refer is certainly a very different affection from laryngismus stridulus. There is constant noisy inspiration—crowing, but rather hoarser than the crow of laryngismus stridulus. There is little evidence of impediment to the entrance of air—I mean, as manifested by the recession of the soft parts. Although it may begin pretty acutely, the disease is a chronic one, and is quickly separated from any of the other diseases of the class to which I am now directing your attention. So far as my experience goes, it is a rare affection. I have seen a few cases. The best marked terminated in extensive cerebral softening, and was, I think, connected with the syphilitic cachexia.

Laryngismus stridulus, this pure spasm of the larynx (if the child dies no trace of laryngeal affection remains), is almost limited to the rickety, and is quite limited to the young child, the infant. But it is not uncommon, nay, I should say it is very common, to have a certain amount of spasm, often a considerable amount, superadded to a catarrhal affection of the larynx in children of a more advanced age, during the first dentition, and occasionally in older children of from five to eight, nine or ten, years of age. This disease is not unfrequently confounded with true croup, and the diagnosis is often very difficult in a first attack, for some time at least; nay, I think I may say that it is almost impossible to be sure at the outset of the affection that you have not to deal with a case of true croup. I say 'in a first attack,' for children who have had one such attack are very liable to a recurrence of the disease, and these are the children who are said to have had 'several attacks of croup.' I say 'these are the children who are said to have had several attacks of croup,' because no child ever has several attacks of true croup, and certainly would not have recovered from several attacks,—true croup being, as we shall see, one of the most fatal diseases of childhood.

This disease, catarrhal laryngitis, accompanied with spasm, begins with a little febrile disturbance and a little hoarseness, perhaps a little cough. The child is supposed to have caught cold. It goes to bed, and, in an hour or two, wakes up with considerable difficulty of breathing. The breathing is not only difficult but noisy, and the child, if it be of any age, is commonly alarmed. You find it more or less feverish, usually sitting up in bed, and with the tracheal breathing. On listening to the chest it is not uncommon to hear a little sonorous rhonchus. It is at this stage of the affection that the diagnosis is difficult—as I say, in many cases impossible. But bear this in mind, that experience

shows that the great bulk at least of cases of so-called croup
are really cases of diphtheria, and that diphtheria commencing in the larynx—*i.e.* the exudation commencing in the
larynx—is exceedingly rare.   Usually, as we shall see
presently, it commences in the pharynx and spreads downwards to the larynx; and although the pharyngeal symptoms may have been most trifling, you will usually find, on
examining the pharynx, unequivocal evidences of the
diphtheritic nature of the disease.   So, if you were called to
such a case as I have just described to you, you would at
once examine the pharynx.

These cases of catarrhal laryngitis with spasm are the
attacks that are so quickly cured by an emetic.   An emetic
acts in such a case, it seems to me, in three ways.   In the
first place, it empties the stomach completely, and in doing
so it removes one source, a common source in the child, of
reflex action; secondly, by the nausea and slight faintness it
produces, it relaxes the spasm; and, thirdly, it promotes free
secretion from the laryngeal and bronchial mucous membrane, and so relieves the catarrhal affection.   The best
emetic is ipecacuanha.   Usually the action of the emetic
is sufficient to make the diagnosis clear.   The patient is at
once relieved, falls asleep, breathes quietly, showing how
large a share spasm played in the affection.   In the morning
the child awakes free from febrile disturbance, and only a
little hoarseness remains to tell the nature of the case.   Persons who have a child subject to this affection have commonly learned the value of emetics, and I have known those
who in travelling always took with them an emetic lest the
child should have an attack of 'croup.'   After the emetic
has acted it is well to clear out the bowels by a brisk purgative, as, for example, a dose of calomel and jalap.   Without
treatment the disease will subside, but then it will last much
longer.   I have seen a case, left to itself, go on, with spasm
varying in degree, for two or three days.

The affection, then, consists in a catarrhal inflammation
of the larynx, with spasm superadded.   It is a local affection,
and when frequently repeated occasionally leaves behind it a
disagreeable hoarseness.   The child's voice is a little changed.
It is probable, certain in some cases, that a little thickening

of the mucous membrane remains from the repeated attacks of catarrhal inflammation.

Children subject to this affection do require considerable care. They are susceptible to cold, and especially to damp cold. A single exposure is often sufficient to induce an attack. So you must urge upon the friends the greatest care to avoid the exciting cause. The strongest children may suffer from it. It is in no way connected with the rickety or other cachexia.

Membranous inflammation of the larynx—inflammation, that is, attended by the presence of lymph on the surface of the mucous membrane of the larynx—is croup. This is a peculiar form of inflammation, as the presence of the lymph proves. If we produce inflammation of a mucous membrane by a direct irritant, we have, as the result, the formation of excess of mucus, or of pus, or of both conjoined; we do not have lymph exuded. If we irritate directly a serous membrane, we may have excess of serum, or we may have pus or lymph produced. There must therefore be some peculiarity in the special inflammation of a mucous membrane which leads to the formation on it of a substance not formed when the inflammation is excited simply by a mechanical irritant. The inflammation is a so-called specific inflammation.

It was once supposed that membranous inflammation of the larynx was peculiar to children. It is now known that it is not so. It occurs, not so very unfrequently, in persons of advanced life. Diphtheria is an acute specific disease attended by inflammation of the pharynx, having as its result exudation of lymph. It is a specific inflammation arising from a specific cause. The specific inflammation in diphtheria has a tendency to spread, to spread over the pharynx in al directions, to pass upwards to the nares, downwards to the larynx, and, in rare cases, to the œsophagus and stomach. From the pharynx it may spread down the trachea and into the bronchi. So that in diphtheria we get, not unfrequently, membranous inflammation of the larynx. But membranous inflammation of the larynx, I have told you, is croup. Is there then a membranous inflammation of the larynx distinct from the acute specific disease diphtheria? Are there a true croup and a diphtheritic croup? Certainly, if you were to place in the hands of the best pathologist the larynx of a child who had died from membranous inflammation of the larynx, the so-called idiopathic croup, and that of one who had died from a true diphtheric inflammation of the larynx, he would be unable to distinguish the one from the other. There is no anatomical character by which he could say, ' This is true croup ; this is diphtheritic inflammation of the larynx.' If, however, the pharynx was also found to be the seat of exudation of lymph he would say, ' This is undoubtedly diphtheritic inflammation of the larynx.' But it is beyond question that true diphtheritic inflammation may be limited to the larynx ; that, in exceptional cases, the pharynx escapes the exudation. Seeing, then, that there are no anatomical characters to distinguish the one disease from the other, are there any clinical characters by which the two affections may be separated ? It has been supposed that the presence of albumen in the urine would be sufficient, and I formerly laid much weight on this distinction. But later years have satisfied me that in cases which present all the characters of true croup, which are sporadic, spread to no other person in the house, come on apparently from exposure to cold and damp,—that in such cases albumen may be present in the urine. It has again been urged that true croup has no tendency to spread ; but this manifestly should no more separate a single case from the diphtheritic croup than should a single case of scarlet fever, because it did not spread, be separated from other cases of scarlet fever. The cause, again—the fact that some cases of croup come on after distinct exposure to cold and wet—cannot be sufficient to separate croup from diphtheritic croup, for it is beyond question that a considerable number of cases of diphtheria do, to all appearance at least, date their origin from exposure to cold and wet. I have seen several solitary cases of true diphtheria thus originating ; not spreading, or spreading, to other persons in the house, as the case may be. So my opinion has undergone some modification, and I am inclined now to the belief that there is no such disease as idiopathic, simple, membranous inflammation of the larynx. I say, I am inclined to this belief. I am not sure that it is true ; but as I formerly thought that the weight of evidence was in favour of their non-identity, I am now inclined, from my further experience, to think that the two diseases are really identical, that the so-called croup is really diphtheria.

Membranous inflammation of the larynx is one of the gravest diseases; it kills rapidly. If the termination be fatal it usually is so within a few days from the outset; rarely does the disease last a week, supposing that the windpipe has not been opened. The disease is usually preceded by uneasiness in the pharynx, sometimes by well-marked evidences of diphtheria; often, however, the pharyngeal symptoms are trifling, and the gravity of the illness is only appreciated when the child wakes in the night with croupy breathing—that is, with rough, hoarse, loud, lengthened inspiration. The difficulty of inspiration is due to two causes. At first it is due to the swollen condition of the mucous membrane, and also largely to the superadded spasm. Subsequently it is due to the false membrane narrowing the passage, and also largely to the superadded spasm. The paroxysms of difficulty of inspiration from which the patient suffers are due to the spasm. The disease is attended by a certain amount of febrile disturbance, and there is a little uneasiness in the larynx, perhaps some pain and tenderness. The lymphatic glands adjacent to the larynx are commonly enlarged and tender. (They require to be felt for.) There is hoarse, rough cough, with expectoration of at first a little glairy mucus, and subsequently pieces of false membrane, —that is, of tough lymph.

The seat and character of the disease are manifested by the severity of the symptoms and their continuousness. That it is diphtheritic in origin is *proved* if one can find any trace of false membrane in the pharynx. Sometimes the pharyngeal membrane is greatly swollen, red, puffy-looking, and a tough mucus is spread pretty evenly over the surface. In other cases, whilst the pharynx exhibits no unequivocal false membrane, there is a discharge from the nose of serous acrid fluid, and on inspecting the nares you may see false membrane on the inflamed surface. But, believing as I do now that all croup is but a local manifestation of the general disease diphtheria, it would matter but little, as regards the diagnosis, whether the pharynx were the seat of membranous inflammation or not.

The child usually gets a little sleep towards the first morning, and seems rather better during the day, i.e. its breathing is less distressing. Its voice, however, never ceases to be hoarse, the cough never loses its clang, the impediment to the entrance of air never disappears. The recession of the soft parts of the chest walls never ceases to occur at each inspiration. It is only a question of more or less. As night comes on the patient is usually again worse, and although there may be again a little remission the following morning, there is, on the whole, a steady advance. When death occurs, it does so from one of several causes. It may be that the patient dies in a paroxysm of difficulty of the entrance of the air. There has been a certain amount of lividity, considerable recession of soft parts, and then, either during a paroxysm or in the interval between the paroxysms, death occurs in an instant. In some of these cases the final occlusion of the larynx is the result of spasm. In other cases, a portion of false membrane partially detached blocks the way, and the patient may also die in an instant. The portion of false membrane does not permit, or only partially prevents, the escape of the air, but forbids its entrance ; it acts as a valve. Again, the patient may die from the extension downwards to the bronchi of the inflammation, the narrowing of the bronchi, the extension perhaps of the false membrane even into the capillary tubes. Again, the patient may die from pneumonia, lobular or lobar, the pneumonia arising from the patient inspiring small particles of false membrane or acrid matter into the finer capillaries of perhaps the air-cells themselves, and the matter thus inhaled setting up local inflammation. These cases are analogous to the cases of lobular pneumonia secondary to the spread through the circulation of pus or of minute particles of fibrine, etc. In the latter case an irritant is carried hy the blood, becomes arrested by the capillaries of the lung, and each particle becomes the centre of a patch of pneumonia. In the former case it is the acrid matter exuded into the larynx and bronchi which passes down the air-tubes, is arrested at their termination, and becomes the centre of a local inflammation. The facility for the occurrence of this blocking up of the lung by inspired particles is the greater because the patient loses considerably the power of coughing. He is unable to close his larynx sufficiently to cough effectually. His cough is rather a hawking-up than a true cough. For a true cough to occur, you know that the lungs must be filled with air, and then the glottis closed, so that the air in the substance of the lung may be compressed violently, and then the glottis be suddenly opened. But the patient who cannot close his glottis well cannot cough perfectly, and substances inspired are drawn in a little way at each inspiration, further than they can be expelled by the imperfect expiratory cough.

To avert death in cases of membranous exudation into the larynx we open either the larynx or the trachea; the trachea in a child; the larynx in an adult. We select the larynx in an adult because of the facility with which it is reached. We are driven to open the trachea in a child because the larynx is too small to admit the tube. The opening into the windpipe still further interferes with the power of coughing. The patient in croup is, as I have said, unable to close his larynx well; still he can close it to a certain degree, and he is able to cough to that degree. The tube, of course, he is unable to close, and hence acrid matters about the tube are more liable to be drawn downwards, and therefore to become impacted in the lung, to produce pneumonia, and in their passage downwards—so acrid is the matter—to produce bronchitis. It must be remembered that the inflammation extends downwards, not merely because the inflammation itself has a tendency to spread, but because the matter thrown out is acrid, and has a tendency to produce inflammation, which, in the constitutional state of the patient, will be a membranous inflammation. Thus, in some cases of diphtheria, the ear is the seat of membranous inflammation, and acrid matter as well as lymph is poured out. It runs down the outer side of the ear. As it passes down it excites inflammation, and the inflamed surface becomes covered with a false membrane. That this false membrane is not the result merely of extension of the inflammation is probable from the fact that if a blister is applied to a person suffering from diphtheria the raw surface frequently becomes covered with lymph, with a false membrane, with a diphtheritic exudation. You will thus understand that the fluid exuded is an irritant; that this irritant produces inflammation; that the inflammation, in the constitutional condition, is attended with an exudation of lymph. It is a specific inflammation, because the person is suffering from a specific disease, just as, when a person is the subject of constitutional syphilis, the local inflammations assume frequently a syphilitic character, or, in the subject of cancer, local injury may cause changes of texture cancerous in nature.

This leads me to a point of some practical importance in regard to tracheotomy. It is commonly stated that the bronchitis which so frequently follows tracheotomy in diphtheria is the result of the entrance of the cold air through the tube. It is said that in ordinary breathing the air is warmed as it passes through the mouth and nose, and the pharynx and larynx, and so it is warmed air only which comes in contact with the bronchial tubes; that the entrance of cold air excites inflammation, and hence that many patients operated on for tracheotomy in croup die from bronchitis. To prevent this entrance of cold air, and I should say also of dry air, the patient's bed is surrounded with blankets, and a tube discharging moist vapour is introduced within the blanket curtains, so that the patient may breathe a warm and moist air.

It seems to me that, if the explanation I have given you be correct, there is no need for these special means—for these blankets and hot vapour. We know that if the larynx be opened for any other affection—for example, such a case as we have now in the hospital—there is no tendency to the occurrence of bronchitis, and the patient walks about and breathes the ordinary air, with very little protection and without danger. A little protection may be necessary. Not only are these special means unnecessary, but in the disease diphtheria they are most injurious. They are most injurious because they tend to produce that exhaustion which is the cause of the fatal termination in so many cases during the second week of their illness. The relief which the patient experiences when you remove all this apparatus is marked. You must have seen it in the woman to whom I have referred. Thus you will understand that I think it most important for the success of the treatment of croup, should tracheotomy be performed, that the patient should be kept in a moderately warm atmosphere, a moderately moist atmosphere, but an atmosphere only so moist as may be produced by a kettle on the fire throwing a little moisture into the room, only so warm as shall be agreeable to the patient. I am sure that I have seen cases terminate fatally that would have recovered had they not been thus over-nursed, over-cared for; had, that is to say, the origin of the bronchitis been properly appreciated.

Holding the views which I now do, you will see at once that I should discard from the treatment of croup all those heroic remedies that were formerly regarded as indispensable —leeching, mercurialising, antimonising; and I should advise you to treat them on the same principles as you would treat diphtheria with exudation commencing in any other part—opening the larynx, however, if death is threatened by its occlusion.

Œdema glottidis, effusion of serum into the cellular tissue of the larynx, and especially of the arytæno-epiglottidean folds, although it may come on and does come on as an acute illness, is always secondary to some other affection, commonly to the chronic disease of the larynx. If life be threatened by it, and the part be not relieved by puncture with the nail, or, if well within reach, by a lancet, then laryngotomy in the adult, tracheotomy in the child, is the remedy. Usually the part is well within sight, and by the use of a tongue depressor and by the aid of the finger there is not much difficulty in the diagnosis. The rapid, sudden development of extreme dyspnœa leads you at once to examine the part. You have only to be aware of the possibility of its occurrence to avoid an error in diagnosis, and you have only to know of its existence to determine its treatment. There is a large quantity of fluid accumulating about the entrance to the larynx; it is within reach of the finger, and can in many cases be let out. If it cannot, drugs are useless, and you must avert death by letting in the air below the point of obstruction.

In regard to an inflamed cyst, the finger and the eye are the aids to diagnosis. The finger will at once give you every necessary information. You feel a rounded smooth surface; you feel its connection with the margin of the epiglottis; you feel it extending backwards: you can trace, in fact, with the finger, all its relations, without difficulty. The smooth elastic swelling and the feeling of fluctuation communicated to the finger are not, so far as I know, simulated by any other affection. The remedy is as certain as the diagnosis. With a lancet or a bistoury open the cavity, and the escape of the fluid affords immediate relief. Here, again, the great point is to be aware of the existence of such a trouble. Suspect, and there is no difficulty in the diagnosis.

A collection of pus in the cellular tissue on one side of the larynx I have seen cause very great distress to the breathing by compressing the larynx. I have seen a child brought within a few hours of death from this cause. The diagnosis is not always easy. There may be no redness of the surface, and the general restlessness and distress render, in the child, the presence of pain doubtful. There is, perhaps, a little general fulness of the part; and it requires careful examination, careful manipulation, to determine the nature of the trouble. The larynx is pushed over a little to one side, and this should at once arrest attention and direct the physician to the seat of the disease. Once having his attention fixed on the seat of the disease, the rapidity of the development of the trouble, the uneasiness and tenderness in the region before the difficulty of breathing commenced, will render the nature of the case probable; and a careful handling of the part will make the diagnosis certain. To overlook the abscess, to leave it unopened, may lead to the patient's death; the relief on opening is instantaneous.

INDEX

MESSRS.

RIVINGTON, PERCIVAL & Co.'s

LIST OF

Medical Works

IN SEPTEMBER

Demy 8vo.   21s. net

LECTURES AND ESSAYS
ON
FEVERS AND DIPHTHERIA
1849 TO 1879

By SIR WILLIAM JENNER, BART., G.C.B.

M.D. Lond. and F.R.C.P., D.C.L. Oxon., LL.D. Cantab. and Edin., F.R.S.,
President of the Royal College of Physicians from 1881 to 1888
Physician in Ordinary to H.M. the Queen and to H.R.H. the Prince of Wales
Consulting Physician to University College Hospital

SEVERAL years since I collected from the Journals to which I had originally sent them my papers on Fever. I now publish together all the papers I have written on Fever, because many of my medical friends have from time to time urged me to do it, and also because all the facts detailed and analysed were observed and recorded at the bedside and in the dead-house by *myself*. While collecting some of these facts in 1847 I caught typhus fever, and three or four years later typhoid fever. I mention this because it was said at the time, 'Before typhus and typhoid fevers can be said to be absolutely different diseases, some one must be found who has suffered from both,' and I was the first, so far as I know, who at that time could be proved to have suffered from both. Dr. E. A. Parkes attended me in both illnesses, and had no doubt about the diagnosis in each case. . . .

The papers I am now publishing are identical with those I originally published in various Journals and in the Transactions of Societies. The only alterations or additions I have now made are contained in a brief note or two appended to some of the pages.—*Extract from the Preface.*

CONTENTS

VII. 93.   **London : 34, King Street, Covent Garden**

Demy 8vo.   21s. net.

THE HYGIENE, DISEASES,
AND MORTALITY OF OCCUPATIONS

By J. T. ARLIDGE,

M.D. and A.B. (Lond.), F.R.C.P. (Lond.).

Consulting Physician to the North Staffordshire Infirmary ;
late Milroy Lecturer at the Royal College of Physicians, etc., etc.

"Dr. Arlidge's work should be welcomed by legislators and philanthropists as well as by the members of the medical profession, whose duty it is to be specially acquainted with those causes which affect the health of the different sections of the industrial community. . . . It only remains for us to say that, having gone carefully through the book, we can confidently recommend it as a valuable work of reference to all who are interested in the welfare of the industrial classes."—*Lancet.*

"A novel and important work dealing with a subject of great public as well as medical interest."—*Times.*

"We have already briefly noticed Dr. Arlidge's interesting work ; but the importance of the questions with which it deals is sufficient to justify a more complete account of the conclusions at which the author has arrived, and of the principal *data* upon which these conclusions have been founded."—*Times.*

"From what we have quoted it will be seen that the researches undertaken by Dr. Arlidge, for his Milroy Lectures, and embodied in the volume before us, are, from a practical as well as a scientific point of view, of the most suggestive character to all who are concerned that wealth shall not increase while men decay."—*Standard.*

"A book of great value and interest." —*St. James' Gazette.*

"This valuable treatise."—*Birmingham Daily Gazette.*

"Dr. Arlidge has given us a highly creditable and useful collection of material on this important subject."—*Scottish Leader.*

"Will be considered the standard authority on the subject for many years to come."—*Glasgow Herald.*

"This masterly work. . . . Dr. Arlidge in the preparation of this work has rendered a signal public service."—*Aberdeen Journal.*

"This invaluable work."—*Daily Telegraph.*

"Few, if any, British men have a better right than Dr. Aldridge to be heard on this particular subject. . . . (The volume is) crammed from cover to cover with most interesting and important information, given with a plainness of speech and a freedom from technical pretence that make it delightful reading for those without a smattering of medicine."—*National Observer.*

"It should be quite invaluable. Perhaps, too, it may render a service to the community in its obvious moral— that special dangers on the part of workmen or workwomen should be met by special precautions."—*Yorkshire Post.*

Demy 8vo. 16s. net.

With Map and Three Plates.

LEPROSY

By G. THIN, M.D.

The work contains chapters on the History, Geographical Distribution, Symptoms, Course, Pathology, and Treatment of Leprosy, with references to the legislative enactments which have been proposed and put in force in different countries in which the disease has prevailed.

" Is a work of wide scope, industry, and research, which as summing up the latest knowledge upon the subject of that terrible scourge, will be extremely valuable to the profession. It is also one of those rare medical treatises which appeal strongly to the general reader."—*Times.*

" We venture to say that his work will rank high amongst the scientific writings on the disease for the thoroughness with which he has entered into all its aspects, and not least for the full presentation of them in the light of its bacillary nature, which throughout Dr. Thin keeps prominently in view."—*Lancet.*

" It is a perfect storehouse of judiciously garnered facts, simple, succinct, and sufficient in themselves to enable a mind of rudimentary training to grasp the subject in its essential bearings, and so interwoven with the unstrained reflections of a convinced and convincing mind, that even lay readers with no training at all can follow the narrative with effortless appreciation." —*Times of India.*

Medium 8vo. 10s. 6d. net.

Limited Edition of 75 copies, numbered and signed.

Reprint of Two Tracts.

1. # AN ESSAY ON GLEETS.
2. # AN ENQUIRY INTO THE NATURE,
   ## CAUSE, AND CURE OF A SINGULAR DISEASE OF THE EYES.

By JEAN PAUL MARAT, M.D.

Edited, with an Introduction,

By JAMES BLAKE BAILEY,

Librarian of the Royal College of Surgeons of England.

London : 34, King Street, Covent Garden

Demy 8vo.   21s.

INFLUENZA,

OR EPIDEMIC CATARRHAL FEVER

An Historical Survey of Past Epidemics in Great Britain
from 1510 to 1890.

(Being a New and Revised Edition of 'Annals of Influenza,'
by THEOPHILUS THOMSON, M.D., F.R.C.P., F.R.S.)

By E. SYMES THOMSON, M.D., F.R.C.P.

Gresham Professor of Medicine and Consulting Physician to the Hospital
for Consumption and Diseases of the Chest, Brompton.

Crown 8vo.   6s. net.

THE ESSENTIALS OF SCHOOL DIET,

or, The Diet Suitable for the Growth and Development
of Youth.

By CLEMENT DUKES, M.D., B.S., Lond.,

Physician to Rugby School; Senior Physician to Rugby Hospital.

Demy 8vo.   1s.

WORK AND OVERWORK

IN RELATION TO HEALTH IN SCHOOLS

An Address delivered before the Teachers' Guild,
at its Fifth General Conference held in Oxford,
April, 1893.

By CLEMENT DUKES, M.D., B.S., Lond.

London: 34, King Street, Covent Garden

Crown 8vo. 2s.

THE ANTISEPTIC TREATMENT
OF WOUNDS

According to the Method of PROFESSOR BILLROTH, Vienna.

Translated from the German Third Edition Improved, of DR. V. HACKER, by

SURGEON-CAPTAIN C. R. KILKELLY, A.M.S.

"**A** handy and carefully prepared book, which seems likely to prove serviceable both as a manual of primary instruction, and as a work of reference on almost every point relating to modern antiseptic surgery."—*Brit. Med. Journ.*

Crown 8vo. 2s.

NEW OFFICIAL REMEDIES

Containing all the Drugs and Preparations contained in the Addendum (1890) to the British Pharmacopœia of 1885, with Pharmacological and Therapeutical Notes, adapted for the use of Practitioners and Students.

By RALPH STOCKMAN, M.D., F.R.C.P.E.

Lecturer on Materia Medica and Therapeutics, School of Medicine, Edinburgh ; Examiner in Materia Medica and Therapeutics in the Victoria University.

Crown 8vo. 1s.

INFLUENZA,
AND
COMMON COLDS

The Cause, Character, and Treatment of Each.

By W. T. FERNIE, M.D.

London : 34, King Street, Covent Garden